Clinical Approaches to Emergent Literacy Intervention

Clinical Approaches to Emergent Literacy Intervention

A Volume in the Emergent and Early Literacy Series

Laura M. Justice, Ph.D.
Editor

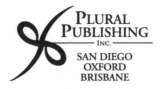

PLURAL
PUBLISHING
INC.
SAN DIEGO
OXFORD
BRISBANE

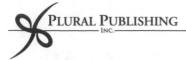

Plural Publishing, Inc

5521 Ruffin Road
San Diego, CA 92123

e-mail: info@pluralpublishing.com
Web site: http://www.pluralpublishing.com

49 Bath Street
Abingdon, Oxfordshire OX14 1EA
United Kingdom

Typeset in 11/13 Garamond by Flanagan's Publishing Services, Inc.
Printed in the United States of America by Bang Printing

Library of Congress Cataloging-in-Publication Data:

Justice, Laura M., 1968-
  Clinical approaches to emergent literacy intervention / Laura M.
Justice.
    p. cm. – (Emergent and early literacy series)
  Includes bibliographical references and index.
  ISBN-13: 978-1-59756-092-4 (softcover)
  ISBN-10: 1-59756-092-8 (softcover)
  1. Reading (Early childhood) 2. Reading–Remedial teaching.
3. Children with disabilities–Education. 4. Speech therapy for
children.   I. Title.
LB1139.5.R43J87 2006
372.4–dc22

                                                    2006032654

This book is dedicated to Dr. Helen Ezell.

Contents

Series Foreword

The purpose of Plural Publishing's Series on *Emergent and Early Literacy* is to provide clinical and educational professionals with usable, practical, and evidence-based resources for enhancing their ability to include literacy as an integral part of their services to toddlers, preschoolers, and school-age children. The books in this series provide professionals with a portfolio of contemporary resources that keep them up to date in theories, scientific findings, and practices relevant to emergent and early literacy.

As the editor of this series, I select topics that represent the pressing needs and interests of clinical and educational professionals and then select authors who can provide an accessible yet expert perspective on these topics. The topics and authors represent the diverse interdisciplinary fields sharing an interest in emergent and early literacy, including education, psychology, speech-language pathology, audiology, and health sciences, to name but a few.

My particular interest as the editor of this series is to provide professionals with timely guidance on theoretically sound and empirically based tools and techniques they can readily use and incorporate into their everyday practice to promote the literacy development of the children and adults with whom they work. For instance, professionals who work with preschoolers exhibiting underdeveloped emergent literacy skills need up-to-date information about effective storybook reading techniques that they can use to accelerate literacy learning. Likewise, professionals who work with school-age children with reading challenges need to know about different assessment tools they can use to evaluate the literacy-learning environment of classrooms in which they teach or consult so that they can enhance these environments systematically. And, professionals who work with adults with limited literacy or those who have lost literacy skills due to illness or injury need to know about effective techniques for remediation. In short, professionals need access to up-to-date information on theoretically sound and empirically based techniques concerning how best to improve the literacy achievements of individuals across the lifespan. Responding to professionals' needs for timely and practical information that is both theoretically sound and empirically based is my foremost goal as the editor of this series, which will take on timely issues of practical import and disseminate these in a reader-friendly manner for the busy professional.

This book, *Clinical Approaches to Emergent Literacy Intervention*, for which I served as editor, is designed specifically for speech-language pathologists and their professional allies—including early childhood educators, special educators, clinical psychologists, literacy coaches, and reading specialists—to promote their ability to meet the needs of children who are struggling with emergent and early literacy development. This book was designed to provide a practical, usable, current, and evidence-based description of exemplary approaches to improving the emergent literacy skills of young children through clinical interventions. I asked the authors who contributed chapters to this book to explicitly describe contemporary methods, approaches, and contexts that can be effectively used to improve the likelihood of reading success among the pupils we serve. It is my hope that this book will provide an important resource to clinical professionals who are vested in promoting the intensity, rigor, and quality of their work with young children in the area of emergent and early literacy.

Laura M. Justice, Ph.D.
Series Editor

About the Editor

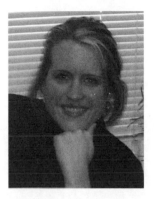 Laura M. Justice, Ph.D., CCC-SLP, is an Associate Professor of Education at the University of Virginia in the McGuffey Reading Center and the Center for Advanced Study of Teaching and Learning. She directs the Preschool Language and Literacy Lab, which conducts basic and applied research on early literacy and language development, home- and classroom-based language and literacy interventions, parent-child storybook reading interactions, and language disorders. She has authored or co-authored five books, including *Shared Storybook Reading* with Helen Ezell and *Scaffolding with Storybooks* with Khara Pence, and more than 50 research articles, several of which have won national recognition, including the 2005 Editor's Award from the *American Journal of Speech-Language Pathology*. In 2006, Dr. Justice was awarded the Presidential Early Career Award for Scientists and Engineers from President George W. Bush, which is the highest honor bestowed on scientists by the U.S. government within the first six years of their career.

Contributors

Karin Boerger, M.S., CCC-SLP
Clinical Faculty Instructor
University of Colorado, Boulder
Chapter 2

Barbara Culatta, Ph.D.
Professor
Associate Dean
Communication Disorders
McKay School of Education
Brigham Young University
Chapter 6

Luigi Girolametto, Ph.D., CCC-SLP
Associate Professor
Department of Speech-Language
    Pathology
University of Toronto, Toronto,
    ON Canada
Chapter 5

Janice Greenberg, B.Sc., D.S.P.
Program Manager
The Hanen Centre, Toronto,
    Canada
Chapter 5

D. Sarah Hadden, Ph.D.
Research Associate
Center for Advanced Study of
    Teaching and Learning
University of Virginia
Chapter 4

Kendra M. Hall, Ph.D.
Assistant Professor
Education
Brigham Young University
Chapter 6

Latisha L. Hayes, Ph.D.
Clinical Assistant Professor
Department of Curriculum,
    Instruction, and Special
    Education
Coordinator
McGuffey Reading Center
University of Virginia
Chapter 11

Sherri M. Lovelace, Ph.D.
Assistant Professor
Communication Disorders
Arkansas State University
Chapter 10

Clara Pérez-Méndez
President
Puentes Culturales
Chapter 2

Amelia K. Moody
Doctoral Candidate
Special Education
Curry School of Education
University of Virginia
Chapter 3

Susan M. Moore, J.D., M.A., CCC-SLP, F-ASHA
Director, Clinical Education and Services
Speech Language Hearing Sciences
University of Colorado, Boulder
Chapter 2

Robert B. Pianta, Ph.D.
Director
Center for Advanced Study of Teaching and Learning
Novartis US Foundation Professor
Curry School of Education
Professor of Psychology
University of Virginia
Chapter 4

Peggy Rosin, M.S., CCC-SLP
Clinical Professor
Department of Communicative Disorders
University of Wisconsin-Madison
Chapter 12

Gloria Soto, Ph.D.
Professor
Special Education
San Francisco State University
Chapter 9

Sharon R. Stewart, Ed.D.
Associate Professor
Division of Communication Disorders
Associate Dean for Academic Affairs
College of Health Sciences
University of Kentucky
Chapter 10

Teresa A. Ukrainetz, Ph.D.
Associate Professor
Division of Communication Disorders
University of Wyoming
Laramie, WY
Chapter 7

Elaine Weitzman, M.Ed.
Executive Director
The Hanen Centre
Toronto, Canada
Chapter 5

A. Lynn Williams, Ph.D.
Professor
Department of Communicative Disorders
East Tennessee State University
Chapter 8

Introduction

Rationale for This Book

Current assessments of educational achievement among America's schoolchildren reveal staggering inadequacies; 38% of fourth graders, for example, fail to read at even basic levels (National Assessment of Educational Progress [NAEP], 2003). Equally disheartening is the finding that there is a markedly disproportionate representation of children who are poor and who are members of ethnic or racial minorities among those who struggle. For instance, 46% and 44% of fourth graders who are African American and Hispanic, respectively, do not achieve even a basic level of reading competence (NAEP, 2003). Researchers, policymakers, and practitioners recognize that no one solution will solve this complicated problem, inasmuch as reading development, reading instruction, and reading disability are complex, multidimensional constructs. Nonetheless, there is consensus across these constituencies that evidence-based educational interventions must utilize preemptive moves through *primary prevention*. Contrasted with *secondary prevention* (entailing interventions to slow or reverse the course of reading problems once they emerge in first grade and beyond) and *tertiary prevention* (entailing interventions to support the affected person's ability to compensate for a reading problem that is serious and persistent), primary prevention focuses on preventing reading difficulties from emerging at the outset, thereby reducing the need for more intensive, expensive, and time-consuming secondary and tertiary interventions. Presumably, an effective primary prevention approach will ease children's transition to the rigors of academic instruction in kindergarten and first grade and provide their first success in a series of accumulating achievements in attaining literacy.

This book was developed in response to this paradigm shift of the last decade that has increasingly emphasized the *emergent literacy period* as the time frame in which solutions to pressing problems concerning reading achievement are most likely to have effect. Research shows the preschool years to be a critical period during which young children develop skills, knowledge, and interests in the code- and meaning-based aspects of written and spoken language. The current emphasis on emergent literacy as an essential aspect of preschool development draws on two growing bodies of research. The first body shows that individual differences among children in emergent literacy skills are *meaningful*, whereby early abilities contribute significantly to longitudinal outcomes in children's reading achievement. Reliable, valid, and sensitive indicators of early individual differences are increasingly used in preschool programs to identify and assist children whose emergent literacy growth trajectory shows vulnerability for later reading difficulties. The second body of research shows that the prevalence of reading difficulties is more likely to be influenced through *prevention*, rather than *remediation*. Once a reading delay manifests for a particular child in elementary school, the odds suggest that a return to healthy progress is quite unlikely. Accordingly, Torgesen (1998) and others advocate the need to "catch children *before* they fall" by allocating resources toward prevention of reading problems.

Speech-language pathologists and their professional allies— early childhood educators, special educators, clinical psychologists, literacy coaches, and reading specialists—all feel the pressure and the urgency to take a close look at their extant practices and boost the intensity and rigor with which these effect children's emergent literacy development. This book is intended as a tool for these professionals to use in these efforts. It provides clear and reader-friendly descriptions of practical, current, and evidence-based approaches to improving the emergent literacy skills of young children through clinical interventions.

Focus and Organization of this Book

This book is organized to provide examples of clinical approaches to designing and delivering emergent literacy interventions that draw on the contributing authors' current research activities and clinical practices. All of the authors are hands-on experts who are actively involved in the design, study, and refinement of clinical approaches to emergent literacy intervention. In approaching these particular authors as contributors to this book, I sought out those who could bring extensive clinical experience incorporating a broad scope of practice in emergent literacy intervention, to include the following:

- A range of **therapeutic contexts**, such as inclusive classrooms, homes, and traditional clinics
- Various **service delivery options**, including direct services and indirect services through consultation and collaboration with other professionals and parents
- Diverse **populations**, including children with identified disabilities, children from culturally and linguistically diverse backgrounds, and children who are reared in poverty
- Different **intervention targets**, such as print awareness, phonological awareness, vocabulary, and writing

I believe that readers of this work, like myself, will be moved to action by the compelling rationales and supporting evidence for the state-of-the-art clinical approaches to emergent literacy presented throughout the chapters. This action is based on recognition of the emergent literacy period as the point in development when we as professionals are most able to affect children's developmental trajectories and improve their chances for becoming lifelong readers.

The book is organized into two sections. Section I, Program Design Considerations, provides foundational information concerning children's emergent literacy development and the design and implementation of quality interventions. Chapter 1 serves as a basic primer for professionals who have not had a great deal of training in emergent literacy or who desire a review of important concepts. This chapter provides a definition of emergent literacy, discusses targets in emergent literacy intervention, and characterizes the essential characteristics of high-quality clinical interventions in emergent literacy. Chapter 2 provides a framework for designing clinical interventions that meet the needs of culturally and linguistically diverse families. Chapter 3 discusses approaches for integrating assistive technology into emergent literacy interventions, such as the use of electronic storybooks. Chapter 4 considers how speech-language pathologists can effectively consult and collaborate with preschool educators to promote the quality of language and literacy instruction within the classroom, which will support the needs of children with communicative impairments as well as their typically developing classmates.

Section II provides detailed information concerning a range of clinical approaches for emergent literacy intervention. Chapter 5 discusses the concept of adult responsiveness and how this facilitates children's developments in both emergent literacy and oral language; this chapter provides important information concerning how speech-language pathologists can collaborate and consult with preschool educators to promote their responsiveness within the classroom. Chapter 6 examines approaches to phonological awareness instruction as part of a classroom-based comprehensive literacy curriculum. It includes careful details concerning how to select targets of instruction and how these may be organized along a continuum to promote children's progress in developing phonological awareness. Chapter 7 illustrates strategies for promoting children's phonemic awareness through the use of scaffolded writing instruction, which simultaneously improves not only phonemic-level skills but also children's emergent writing abilities. Chapter 8 provides an innovative approach to using shared storybook reading as a context for facilitating both literacy and language goals, including phonological awareness. This chapter examines the evidence concerning the use of dialogic reading as a means for supporting oral language achievements, and how to integrate attention to other important literacy goals into dialogic reading events. Chapter 9 describes how storybook reading participation for children with complex communicative challenges can be organized to facilitate more active involvement of these children. This chapter details the importance of looking closely at book reading exchanges to understand how children with complex communication needs are participating and how their active participation can be enhanced during clinical interventions. Chapter 10 provides an informative discussion of how children's print-related skills, including print concepts and alphabet knowledge, can be improved during shared storybook reading using a range of techniques, including print referencing. Chapter 11 describes the techniques and principles of word study, an effective approach for improving children's decoding and spelling skills from the emergent literacy stage onward. Word study can be used within the classroom to organize phonics instruction for children, or it can be used as an important supplement in clinical speech-language programs to ensure a systematic focus on spelling and decoding skills. The final chapter, Chapter 12, provides an excellent description of how to design and implement a comprehensive emergent literacy program serving culturally and linguistically diverse children that includes attention to traditional speech and language goals, as well as specific literacy needs, including alphabet knowledge and phonological awareness.

Together, the chapters in this book provide the clinical professional with a host of possibilities for how to include a more systematic focus on emergent literacy within clinical interventions. The authors of the chapters show how many different methods, approaches, and contexts can be used for the purpose of achieving one end: improving the likelihood of reading success among the pupils we serve.

References

National Assessment of Education Progress. (2003). *The nation's report card.* Retrieved October 10, 2004, from http://nces.ed.gov/nations reportcard

Torgesen, J. K. (1998, Spring/Summer). Catch them before they fall: Identification and assessment to prevent reading failure in young children. *American Educator*, 1-8.

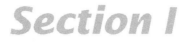

Section I

Program Design Considerations

Chapter One

Emergent Literacy: Development, Domains, and Intervention Approaches

Laura M. Justice

Overview

Young children know a lot about reading and writing. Sometime around their first birthday (and for some children, even before!), children reared in literate households typically begin to play with storybooks, to scribble with crayons, to show interest in print within their environments, and to play happily with the sounds of their language. Although the timeline for beginning these achievements can vary enormously among children and is strongly influenced by the specific sociocultural environments of both family and community, all of these behaviors are indicators of the emergence of early forms of literacy, termed emergent literacy. *Emergent literacy* can be defined as the reading and writing behaviors of young children before they become readers and writers in the conventional sense. Children have become conventionally literate when they can read and write according to the rule-governed system of the alphabetic principle. Before this achievement, however, children engage with reading and writing in many unconventional yet developmentally appropriate ways. Thus, emergent literacy represents a legitimate and important stage in children's achievement of literacy.

In this chapter, emergent literacy is introduced as a developmental construct and as a focus of intervention for professionals who work with young children. Also included are a historical perspective on the evolution of emergent literacy theory and a review of current thought on emergent literacy as a stage of literacy development. The different domains of emergent literacy development and their predictive relationship with later achievements in reading are examined as well, followed by a consideration of characteristics of high-quality emergent literacy intervention. This subject matter provides a foundation for the remainder of the book, which describes various approaches for supporting young children as they develop emergent literacy skills.

Emergent Literacy Development

Typically, in American society, children are viewed as being in the emergent literacy stage of development from birth to about 5 years of age, the latter point corresponding with the transition to kindergarten. During this period, most children will show the following behaviors, all of which are characteristic of the emergent literacy stage of development:

- Displaying a keen interest in print, although they are not able to read
- Viewing themselves as being able to read, particularly with familiar storybooks
- Playing with writing utensils and media, and viewing their written productions as meaningful
- Using and enjoying books as a play or relationship-building activity
- Playing with the phonology of oral language, such as making rhymes or noticing alliterative patterns across words
- Utilizing literacy themes or props within their dramatic play

An important point is that children's interest in print, use of writing utensils, enjoyment of and interactions with books, play with sound structures, and use of literacy themes and props within their dramatic activities have been linked to their later and more conventional achievements in literacy. For instance, the number of nursery rhymes with which a preschool child is familiar is suggestive of how successful that child will be later in the beginning stages of conventional literacy instruction, when he or she begins to read and to spell (Bryant, Maclean, & Bradley, 1990). Likewise, children's enjoyment of and engagement with books—their "orientation to literacy"—also has been linked to later conventional literacy achievements in reading and writing (Fritjers, Barron, & Brunello, 2000). In the past several decades, researchers have conducted numerous studies to theoretically and empirically describe the emergent literacy achievements of young children and, equally important, how these relate to later developments in reading, writing, and general academics (Hammill, 2004; Scarborough & Dobrich, 1994; Storch & Whitehurst, 2002).

Researchers have shown that nearly every discrete, measurable achievement in emergent literacy can be statistically linked to later literacy success, although great variability has been observed in the strength of the relationship between a specific emergent literacy skill, ability, or behavior (e.g., name writing) and a later literacy ability (e.g., spelling). These prediction studies reliably show linkages between emergent literacy achievements and later literacy abilities, showing that literacy development is a continuous process that begins soon after birth (e.g., Storch & Whitehurst, 2002). As an analogy, we recognize that although children's productive use of language does not begin until the second year of life, when they begin to accumulate an expressive lexicon and to combine words to form short phrases, language development begins to emerge at birth, if not before. We also recognize early communicative behaviors, such as babbling, joint attention, and gesturing, as important precursors to language development that exist on the same developmental continuum. Similarly, children's early reading and writing behaviors, although far less readily characterized because of their inherent variability among individual children, exist along the same developmental continuum as later reading and writing achievements. Of importance, studies have shown that children with an early start in literacy are more likely than those experiencing a late start—because of experiential, dispositional, or developmental circumstances—to become successful readers and writers. This connection between early delays in literacy development with increased later risks for poor reading and writing skills has become an important issue in the field of preschool education and early intervention (Snow, 2006). Increasingly, those professionals who work with young children to deliver educational and clinical programs are asked to integrate systematic and explicit attention to helping children develop emergent literacy fundamentals to mitigate their risks for later literacy difficulties (Justice, Invernizzi, & Meier, 2002; Snow, Burns, & Griffin, 1998).

Emergent Literacy Theory

The focus on emergent literacy theory is relatively new, as it has been only within the last few decades that researchers have begun to empirically recognize what many parents and educators already knew to be true: that literacy does not begin with formal schooling. In an important work published in 1986, *Emergent Literacy: Writing and Reading*, William Teale and Elizabeth Sulzby presented a comprehensive portrait of the importance of emergent literacy achievements and envisioned emergent literacy as an important area of scholarly inquiry. Their work was stimulated by several significant papers and books that had already begun to emphasize the importance of children's emergent literacy knowledge, including New Zealander Marie Clay's doctoral dissertation (1966) titled *Emergent Reading Behaviour* and her subsequent seminal text (1979), *Reading: The Patterning of Complex Behaviour*. Many credit Clay as a pioneer in the establishment of emergent literacy as both a field of study and as a focus of education.

Before the concept of emergent literacy took hold, a "reading readiness" perspective persisted in the United States and elsewhere. This perspective viewed children's literacy achievements as emerging only within and as a function of formal instruction. Proponents of a reading readiness model argued that children were not "ready" for reading until they had achieved sophisticated oral language proficiency, and that instruction was needed for children to acquire reading and writing abilities. Thus, this perspective emphasized that reading instruction could be delivered to children only when they are ready. An impact of the reading readiness perspective was that literacy instruction often was withheld until the child was considered "ready" to benefit from it. Likewise, few researchers invested themselves in studying the literacy behaviors of young children because these were not viewed as legitimate or important behaviors that served as precursors to later achievements. Although the reading readiness perspective has been replaced by an emergent literacy perspective, the former still prevails in the minds of some educators, who therefore withhold or delay exposure to key literacy concepts. For instance, a special education teacher who teaches in a self-contained classroom serving only children with moderate to severe disabilities may view the children in her room as "not ready" for phonological awareness instruction and thus not provide this instruction to her pupils. Likewise, an early childhood teacher may view his 3- and 4-year-old pupils as "too young" to engage in writing activities, and thus may not have a writing center in his classroom in which children can experiment with writing on their own or under guidance from others. Nonetheless, as an important antidote to these "readiness" perspectives, considerable research shows that even children who have great difficulty with learning as a result of developmental disabilities and even those who are quite young can benefit from instruction in phonological awareness and other aspects of emergent literacy, including invented spelling (Justice, Chow, Capellini, Flanigan, & Colton, 2003; Justice, Kaderavek, Bowles, & Grimm, 2005; Katims, 1994; O'Connor, Notari-Syverson, & Vadasy, 1996).

Teale and Sulzby's seminal 1986 work presented key characteristics of *emergent literacy theory*, which essentially provides a working model of this early period of literacy development and how educators might go about supporting children's achievements. Much of their theory has made its way into current conventional thought:

- Literacy development begins at birth, and many literacy milestones are achieved before children enter school.
- Literacy development and language are reciprocally related.
- Children are active (not passive) participants in the literacy development process.
- Children acquire much of their literacy knowledge incidentally.
- Children's literacy development is mediated by adults.
- Children's earliest literacy achievements tend to follow a developmental sequence.

Emergent Literacy as a "Stage" of Literacy Development

Like many other aspects of development, children's literacy development typically is conceptualized as comprising a series of stages that unfold from birth forward. In reality, stages tend to blur, and little research is available that provides evidence for the "inflection points" that would need to be apparent to truly represent literacy development as a series of stages. An inflection point is a point in development at which new skills emerge and begin to rapidly develop (Ganger & Brent, 2004), and evidence of inflection points would provide some support for stage theories of development. Without empirical evidence of inflection points, it is likely more appropriate to view development as proceeding along a generally linear pathway in which there are no putative endpoints between stages and achievements characteristic of one stage blur with achievements characteristic of another stage. Nonetheless, it is quite typical to hear experts and practitioners discuss literacy development as comprising a series of stages, and in this chapter, stage terminology is used because it allows categorization of skills and an estimation of where children are along on a continuum of development, real or hypothesized.

The terms *emergent*, *early*, and *conventional* literacy generally approximate the developmental continuum of literacy achievement across the preschool through later elementary years (Snow et al., 1998). In the preschool years, which constitute the emergent literacy stage, children are rapidly developing important precursory skills in reading and writing. Although they are not yet reading in a conventional sense, they have an emerging interest in print and books and have acquired a rudimentary knowledge of the distinctive features and names of individual alphabet letters. They are able to distinguish among an array of written language forms and functions, they show a developing sensitivity to words as units of both print and sound, and they are increasingly aware of the sound segments that make up running speech, such as words and syllables.

Observations of a normal 18-month-old child (my own daughter) showed the following emergent literacy behaviors, which may be familiar to many readers involved in ongoing care of children in this age group:

- Knowledge of the names of several alphabet letters, including O, M, and W
- Enjoyment of storybook reading interactions, including seeking out such interactions unprompted by an adult
- Use of writing media, including paper and any type of available writing utensil, to scribble and draw
- Understanding of how to orient a storybook and how to turn pages from left to right
- Awareness of print as different from other types of stimuli in the environment

Children's emergent skills in these areas and others continue to mature as they enter the early literacy stage. With transition to the early literacy (or beginning reading) stage, they begin to apply the alphabetic principle to decode unknown words and to spell words in their writing. The *alphabetic principle* is, simply put, the basis for the code used in English writing to map speech onto letters through letter-sound correspondences. In the early literacy period, children bring their knowledge of print (print awareness, alphabet knowledge) and sound (phonological awareness) to its end application in the alphabetic principle.

Children typically enter the early literacy stage between the ages of 5 and 7 years, when they begin to use alphabetic information to read and spell, representing their emergent application of sound-symbol correspondences (Chall, 1983; Ehri, 1991; Frith, 1985). Children's early application of the alphabetic code is incomplete, however, and often plagued by "errors," as in reading the word "dock" as "dog" or writing the word "milk" as MK. These errors are entirely normal, similar to the typical developmental errors children make as they develop and refine their phonology (e.g., saying "lellow" for "yellow), grammar (e.g., saying "wonned" for "won"), and vocabulary (e.g., calling a raccoon a possum).

The early literacy stage is often called the "partial phonetic cue" stage (Ehri, 1991), because children do not fully utilize all alphabetic and phonetic information in their decoding and spelling. For instance, when looking at an unknown word, children may attend to only one or two letters in the word—such as the b and t in "boat"—and make an educated guess at the word's pronunciation (e.g., "boot," "boat," "bought"). Thus, children in this stage sometimes are viewed as "deciphering" rather than actually decoding (Snow et al., 1998). Bear, Invernizzi, Templeton, and Johnston (2003) have shown that the kinds of errors children make during this phase offer insights into what they understand about print: " . . . using context as well as partial consonant cues, a child reading about good things to eat might substitute *candy* or even *cookie* for *cake* in the sentence 'The cake was good to eat' " (p. 22). In this example, the child obviously is using some phonetic cues to decipher print, specifically the beginning and the final consonants of words, with a heavy reliance on contextual support.

This pattern of deciphering (or making educated guesses about words based on partial phonetic or alphabetic information) also is seen in children's spelling during this period. Whereas a child in the emergent literacy stage may write the word "fun" as a scribble or with totally random letters, the child in the early literacy stage begins to produce some correct consonants in his or her spelling, but typically only at the beginning and the end of words that have not already been memorized by the child as "sight" words (e.g., the child's first name, familiar words in the environment). Vowels usually are not produced at first, so "fun" would be written as FN and "milk" might be written as MK. This stage of spelling has been called the "letter-name spelling stage" because children rely on the names of letters in their spelling of words (Ganske, 2000, p. 12):

> Approaching each word one sound at a time, they seek out the letter name that most closely matches the sound they are trying to reproduce. Some sounds have a more direct match than others. Consider, for example, the word "bake." The "buh"—*b*, "aye"—*a*, and "kuh"—*k* are much more straightforward for these young spellers than are the sounds in "drip." In the latter word, there is no direct letter name match for either the jr sound of the "dr" or for the short i vowel sound. When this happens, children choose the letter name with the closest "feel" (place of articulation) . . . although spellings like JEP, GEP, HEP (or even JP, GP, or HP at the beginning of this stage) for "drip" are certainly nonstandard, they are well-reasoned attempts by novice writers seeking to make sense of our English spelling system.

As children move through the early literacy stage, they progress from using partial phonetic and alphabet cues to making more complete use of phonetic cues to read and spell by the end of the kindergarten year, and they continue to refine their skills through the first grade in the context of formal skills-based reading instruction. This stage of literacy development often is termed *learning to read*, to emphasize its correspondence with the focus of instruction occurring in schools. During first and second grade reading instruction, children increasingly become more automatic in their decoding and spelling and rely less on grapheme-phoneme knowledge and more on a sight word vocabulary developed through reading and instruction, as well as by "chunking" parts of words (e.g., onsets and rimes) so that words can be processed more quickly (rather than figuring out one letter at a time). Children's spelling of words also reflects this increased knowledge of phonology, orthography, and automaticity, and their spelling moves from the Letter-Name Stage to the Within-Word Pattern Stage (Ganske, 2000). Within the Letter-Name Stage, children work in a letter-by-letter and sound-by-sound manner, trying to represent each phoneme in a word within a letter; by contrast, in the Within-Word Pattern Stage, children are much more familiar with the orthography of their written language and thus begin to develop and apply knowledge of patterns and rules governing the internal structure of words, such as rules concerning the depiction of long vowels.

Truly productive or conventional literacy is achieved when children are able to automatically process a large corpus of words, thereby freeing precious cognitive resources from a focus on decoding and word recognition to reading comprehension, or reading for meaning (Chall, 1983; Frith, 1985). Children's reading skills have become increasingly automated with ongoing exposure to the orthography of their language during the early literacy stage, acquired through the act of reading and the "self-teaching" that occurs by repeated engagement in reading activities. When children are able to read many words encountered automatically, they are able to shift important processes to the act of reading for meaning; thus, this phase of literacy corresponds to a focus on *reading to learn*.

Emergent literacy thus can be appropriately viewed as the starting point on a continuum of literacy development or, alternatively, as the bottom of a pyramid in which early achievements support later achievements. Clearly, supporting children's emergent literacy achievements is critical to their later success in early and conventional literacy, and this important time frame is the subject of this book. As speech-language pathologists (SLPs) and other professionals who work with young children, we must take an active role in supporting children's development of foundational literacy skills, recognizing that these achievements provide a significant and unique contribution to all else to come.

Domains of Emergent Literacy Development

As noted earlier, children's earliest achievements in literacy are both remarkable and numerous. Around the time of the second birthday, many children will exhibit some readily observable emergent literacy behaviors, such as enjoying and seeking out storybook reading interactions, understanding how to hold a storybook, attending to nursery rhymes, and being aware that print is a specific type of visual stimulus. By the age of 3 years, many children know the names of several storybooks, can point to words on pages of books, can recognize a few capital letters, can scribble using crayons and paper, will sit alone and look at books (perhaps even pretending to read), and so forth. By the age of 4, a child may write his or her own name, recognize a few words in environmental print, "write" letters to friends and family members, and sing the entire alphabet song.

In view of the many areas of knowledge associated with emergent literacy, an important consideration of particular interest to clinical SLPs and other professionals who work with young children is *target selection*, or identification of those skills and behaviors on which interventions should be focused. Selecting targets for intervention can be just as important as selecting a particular intervention approach. In the area of emergent literacy, the most desirable targets are those that (1) directly contribute to and are predictive of later reading and writing achievements, and (2) are amenable to change through intervention (National Early Literacy Panel, 2004)

Particularly useful to helping us identify these important emergent literacy targets are the results of *meta-analysis*. A meta-analysis is a specific type of research design that involves aggregating data from many studies on a similar topic to study convergence of findings. As one example, The National Early Literacy Panel (2004) was commissioned by the National Center for Family Literacy to conduct a meta-analysis that answers, among others, the following question: What are young children's (ages birth through 5 years) skills and abilities that best predict later reading, writing, and spelling outcomes? The panel's review of several hundred studies identified those emergent literacy skills that consistently and most strongly related to later literacy achievement, with these being among the strongest:

- Alphabet knowledge: receptive and/or expressive knowledge of the individual letters of the alphabet
- Concepts about print: knowledge of the rules governing how print is used and organized across various genres, including books and environmental print
- Phonological awareness: sensitivity to the sound structure of spoken language
- Invented spelling: representation of the orthography of written language
- Oral language: grammatical, lexical, and narrative abilities
- Name writing: representation of one's own name in print

These six areas of emergent literacy development can be organized into four general domains:

1. *Print knowledge* (alphabet knowledge, concepts about print)
2. *Phonological awareness*
3. *Writing* (invented spelling, name writing)
4. *Oral language* (grammar, vocabulary, narrative)

For professionals working with young children to promote their emergent literacy skills, the National Early Literacy Panel recommends maintaining vigilance to ensure achievements across all four of these domains. The important question, of course, is whether skills in these domains are amenable to change through intervention. The available evidence confirms that they are—and also supports the potential for early interventions to reduce children's risk for later literacy difficulties (see the 2003 review by Justice and Pullen). Several approaches using such interventions are presented in this book. Chapter 5, for instance, details ways to promote children's language skills; Chapter 6 discusses an approach for promoting phonological awareness; Chapter 10 discusses ways to facilitate print knowledge; and Chapter 11 provides details on an approach for improving children's invented spelling skills.

In selecting targets for intervention with young children, it is important to bear in mind that there is no evidence suggesting that exposing children to emergent literacy intervention is harmful and that no research supports withholding intervention until children are sufficiently "ready." I make this point in an attempt to alleviate concerns of professionals who may fear that emergent literacy intervention is not developmentally appropriate for some young children. What does warrant consideration, of course, is the issue of *how:* how intervention is delivered so that it is sensitive to children's needs and interests. Of particular import is ensuring that children receive high levels of support to acquire skills that are particularly difficult for them, with decreasing levels of support over time to support movement toward mastery. For example, rather than deciding that a 4-year-old boy with developmental delay is "not ready" to learn to write his name, the skillful interventionist will provide high levels of support in the early stages of instruction when this objective is particularly challenging to the child. An appropriate intervention may be to give hand-over-hand assistance to the child in holding a crayon to make a mark on his drawing, and then to assign meaning to the mark for the child: "Look, you wrote your name! You signed your name on your art so now we all know it is yours." Over time, the child will become more independent in writing his name (Justice et al., 2003) and develop more understanding about the print and sound structures of written language.

Thus, an important component of emergent literacy intervention is ensuring that children have ongoing exposure to high-priority targets of instruction (those predictive of later literacy achievements) within the context of high-quality instruction through adult mediation. Although many children may explore print and sounds on their own, without adult mediation their explorations may not be adequate for timely acquisition of sophisticated levels of emergent literacy skills. Adult mediation—or *scaffolding*—is the key to supporting children's emergent literacy achievements and ensuring timely development of high-priority skills. The term scaffolding has its roots in the theories of Lev Vygotsky, who argued that children's learning occurs along a social to psychological plane (Vygotsky, 1978). By this perspective, emergent literacy skills are introduced to the child by a sensitive adult within a scaffolded social-interactive context; over time, as the adult withdraws support, the skill works its way inward to psychological ownership (i.e., internalization) by the child. This theory advocates the sensitive use of supports to move a child from dependence to independence in a particular skill or behavior. In achieving a new skill or behavior, such as the ability to write their name, children initially may require extensive supports. Children may develop a modicum of name-writing skill by watching and imitating adults around them, but they may be unlikely to progress far without explicit guidance. With scaffolding, adults provide whatever supports are needed for children to achieve competence in an activity; gradually, these supports are removed until the child is able to perform independently.

Characteristics of High-Quality Emergent Literacy Intervention

High-quality emergent literacy intervention thus involves scaffolding children's achievements in print knowledge, phonological awareness, writing, and language abilities. This scaffolding is most effective when grounded in instructional contexts characterized as *explicit*, *systematic*, and *purposeful*, which represent three key features of high-quality emergent literacy intervention.

Explicit Intervention

Explicit refers to the act of making very clear what the teacher or SLP expects the child to learn from an activity. Rather than leaving the intended goal vague, unstated, or *implicit* to the child, explicit intervention involves identifying for the child what it is he or she is to focus on and think about during an activity. Perhaps the concept of explicitness is best illustrated by an example based on personal observation: An SLP working with a preschooler repeatedly reads aloud a book that features large and bold narrative print, with few words on each page, and characters pictured with speech bubbles coming out of their mouths with words in them. This activity seems like an ideal way in which to promote the child's print-related knowledge, including alphabet knowledge and print concepts (see Justice & Ezell, 2002). In fact, the SLP has included "to improve print-related skills" as a short-term objective for this child, with "read print-salient books during each session" as a means for achieving this goal. However, if the reading sessions are conducted without clarification of what the child is expected to learn about print (e.g., the names of some letters, how print moves from left to right), then this activity not only fails to achieve the characteristic of explicitness but also is unlikely to improve the child's print-related skills. This is because the learning goal is implicit, and the SLP has not explained to the child the focus of the learning activity.

To make this approach to intervention more explicit, the SLP should identify specific print-related goals to address before, during, and after the book reading session. In the following example, the SLP clarifies for the child that the focus of the reading session is on two specific letters:

> *Before reading*: "When we read, we'll listen to the story and also look at some letters. Let's look for the letters S and P, which are both in the word 'spot.' This is an S and this is a P . . . . "

> *During reading*: "Do you see any of our letters on this page? I saw an S but no P. Can you help me find them? That's right, this is an S and it's the first letter in the word 'see.' But there are no Ps on this page. Let's keep looking for them . . . . "

> *After reading*: "That was a great story. I also liked how you helped me find some of our letters in the book. We found some Ss and some Ps. Let's make a list of some of the words in the book that had these letters in them . . . . "

What the child is expected to learn from participating in the storybook reading exchanges is sufficiently explicit—the SLP clarifies the goals of the activity and also the print-related features on which the child is expected to focus.

The same principles are applied to any literacy-related activity in which learning or applying a new concept is the SLP's goal for the child. For instance, for work on vocabulary goals, the concept of explicitness implies that the SLP will not merely expose the child to a few new words but will very specifically guide the child's attention toward the learning goals of the activity. In the intervention context of shared storybook reading, the SLP may make explicit these word-learning goals as follows:

> *Before reading*: "We'll be learning a few new words in this book. The words are 'gigantic,' 'marsh,' and 'racket.' Let's talk about what these mean, and then when they appear in the story, we can talk again about what they mean . . . . "

> *During reading*: "There's that word 'marsh.' Do you remember what 'marsh' means?"

> *After reading*: "Let's talk about those new words we heard in this story . . . . "

Systematic Intervention

A second feature of high-quality emergent literacy intervention is that it is systematic. *Systematic* means that intervention activities follow a specific sequence of instruction to move along a continuum of skill or goals. Being systematic has two advantages. First, it allows the SLP to link a current learning goal to a previously learned goal or activity. For instance, in teaching a child how to produce rhymes, the SLP can point out: "Last week, we listened to rhymes to decide if two words rhymed or not. Today we're going to do something a little different. It might even be a little harder . . . " Second, it allows the SLP to establish the means for achieving a specific high-priority end. To illustrate, if a goal is set for a child to "write his/her own name independently," the SLP establishes a systematic sequence to follow to achieve that end.

Many SLPs are well trained to be systematic in their design and delivery of interventions; thus, this concept is not new. What may be relatively unfamiliar, however, is how to select a sequence of intervention for specific emergent literacy targets, such as alphabet knowledge and phonological awareness. There is no consensus on how to set up a particular sequence of instruction, with some experts contending the need to follow a developmental sequence and others supporting alternative approaches. As an example, let's take the case of phonological awareness. Phonological awareness emerges in children in a developmental sequence by which they first become aware of larger segments of speech such as words and syllables and later become aware of smaller segments of speech—namely, the phoneme. Two possible approaches to sequencing phonological awareness intervention are:

1. *Developmental sequence*: Follow a continuum that reflects how phonological awareness typically unfolds (from larger to smaller units of speech), and sequence instruction on a developmental ordering of targets (words, syllables, rimes, onsets, phonemes in all positions).
2. *High-priority focus*: Target instruction toward smaller units of speech only (phonemes), and sequence instruction to move across different types of tasks (e.g., blending phonemes in consonant-vowel-consonant [CVC] words, segmenting phonemes in CVC words, re-organizing phonemes in CVC words).

Currently, although the available evidence shows that participation in phonological awareness intervention is advantageous for children with needs in this area, the research base is not sufficient to characterize whether one sequence of instruction is better than another (National Reading Panel, 2000). What is clear is that skills in one area of phonological awareness (e.g., rhyme awareness) do not necessarily generalize to other areas (e.g., beginning sound awareness) (O'Connor, Jenkins, Leicester, & Slocum, 1993), and that the time spent in phonological awareness intervention need not be excessive (National Reading Panel, 2000). Rather, what seems important is for professionals to set an end goal for phonological awareness instruction that involves some level of phonemic-level awareness (e.g., ability to analyze phonemes) and then deliver intervention that is designed to systematically achieve this end goal, with a variety of sequences possible.

In some aspects of emergent literacy intervention, it can be very difficult to determine a sequence of instruction to ensure its systematicity. For instance, in the area of alphabet knowledge, should a specific order of letters be followed in intervention? Presently, there is no clear answer to this question. One possibility is to teach the letters to follow the alphabet string (A, B, C . . .), as many curricula do. Another possibility is to teach first those letters that are meaningful to the child (e.g., letters in the child's name or in a peer's name), as other curricula do. Another question one might ask is: should lowercase letters be taught first and then uppercase letters next, or vice versa? Again, no currently available evidence is sufficiently specific to guide these sorts of decisions. Although there is evidence showing that children learn first those letters in their own names (Justice, Bowles, Pence, & Wiggins, 2006), such findings could be interpreted in two ways in their application to sequencing instruction. It could be argued, for example, that intervention should teach first the letters in a child's own name, because that these emerge first (a developmental approach); conversely, perhaps intervention should teach anything but those letters in a child's own name, in view of the fact that these will tend to emerge on their own. The important point here is that the science available to professionals is somewhat unclear about the most *effective ways* to promote different emergent literacy skills, and arguments made to support one approach over another are typically based on theory and philosophy rather than hard evidence. What we do know, however, is that alphabet knowledge is an important goal of emergent literacy intervention, and that SLPs ought to design some sort of systematic way to ensuring that all children learn the letters in an efficient manner. How they go about achieving this goal should be done as systematically as possible, but there are many ways to do so. In setting a particular sequence of instruction, whatever it may be, systematicity allows the SLP to link a current goal to a previously learned concept: "Today we are going to learn about the lowercase P; last week we learned about uppercase P, and they are very close friends . . . Let's review what we know about uppercase P . . . . " Just as important, systematicity allows us to ensure that a child is moving along a set path to mastery, and that we always have the end goal in mind.

Purposeful Intervention

High-quality emergent literacy intervention involves ensuring that it is *purposeful*—that a given activity or goal has some linkage to the end purpose of reading, which is to comprehend (Ukrainetz, 2005). In emergent literacy intervention, much of the SLP's time will be devoted to helping children develop code-related skills across the domains of print knowledge and phonological awareness, because these directly promote a child's later transition to becoming a decoder. Becoming a good decoder is simply a means to an end, however, as is instruction that focuses on developing print knowledge and phonological awareness. The end goal is always to ensure a child's ability to ultimately be able to read to learn and to be a good comprehender. If this were not the end goal, we would simply be training children to call out words that they read.

The following example illustrates the relevance of purposeful intervention as applied to speech intervention. The SLP has been called in to work with a 3-year-old child who is severely unintelligible and who has a very limited repertoire of speech sounds. During intervention, the SLP focuses on increasing the child's inventory of speech sounds and suppressing certain processes that are adversely affecting intelligibility. Although improving articulation of specific speech sounds is a reasonable goal, it is a means to an end, which is ultimately to improve the child's ability to communicate well with others. Simply improving a child's intelligibility is a short-sighted goal, and one that fails to appreciate the purpose of intelligible speech. Thus, an experienced SLP will be sure to address speech sound goals within functional activities that promote the use of speech for meaningful and purposeful communication—which is, ultimately, the long-term goal of the intervention with this child.

In working with children to develop early code-related literacy skills, such as phonological awareness, the long-term goal to be kept in mind is for the child to one day be sufficiently able to "read to learn." To keep this focus in mind, it is useful for the SLP to link code-related activities to more purposeful aspects of literacy, to ensure that (1) the child recognizes and appreciates the purposes or functions of reading and writing, and (2) the child has ample opportunity to engage in these purposes and functions.

There are many ways to link code-based activities to the purposeful and meaningful aspects of reading and writing. For instance, an SLP could engage a child in a rhyming activity and then afterwards read a storybook with the child that features rhyming patterns; during the reading activity, the SLP can point out how the rhymes make the story fun, and how being able to listen carefully to words ultimately helps the child to be a better reader. Alternatively, in an activity focused on teaching a child several letters, rather than instructing the child to sit and write these letters rotely, the SLP can help the child generate a list of words related to friends or family members containing the target letters. The child can dictate the words to the SLP, who writes them down and points out the target letters; then the child and the SLP can read the words together. Again, by including a focus on the purposeful aspects of reading and writing, the SLP not only can create a more motivating context of learning but can also prime the child for recognizing that being able to rhyme and to name letters are part of one and the same skill set—the immensely important reading and writing skills that later in life will serve a range of purposes.

Emergent Literacy and Primary Prevention

The emphasis thus far has been on emergent literacy skills as critically valuable achievements on a continuum of literacy development and more specifically on those emergent literacy skills that are considered high-priority targets. As noted in the previous section, high-quality emergent literacy intervention should be explicit, systematic, and purposeful. The third characteristic, *purposeful*, reminds us that emergent literacy intervention is a means to an end. That end is to increase a child's likelihood of becoming a successful reader and writer. As was pointed out in the Preface to this book, the statistics concerning reading achievement among American schoolchildren are abysmal, with roughly 37% of fourth graders failing to attain even basic levels of reading performance (National Assessment of Education Progress, 2003). Presumably, none of us would find that statistic acceptable for our own children, and if our children were attending a school that reported a "63% success rate" in the area of reading, we would promptly find another school for our children.

Such statistics make it clear that the educational community, including SLPs who work in schools, needs to identify effective proactive solutions to shift children's odds toward healthier outcomes in the area of reading and then collaborate to ensure that these solutions are rigorously applied within our schools. Research has shown that reading and writing development begins much earlier in life than was previously recognized and that differences among children are predictive of their later likelihood for succeeding as readers; this evidence has opened the door to thinking about prevention as a viable solution for improving children's chances for becoming readers. Early identification of children who are not achieving well in emergent literacy development raises the possibility of being able to prevent (or at least ameliorate) the likelihood of their later experiencing a reading disability. For this reason, increased efforts are being directed toward early identification of children who are struggling in emergent literacy, and to provision of effective and rigorous emergent literacy interventions for children who are so identified.

Designing and delivering interventions that strengthen children's emergent literacy skills in print knowledge, phonological awareness, early writing, and oral language is consistent with a concept called *primary prevention*. Interventions for primary prevention can be differentiated from those for secondary and tertiary prevention, which are the traditional avenues for addressing reading and writing difficulties among children. Whereas primary prevention interventions focus on averting a disorder from ever emerging, secondary interventions focus on slowing the progression of a disorder once it has emerged, and tertiary interventions focus on compensating once a disorder has progressed. Secondary and tertiary interventions are focused on problems that not only are present but also already are exerting negative consequences.

Much of the school-based SLP's work involves secondary and tertiary interventions, because the typical caseload in this practice setting comprises children with identified disabilities who are eligible for special education services. Helping children develop emergent literacy skills requires a different model of practice from that of the secondary and tertiary interventions with which SLPs are most familiar and that they deliver to children who exhibit clinically depressed performance on some language or literacy measure. Although we may want to identify a child as having an "emergent literacy disorder," which therefore requires secondary-type intervention, the child who is slowly progressing in emergent literacy development should not be viewed as having a "disorder." In fact, most children who exhibit relatively slow development of emergent literacy skills can readily catch up with their better-achieving peers with adequate high-quality emergent literacy intervention, thereby mitigating their need for subsequent secondary and tertiary intervention (Justice & Pullen, 2003). Thus, there is no need to identify early differences or delays in emergent literacy development as "disordered" as a means for a child to warrant special services; rather, emergent literacy intervention ought to be conceived as a primary prevention practice that is designed to avert or thwart a disorder from ever emerging.

To illustrate the differences among primary, secondary, and tertiary interventions and how emergent literacy intervention is best characterized as primary prevention, an analogy can be drawn between literacy supports and dental care. Very early on, all young children learn to brush their teeth as a matter of good hygiene and to prevent the occurrence of tooth and gum disease. Some people may be particularly vulnerable for teeth and gum decay as a result of eating and cleaning habits as well as genetics. Nevertheless, tooth brushing is advocated as "best practice" for *everyone*, because early on, when children are very young—it is difficult to predict who is most likely to later experience teeth and gum decay. Some children may be particularly prone to dental hygiene problems because of environmental circumstances (e.g., limited family resources to pay for dentist visits) and developmental circumstances (e.g., cleft palate). For these children, primary prevention is even more important and valuable than it may be for other children without such risks. Especially in this population of children, good dental hygiene during the early years is considered to be a preventive strategy that may well prevent serious dental disease in adulthood.

Likewise, emergent literacy intervention can serve as a strategy to prevent serious problems later in life. The current emphasis on emergent literacy interventions is a highly favorable development that parallels the nationwide emphasis, by now taken for granted, on good oral hygiene. Children need to be supported in their earliest literacy achievements—even before they begin to read—to keep a reading disability from manifesting itself or at least to mitigate its severity if the disability truly cannot be avoided. When children are young, it is hard to tell which ones will later experience reading disability; although some risk factors may be indicators of subsequent literacy difficulty, a number of children will struggle with reading for no known reason. Thus, all children should be provided with implicit and explicit supports to develop emergent literacy foundations that presumably will decrease the occurrence of reading disability among the nation's schoolchildren. The posters that hang in physicians' offices urging parents to read to their children constitute a primary prevention approach. Playing phonological awareness games in the preschool classroom also is consistent with primary prevention. The historical approach to addressing reading disabilities did not emphasize primary prevention. The only model of intervention was secondary and tertiary: Supports were delivered only after problems manifested. Thus, today's emphasis on emergent literacy interventions is truly revolutionary.

Giving weight to the importance of primary prevention in the area of reading is the understanding that when reading difficulties are allowed to progress, their remediation not only is quite difficult but also can be very expensive. Secondary interventions focus on slowing the course of reading difficulties in children who show problems in early literacy, in the "learning to read" stage. Interventions at this stage include, for instance, Reading Recovery and Book Buddies, both of which involve small-group or one-on-one tutoring to kindergarten and/or first-grade students showing signs of reading difficulty. These programs are akin to filling a cavity: Difficulties are noted in the area of reading, but with appropriate measures these difficulties can be halted. Of course, for some children, filling the cavity does not save the affected tooth; correspondingly, reading difficulties will continue to progress. However, this will be the case for far fewer children than if the secondary approach had not been provided. By about the third and fourth grades, when children begin to "read to learn," tertiary interventions are needed for those children who are truly struggling. If these children receive primary and secondary interventions, their manifestation of reading disability in the later elementary grades will not be as grave as if those early preventive approaches had not been provided. Likewise, it is plausible that far fewer children will be affected than if the primary and secondary approaches were not implemented. Presumably, with these multiple tiers of reading difficulty prevention in place, the rate of reading disability in the United States can be reduced from strikingly grave levels (40% to 50%) to very low levels (2% to 5%). Nevertheless, once a bona fide reading disability manifests and is present in the later elementary grades, the consequences are significant. Not only are interventions at this level expensive and intensive, but children do not have the reading skills that are needed to achieve across content areas such as history, literature, and mathematics.

For children with language impairment, the rates of reading failure are exceedingly high. Catts, Fey, Tomblin, and Zhang (2002) reported that 53% of children with language impairment exhibited depressed reading performance in second grade, and 48% exhibited poor performance in fourth grade. By comparison, the rates of poor reading performance were 8% in second and fourth grades for typically developing children. Those children with nonspecific language impairments (characterized by generally low intelligence) had the greatest risk for reading difficulties, with 64% of these children meeting the criteria for reading disability at fourth grade.

These data unequivocally show the need for SLPs to take a proactive role in preventing reading difficulties among the children with whom they work, as well as in the more general population of at-risk children for whom emergent literacy intervention may serve as the most powerful mechanism for improving the likelihood that they will become lifelong readers.

References

Bear, D. B., Invernizzi, M., Templeton, S., & Johnston, F. (2003). *Words their way*. Upper Saddle River, NJ: Prentice Hall.

Bryant, P., Maclean, M., & Bradley, L. (1990). Rhyme, language, and children's reading. *Applied Psycholinguistics, 11*, 237–252.

Catts, H. W., Fey, M. E., Tomblin, J. B., & Zhang, X. (2002). A longitudinal investigation of reading outcomes in children with language impairment. *Journal of Speech, Language, and Hearing Research, 45*, 1142–1157.

Chall, J. S. (1983). *Stages of reading development*. New York: McGraw-Hill.

Clay, M. M. (1966). *Emergent reading behaviour*. Unpublished doctoral dissertation, University of Auckland, New Zealand.

Clay, M. M. (1979). *Reading: The patterning of complex behaviour*. Exeter, NH: Heinemann.

Ehri, L. (1991). Learning to read and spell words. In L. Rieben & C. A. Perfetti (Eds.), *Learning to read: Basic research and its implications* (pp. 57–73). Hillsdale, NJ: Lawrence Erlbaum Associates.

Frijters, J. C., Barron, R. W., & Brunello, M. (2000). Direct and mediated influences of home literacy and literacy interest on prereaders' oral vocabulary and early written language skill. *Journal of Educational Psychology, 92*, 466–477.

Frith, U. (1985). Beneath the surface of developmental dyslexia. In K. Patterson, J. Marshall, & M. Coltheart (Eds.), *Surface dyslexia: Neuropsychological and cognitive studies of phonological reading* (pp. 301–330). London: Lawrence Erlbaum Associates.

Ganger, J., & Brent, M. R. (2004). Reexamining the vocabulary spurt. *Developmental Psychology, 40*, 621–632.

Ganske, K. (2000). *Word journeys*. New York: Guilford Press.

Hammill, D. D. (2004). What we know about correlates of reading. *Exceptional Children, 70*, 453–468.

Justice, L. M., Pence, K., Bowles, R., & Wiggins, A. K. (2006). An investigation of four hypotheses concerning the order by which 4-year-old children learn the alphabet letters. *Early Childhood Research Quarterly, 21*, 374–389.

Justice, L. M., Chow, S. M., Capellini, C., Flanigan, K., & Colton, S. (2003). Emergent literacy intervention for vulnerable preschoolers: Relative effects of two approaches. *American Journal of Speech-Language Pathology, 12*, 320–332.

Justice, L. M., & Ezell, H. K. (2002). Use of storybook reading to increase print awareness in at-risk children. *American Journal of Speech-Language Pathology, 11*, 17–29.

Justice, L. M., Kaderavek, J., Bowles, R., & Grimm, K. (2005). Phonological awareness, language impairment, and parent-child shared reading: A feasibility study. *Topics in Early Childhood Special Education, 25*, 143–156.

Justice, L. M., Invernizzi, M. A., & Meier, J. D. (2002). Designing and implementing an early literacy screening protocol: Suggestions for the speech-language pathologist. *Language, Speech, and Hearing Services in Schools, 33*, 84–101.

Justice, L. M., & Pullen, P. (2003). Early literacy intervention strategies: A review of promising findings. *Topics in Early Childhood Special Education, 23*, 99–113.

Katims, D. (1994). Emergence of literacy in preschool children with disabilities. *Learning Disability Quarterly, 17*, 58–69.

National Assessment of Education Progress. (2003). *The Nation's report card*. Retrieved October 10, 2004, from http://nces.ed.gov/nations reportcard/

National Early Literacy Panel. (2004, November). *The National Early Literacy Panel: A research synthesis on early literacy development*. Presentation to the Annual Meeting of the National Association of Early Childhood Specialists, Anaheim, CA.

National Reading Panel. (2000). *Teaching children to read: An evidence-based assessment of the scientific research literature on reading and its implications for reading instruction*. Washington, DC: U.S. National Institute for Literacy.

O'Connor, R. E., Jenkins, J. R., Leicester, N., & Slocum, T. A. (1993). Teaching phonological awareness to young children with learning disabilities. *Exceptional Children, 59*, 532–546.

O'Connor, R. E., Notari-Syverson, A., & Vadasy, P. (1996). Ladders to literacy: The effects of teacher-led phonological activities for kindergarten children with and without disabilities. *Exceptional Children, 63,* 117–130.

Scarborough, H. S., & Dobrich, W. (1994). On the efficacy of reading to preschoolers. *Developmental Review, 14,* 245–302.

Snow, C., Burns, M. S., & Griffin, P. (Eds.) (1998). *Preventing reading difficulties in young children.* Washington, DC: National Academy Press.

Snow, K. L. (2006). Measuring school readiness: Conceptual and practical considerations. *Early Education and Development, 17,* 7–41.

Storch, S. A., & Whitehurst, G. J. (2002). Oral language and code-related precursors to reading: Evidence from a longitudinal structural model. *Developmental Psychology, 38,* 934–947.

Teale, W. H., & Sulzby, E. (1986). *Emergent literacy: Writing and reading.* Norwood, NJ: Ablex.

Ukrainetz, T. A. (2005). *Contextualized language intervention.* Eau Claire, WI: Thinking Publications.

Vygotksy, L. (1978). *Mind and society.* Cambridge, MA: MIT Press.

Chapter Two

Meeting the Needs of Culturally and Linguistically Diverse Families in Early Language and Literacy Intervention

Susan M. Moore
Clara Pérez-Méndez
Karin Boerger

Overview

Children of immigrants constitute the fastest-growing component of the child population of the United States (Matthews & Ewen, 2006; U.S. Census, 2000). In fact, one in every five children in U.S. schools comes from a home in which the family speaks a language other than English, and many children of immigrants (56%) live in families with low incomes or have parents with low education levels and limited English proficiency (Capps, Fix, Passel, Ost, & Reardon, 2005). Paradoxically, there is a documented long-term tendency for both over referral and under-referral of children who are English language learners (ELLs) to special education services (Artiles & Ortiz, 2001). This is attributed in part to a long-existent difficulty among professionals in distinguishing language *disorders* from language *differences* (Goldstein, 2004; Kayser, 1993; Roseberry-McKibbon, 2003), as well as a sociohistorical perspective that children whose first language is other than English frequently will exhibit problems in learning (Goldstein, 2004).

Currently, there is a significant need for proactive, preventive programs that facilitate positive developmental outcomes for children who are ELLs, while simultaneously supporting their families' specific needs and strengths. Speech-language pathologists (SLPs) and other professionals can play a key role in such activities, as they do in *El Grupo de Familias*, a parent education and support program that includes a focus on children's language and emergent literacy development. El Grupo de Familias was developed in 1995 through funding by a personnel preparation grant designed to expand clinical educational opportunities for bilingual master's degree candidates in speech-language pathology as they prepared to serve linguistically diverse populations. The program was developed in response to an increasing population of children from Spanish-speaking families in Boulder, Colorado. At the time, there was a paucity of services available for families of young children with identified challenges in language development, and these families were struggling with decisions regarding which languages their children should learn (i.e., English versus Spanish). This provided the impetus for developing a prevention program focused on improving the language and emergent literacy development of children learning English as a second language (ESL) through parent education. El Grupo focuses on family members' use of high-quality interactive strategies during everyday routines and activities, including storytelling and shared storybook reading. Beyond its focus on promoting home-based parent-child interactions, this program also emphasizes provision of information and supports to parents, with goals that include helping them make informed decisions about which languages their children should learn and fostering connections to community supports to enhance their own learning.

This chapter presents an overview of El Grupo de Familias as a model prevention program that SLPs throughout the country may adapt for their own activities with culturally and linguistically diverse (CLD) families. The chapter is organized to first provide background information concerning service challenges and needs in working with CLD families, particularly as they make decisions concerning their young children's language development. The specific design principles utilized in developing El Grupo de Familias are reviewed next. The final section presents approaches incorporating specific activities used in parent education to support the goals of the program.

Service Challenges and Needs: Supporting CLD Families in Language-Learning Decisions

As noted by Goldstein (2004), "the rapid growth of . . . ELLs . . . has greatly challenged our present system for assessing and treating ELLs with communication disorders" (p. 5). Such challenges include the following:

- An inadequate supply of educators and health care providers with knowledge of cultural and linguistic factors that influence communication development
- A paucity of speakers of languages other than English in the provider workforce, along with a lack of trained interpreters and translators
- Health care and early education systems that often are difficult to access for low-income and/or diverse families
- Inadequate assessment tools appropriate for CLD children, resulting in over- and under-identification of disabilities
- Mismatches between the cultures of families and teachers, with the latter expecting children of these families to fit the dominant culture's expectations

As might be expected, such system-specific challenges can influence the decisions that parents make when confronted with choices concerning their children's language development. Native Spanish-speaking parents who are learning ESL must decide whether to raise their children as English speakers, Spanish speakers, or bilinguals, and too often families base their choices about the languages their children will learn on fear of discrimination, limited information about the benefits of bilingualism, and other negative sociocultural considerations and concepts (Hammer, Miccio, & Wagstaff, 2003; Pérez-Méndez & Moore, 2003; Sanchez, 1999). Of importance, what they want most is for their young children to succeed; therefore, a common assumption among family members is that they often have to choose English over their home language. At least for some children, this results in a loss of the home language. Wong Fillmore (1991) highlights the negative consequences for any child who loses his or her first language, which typically is the case when families are counseled or decide to focus on learning only the dominant language of English. Some of these negative consequences include loss of identity, self-esteem, connection to family and heritage, and potential for native language proficiency.

Although learning the "dominant" language of a community may have some perceived benefits, a loss of bilingual opportunity has been correlated with lower levels of performance later in life, in comparison with well-developed bilingualism. Research indicates that students with highly developed bilingual skills reach higher levels of academic and cognitive functioning than those attained by monolingual students or students with poor bilingual skills (Hakuta & Garcia, 1989). Kessler and Quinn (1987) found that bilingual children performed better than monolingual children did in creativity and problem-solving tasks, showing more complexity and sophistication in their performance. Children who are proficient in speaking their first language and are literate in their first language may have an easier time learning ESL (Artiles & Ortiz, 2002; Genesee, Paradis, & Crago, 2004; Goldstein, 2004; Lindholm-Leary, 2005), because exposure to more than one language in a systematic way allows use of strengths in the first language to enhance proficiency in a second language (Tabors, 1998; Thomas & Collier, 1997–1998). Additionally, within the increasingly global economy, bilingualism carries even more advantages beyond its facilitating effects on language and cognition. As noted by August and Hakuta (1997), students who are bilingual will have skills that in adulthood will enable them to take advantage of more career opportunities, making them increasingly competitive in the global market.

As is emphasized in El Grupo de Familias, parents and family members need access to information about bilingualism as they make decisions regarding their children's language development. It is critical that they have all of the available information regarding benefits of bilingualism to help them engage in a decision-making process about which languages their children will learn. Information that supports their decision to preserve home language and culture is especially appropriate in view of the current sociopolitical environment in the United States. At least in some communities, a "subtractive" attitude that devalues bilingualism and preservation of home language learning prevails, in contrast with an "additive environment" in which linguistic diversity is valued. Thus, families often are told that giving up their first language at the expense of learning a second language is necessary or preferable for their children to succeed. Unfortunately, many educators and professionals continue to discourage use of a child's home or first language and recommend that young learners focus on learning English to the exclusion of the language of the home.

For children who have developmental weaknesses in language, reflecting a general or more specific language impairment, it is particularly important that parental decisions concerning language development are made in an informed and timely manner. Some parents of children with language impairment may be counseled to support the child's development of only one language. However, with sufficient exposure, interaction, and an "additive environment," wherein linguistic diversity is valued, young children with identified language impairments clearly have the capacity to learn two languages (Genesee et al., 2004). Genesee and colleagues recently studied bilingual children with specific language impairment (SLI) who were exposed to two languages from birth. Their study results showed that children with SLI exhibited difficulties in both languages but could become well-balanced bilingual speakers. They also reported that rates of language learning did not differ significantly between children with SLI exposed to two languages and those exposed to only one language. In another study by Bird and colleagues (2005), the language abilities of eight children with Down syndrome (DS) who were raised in bilingual environments were compared with those of three groups of children matched on developmental level: monolingual children with DS, monolingual typically developing children, and bilingual typically developing children. Results showed there to be no detrimental effect of bilingualism.

As these findings suggest, counseling parents of children with SLI to expose their children to only one language is not consistent with the available empirical evidence. Indeed, there is enough persuasive research showing that professionals need to refrain from automatically assuming that having two languages is the exclusive domain of children with typical development (Genesee et al., 2004). The research on children with SLI shows that these youngsters will be challenged in learning two languages, just as they are challenged in learning one language, but that learning two languages does not necessarily compromise language development (Genesee et al., 2004). As Restrepo (2005) has pointed out, those children with and without SLI who speak Spanish as their first language experience less language loss with entry into a second language environment if their first language is supported. Of course, it is critical that researchers continue to investigate the impact of an identified language disability on learning two languages. At present, information regarding how young children learn languages applies regardless of the presence of a challenge or disability (Moore & Perez-Mendez, 2006). Thus, it can be asserted that bilingual children with SLI will experience difficulty associated with their language impairment, but no more than that experienced in a monolingual environment. Opportunities and exposure to two languages can result in successful bilingualism and should not be automatically denied on the basis of an identified disability.

Factors, Phases, and Processes Influencing Second Language Learning

Myriad factors can influence how children learn two languages, as shown in Table 2-1. These include the age and timing of exposure to the second language, environmental factors, and intrinsic characteristics of the child, such as motivation, language aptitude, and learning styles/personality. Examining these factors helps professionals to understand individual variation among learners and to recognize that children will display individual differences in their pattern of language development consistent with their circumstances. As is emphasized in El Grupo de Familias, family members need to understand what factors influence their children's learning of more than one language and consider this information as they make decisions about which languages they will speak at home. Family members also benefit from information regarding influences that are inherent in different stages and phases of second language learning, especially how children will use bilingual processes (e.g., code switching) that are typical in the second language acquisition process. Often, these typical bilingual processes are mistaken as signals of a disorder, versus a difference, by persons who do not understand the different factors that influence second language acquisition.

There are many resources available that can help family members and professionals understand those factors that influence the language acquisition of children learning two languages. For parents whose children are learning a second language sequentially (see Table 2-1), which often is the case for CLD families, in which

Table 2–1. Influencing Factors in Second Language Acquisition

---

Age/Timing:

Simultaneous: Learning two languages from birth

Sequential: Learning second language after degree of proficiency is reached in first language

Environment:

Subtractive bilingual environment: When children are expected to learn the dominant language and to give up their native language

Additive bilingual environment: When there is substantial support for children to maintain their native language as they acquire a second language

Degree of exposure: Quality and quantity of language inputs in both languages

Child Characteristics:

Motivation

Language aptitude

Learning styles and personality

Source: Adapted from Moore et al., (1995) *Developing Cultural Competence in Early Childhood Assessment*, UCB Boulder, Co.

children learn a second language when entering preschool or elementary school, it is helpful to identify for the parents how their children will use language as they move through stages or phases of second language acquisition; Tabors (1997) and Krashen (1982) provide excellent resources. For example, both authors point out that young preschool-age children who are sequential rather than simultaneous learners of two languages from birth typically experience a nonverbal or "silent period" when they first enter a second language learning environment. Many teachers have observed this behavior and mistakenly construed it to mean that the child has a language disability or delay. It is important to distinguish this behavior from language impairment, because young children who are learning two languages will continue to watch, use gesture, mimic their friends, and eventually take the risk of speaking the second language if they are in an additive situation wherein their first language is respected and valued. Sanchez (2005) explains the critical importance of offering support during this time and refraining from criticizing, punishing, or correcting the young language learner for using a first language. She emphasizes that children need to feel safe as they venture out and begin to use their second language.

After a silent period, sequential language learners may then begin to use single words or formulaic phrases (e.g., "my turn") to communicate their needs and ideas (Tabors, 1997). As their comprehension of the second language develops, children will continue to develop longer and more complex expressive language if supported to do so. During this phase, a variety of bilingual processes may be served, including code switching or code mixing, in which vocabulary from both languages is used in one utterance (e.g., "I missed my abuelo mucho") or when the rules of one language for word order are carried over to the second language (e.g., "the boy tall" versus "the tall boy"). These patterns as well as those of language loss and reduced exposure all are explained in the literature and are very typical for ELLs (Genesee et al., 2004; Goldstein, 2004; Krashen, 1982; Tabors, 1997).

It is important for family members to understand that such behaviors are typical and can be expected as part of the language learning process for children exposed to two or more languages. If parents understand the process of second language learning, they can better support their children to learn two languages and become proficient bilingual speakers. They also can acquire understanding of why their children may behave in particular ways at certain times, and whether these behaviors are typical or not. For example, as children get older and are exposed to persons who devalue their language, they may refuse to speak their home language at school and at home with their parents. This is a commonly reported occurrence among CLD children growing up in an English-dominant community that holds a subtractive view of bilingualism.

Literacy Learning in Two Languages

Thus far, the discussion has focused on issues associated with language development for children of CLD families, particularly the importance of supporting families' access to information concerning bilingualism. Another important consideration is supporting families to ensure their children's timely development of emergent literacy skills through high-quality home activities. This is particularly relevant in working with parents who may have had few, if any, home literacy experiences themselves as children. In El Grupo de Familas, a key goal is supporting the frequency of home-based shared reading between parents and their children, identified as a key predictor of later reading abilities (Adams, 1990; Dickinson & Tabors, 2001; Kaderavek & Sulzby, 1998; Wells, 1985). More recently, the literature has suggested that researchers need to look beyond *frequency* as a predictor of later reading abilities and spend more time investigating the *quality* of interactions when parents read with young children (Snow, Burns, & Griffin, 1998). Thus, in El Grupo de Familias, parents also are assisted to engage their children in high-quality reading experiences.

Families benefit from understanding that both frequent shared story-book reading and how they read with their children can directly influence how their children learn about the meaning of print and develop an understanding of new vocabulary and alphabetic knowledge in their first or second language. Parents appreciate learning how their practices with their children at home can foster their children's short- and long-term achievements, because many of the parents served in the El Grupo program have high expectations for their children:

> "I want for my son to study, to graduate, and to choose a career to follow what he wants to study."—A father from El Grupo de Familias

> "I would like my daughter to learn what I never learned. I want her to go to university . . . all the way."—A mother from El Grupo de Familias

El Grupo de Familias: Design Principles

El Grupo de Familias uses a prevention model focused on enhancing the early language and emergent literacy development of children from CLD families. A principal feature of the program is the direct involvement of parents in the program, who meet in a series of ten 2-hour sessions using a triadic model of implementation, meaning that both children and parents or family members are involved in each session. An overview of session topics is presented in Figure 2–1.

EL GRUPO DE FAMILIAS
Primavera 2005

9 de FEBRERO
de 4:30 a 6:00 PM
En la Escuela del Centro
de la Universidad
"La Barita que Habla"

16 de FEBRERO
de 4:30 a 6:00 PM
En la Escuela del Centro
de la Universidad
"El Desarrollo de
la Lectura"

23 de FEBRERO
de 4:30 a 6:00 PM
En la Escuela del Centro
de la Universidad
"¿Quién Manda
en Casa?"

2 de MARZO
de 4:30 a 6:00 PM
"Visita a la
Biblioteca"

9 de MARZO
de 4:30 a 6:00 PM
En la Escuela del Centro
de la Universidad
"Preservación de la Cultura
y del Lenguaje"

16 de MARZO
de 4:30 a 6:00 PM
"Visita al Museo
de los Niños"

6 de ABRIL
de 4:30 a 6:00 PM
En la Escuela del Centro
de la Universidad
"Navegando el Sistema
Escolar"

13 de ABRIL
de 4:30 a 6:00 PM
En la Escuela del Centro
de la Universidad
"Fiesta de Graduación y
Cajas de Literatura"

Figure 2–1. Schedule of Spring 2005 sessions for El Grupo de Familias.

El Grupo participants are parents and their children between the ages of 2 years 6 months and 3 years 6 months who attend the Child Language Center (CLC) preschool classroom at the University of Colorado. Eight children participate at a given time, and typically at least three of the eight have been identified as having a language disability or are at risk for language difficulties. Families are referred to El Grupo from a variety of persons and agencies or institutions. Child Find Español and Part C services in the city of Boulder often recommend that parents enroll in El Grupo because of concerns about the child's development. Many other children are referred by family members, pediatricians or other health care providers, or neighbors. Inclusion is considered best practice to building community at this level. Throughout the 10-session parent education program, parents or family members observe their children in interactions with peers and meet for selected topic discussions in a comfortable room upstairs.

El Grupo is coordinated by a cultural mediator who is both bilingual and bicultural, which helps to ease the enrollment process. In scheduling the weekly sessions, parents' work schedules and other obligations are taken into consideration for determining a specific time and day. There is an attempt to be flexible to meet the needs of single parents as well as families in which both parents are working, sometimes on two different schedules. Also, parents can invite family members and friends to participate in the program sessions, including peers, mothers, fathers, grandparents, aunts, and uncles.

Before beginning the program, parents often are introduced to the purposes of the group during home visits with the cultural mediator and a bilingual graduate student or staff member. The initial session of the series serves as an opportunity for participating children and parents to meet each other and for completion of paperwork. At this first session, general questions are asked and answered, transportation arrangements are confirmed, and input regarding specific topics for desired discussion is collected. A video camera allows parents to observe their children in the classroom from the comfortable rooms upstairs. They also can use an observation booth with a one-way mirror, or they may be encouraged to join the children in play activities in the classroom.

The program design of El Grupo carefully attends to the accumulated scientific and theoretical evidence concerning parent education programs and early intervention. Thus, the following principles were selected to guide El Grupo:

- Family-centered practice
- Authentic experiences
- Culturally resonant practices
- Linguistically and culturally responsive relationships
- Prevention

Specifics of how these principles are applied in the El Grupo program are presented next.

Family-Centered Practice

Early language and literacy learning is strengthened when parents are listened to and involved in the process early on, especially for children identified with SLI or considered to be "at risk" for learning two languages. Parents benefit from talking with professionals and other parents about their concerns and questions regarding their child's development. Consistent with the proven benefits of early intervention, a key program tenet is "the earlier the better," especially for children with developmental concerns. When parents or family members share their story, they provide critical information that helps professionals know and understand their child. When the participants are listened to and respected, they become more invested in the intervention process because they perceive that their feelings and values are understood and appreciated. As they become more comfortable, they are willing to become involved and participate in activities that enhance and promote their child's early communication, language(s), and preliteracy development. They feel listened to when a cultural mediator who is both bilingual and bicultural visits them at home, explains the goals and purposes of the program, and seeks their input on what information they feel they need to support their child's learning. Use of open-ended questions to facilitate parents' sharing of priorities, concerns, what they know about their child, and what they want more information about promotes trust and participation in a process that often is new to them.

Authentic Experiences

Children learn languages and build foundations for literacy by being exposed to language in everyday routines and interactive activities, as well as in shared storybook reading. From birth onward, young children learn vocabulary and develop oral language abilities by being read to and talked to throughout the day (Hart & Risley, 1995). They learn through constructing meaning in their world. Exposure to and interactions in one or both languages are critical in building early language abilities and foundations for conventional literacy. Activities that incorporate a focus on vocabulary learning, phonological awareness, alphabetic knowledge, and print awareness are embedded and modeled in the classroom during group play and storybook reading with peers. Parents enjoy observing their children and engaging in activities that they can bring home. They watch and learn how their children respond. They learn why it is important to embed learning opportunities into daily routines and activities, and to read with their children on a daily basis.

Culturally Resonant Practices

Preservation of home language and culture involves the recognition that all children with or without identified language challenges have the potential to learn more than one language. It can no longer be assumed that just because a child has an identified language challenge, he or she cannot learn more than one language (Genesee et al., 2004). Family members need this information so that they can make informed decisions about which languages their child will learn. Family members need information about how children learn their first and second languages and how this affects later learning and development of conventional literacy in both languages. Families develop knowledge through dialogue and interactions when they have access to all of the information, including the benefits of bilingualism. They are encouraged to make decisions based on their newly acquired knowledge in the context of what they value and want for their child.

Linguistically and Culturally Responsive Relationships

Practices that are linguistically and culturally responsive build trusting relationships with family members based on cultural understanding and individual consideration. The ability of the professional to communicate in a preferred language with all participants obviously helps family members gain a level of comfort needed to share their stories and to discuss any issues and concerns about their child's development of language(s). Communicating in the preferred language of the home also provides a model for children that their language is valued and respected. The language of El Grupo is Spanish, although many of the family members are emergent bilingual and speak some English. Cultural activities and ways of sharing that celebrate and honor the values and beliefs of those represented in a group instill trust and cultural understanding without stereotyping the participants. Understanding what is culturally responsive for a particular group is determined by knowing and understanding the particular people who make up that group. Stories about lifeways, previous educational experiences, what the family members consider important, and what families want for their children help develop understanding and are not necessarily assumed to be the same for all families. Differences among families are respected. Diverse perspectives on expectations, educational options, and how children learn are discussed and shared among members of the group.

Prevention

Overrepresentation and underrepresentation of CLD children in special education is a continuing issue that parents are concerned about and that is a reality for many children from diverse backgrounds in today's schools. Many parents are concerned that if their children are labeled as ELLS, they will not have the same educational opportunities as those for other children and may end up in special education classes. Other families are hesitant to access the services and supports that are available to children identified with special needs. Sometimes they do not even know that these services and supports exist. It is important for families who are CLD to understand how the educational system works and how they can gain access to resources that are best for their child. Learning about what they can expect when their child is young prevents later misunderstandings and conflicts. Dialogue and discussion about educational options, what can be expected as children enter school, and how to access appropriate resources can help families to understand the system and advocate for their child.

A Developmental Model for Working with Families

In addition to the design principles just outlined for El Grupo, a transactional model of information sharing that views parents' growth from a developmental perspective also was incorporated into program design. Just as children grow and change in response to direct literacy interventions, parents also can be supported to grow and change through effective interventional activities, particularly concerning their own sense of efficacy in influencing their children's lives. Accordingly, we adapted a developmental model based on work by Erikson (1959) to represent the growth of parents as they developed their own identity as instrumental in influencing their children's lives. This model assumes a parallel process between Erickson's initial developmental stages of child growth and development and a parent's developmental process in obtaining the necessary knowledge and information to successfully support the child's learning and education. An overview of Erikson's three stages, related to how El Grupo supports parents' movement through these phases, is presented next.

Establishing Trust and Mutual Understanding

Trust involves feelings of safety, knowledge of what to expect, and mutual understanding between family members and those involved in providing support and information. In order to establish trust, professionals working with families benefit from examining differences in expectations that may be associated with a family's background or cultural heritage. This demands individual consideration of each person and each family and moving beyond assumptions based on backgrounds and culture. Understanding of role differences in parenting and lifeways leads to respect even though they may differ from those of the dominant culture or those of the professional. As previously noted, trust evolves when parents are listened to and are provided the information they need in a nonjudgmental way so they can make informed decisions about their child and family. Reciprocity and conversations are key. These values are basic tenets of family-centered practice in that parents are recognized as the primary decision makers for their children; the professional's role becomes one of consultant.

Promoting Confidence and Autonomy

Establishing trust leads to increasing confidence and autonomy on the part of participating family members that is marked by feelings of competence and confidence based on experience, affirmation, and respect. Families develop the skills to interact with professionals and advocate for their children only when they trust in the responsiveness of the system, are knowledgeable about the system, and have enough information to make appropriate choices for their child and family. El Grupo provides opportunities for family members to participate as respected members of the team and to advocate for their child. The strengths of family members are emphasized and affirmed. El Grupo creates opportunities for families to organize, participate, and initiate, and participating professionals are responsive to family initiations. There is a focus on support for family-to-family connections and shared experiences.

Affirming Initiative and Independence

The third stage involves increasing initiative based on motivation, feelings of adequacy, and decision making that leads to advocacy and empowerment and independence. This is consonant with a proactive empowerment model of parent education and support, as articulated by Dunst, Trivette, and Deal (1988) and Turnball and Turnball (2001). As parents are supported to move into and through this stage, the emphasis is on affirming parents' questions and concerns, building reliable alliances between parents and community members and organizations, and connecting parents to other parents.

Guiding Principles in Working With Families

For SLPs to work with CLD families in programs such as El Grupo, they must promote parents' developmental progress through the three stages discussed previously. The efficacy of professionals' work with parents is grounded in their ability to be culturally competent, which is a particularly important concern when program leaders differ in cultural and linguistic background from the program participants. The El Grupo program emphasizes six principles and practices of which professionals must be particularly aware. These principles, listed in Table 2–2, are briefly described next.

Table 2–2. Guiding Principles and Practices for Professionals Working with Families in the El Grupo de Familias Program

---

Connecting With Families: El Grupo Principles

- Examine your own culture, beliefs, values, and bias
- Avoid assumptions
- Move beyond stereotypes
- Adopt ethnographic interviewing strategies
- Recognize barriers to communication
- Make effective use of cultural mediators, translators and interpreters
- Remember always that culturally competent, relevant, and meaningful interactions build the foundation for relationships with families

---

Source: From Moore, S. M., & Perez-Mendez, C. (2006). *A Story about El Grupo de Familias.* Boulder, CO: Landlocked Films. Available at: http://www.landlockedfilms.com

Examining One's Own Culture, Beliefs, Values, and Bias

This is the first step in developing cultural competence according to Lynch and Hanson (1998, p. 87). These authors outline a cultural journey that leads professionals to examine their own cultural background and heritage and promotes an awareness of the ongoing reality of racism and prejudice in today's world. They recommend that, for each professional, the process of self-examination should begin with a process of self-reflection about personal origins, knowledge of ancestors, family traditions, celebrations, and ceremonies or stories that reflect some aspect of personal heritage. Through this process of self-reflection, professionals come to realize the impact of background and culture on personal values and beliefs, and how this "cultural lens" can lead to judgments of adequacy of others' values when compared with one's own. The journey continues with reflections about negative comments or attitudes toward one's own culture, religion, or ethnicity. These authors suggest that only through self-reflection about one's own background can an awareness and respect for differences of others be developed.

Turnbull and Turnbull (2001) also affirm that a first step in developing reliable alliances with family members is developing self-knowledge. Understanding one's own values and beliefs is prerequisite to understanding another's perspective. Knowing one's own biases increases awareness of how to handle perspectives different from one's own. These authors also emphasize the importance of gaining knowledge about other cultures that differ from one's own. Reading about different cultural beliefs, lifeways, perspectives on child rearing, or beliefs regarding disability provides the background knowledge necessary to understand why families may make decisions or act as they do, as well as respect for those decisions. For example, a book by Anne Fadiman, *The Spirit Catches You and You Fall Down*, is highly recommended reading for anyone working in health care or education. This poignant story of a young child with a seizure disorder and her family's conflicts and misunderstandings with her health care providers opens up the reader's understanding of how culture influences all aspects of life. Listening to family stories about previous experiences or the lifeways of a family's country of origin builds an appreciation for cultural differences and an understanding of what might be considered culturally responsive practice.

Avoiding Assumptions

Despite the fact that a family may use a particular language (e.g., Spanish) or identify itself as part of a particular culture (e.g., Hispanic), culturally competent professionals avoid making generalizations based on language and culture. Such professionals recognize that "all families, in fact, vary greatly in the degree [to] which their beliefs and practices are representative of a particular culture, language group, religious group, or country of origin" (Thorp, 1997, p. 261). Culturally competent professionals also avoid making assumptions based on their own intentions and beliefs. For example, instead of assuming that absence from parent meetings or IEP meetings means lack of interest, educators must understand the barriers that hinder some parents from participating in their child's education. Instead of assuming that children are passive and quiet, teachers need to understand that many families want and tell their children to behave, respect, and obey what teachers say to them.

Sometimes children may even be instructed not to ask questions in class, because this may be considered a sign of disrespect.

Assumptions can be dangerous in attempts to develop trust with a family. The skill of *reframing* (Barrera, 1993) is useful in all of life's endeavors because it helps us reflect on the judgments we may automatically make and to "rethink" them. Reframing means rewording what one is thinking or assuming in a positive way that can lead to a workable solution to a dilemma. For example, an educator may comment, "Those parents never show up to meetings. They just don't seem to care." Reframing this statement may lead to better understanding of what is truly happening: "I wonder what is preventing Jose's parents from coming to meetings? Maybe I should try talking with them."

Moving Beyond Stereotypes

Respect for and recognition of individual differences in levels of acculturation, perspective, values, and lifeways allow professionals to avoid stereotyping individual people and families. As Bateson notes (1999), stereotyping often is used by professionals to make sense of complex issues:

> Prejudice and stereotyping are ways of making intellectual and emotional sense of a puzzling world, easy solutions to the challenges of difference. They offer the assumptions of commonality with one group, denying the differences that are there. (p. 57)

Although there are frequent commonalities among groups of people, extreme variations are common among individuals of similar backgrounds. It is easy to lump people together and to stereotype, but such attitudes typically are not informative or helpful in professional practice. For example, in special education, labeling according to etiology often is misleading in understanding a particular child's needs or abilities. Among children with autism, for instance, there is considerable variation in learning styles, temperament, interests, and communication abilities. The same can be said about labeling families. Not all Latino families have similar experiences or feel the same way or hold the same perspectives. Native American families come from very diverse backgrounds based on tribal heritage, as well as life experiences in cities versus reservations. Moving beyond stereotypes is critical to building authentic relationships with families, especially those from CLD backgrounds.

Adopting Ethnographic Interviewing Strategies

"Asking the right questions, to the right people, in the right ways, and at the right time," as articulated by Westby (1990), is a way to create trusting and respectful relationships as the professional gathers and shares information with family members (Westby, Burda, & Metha, 2003). For ethnographic interviewing, it is important to use strategies that promote conversational interaction, rather than professional-to-parent interviews. Strategies include use of open-ended questions, "grand tour" questions such as "Tell me about your day," and "mini-tour" questions such as "What happens when he is getting ready for bed?" Letting the family do the talking by asking authentic, open-ended questions, with lots of pauses, helps professionals to focus on family strengths and successes and encourages sharing of different views without judgment. These strategies prove effective in learning "who" the family is and what the family's priorities are, as well as about their lifeways that affect their child's development and learning; such strategies also help to keep interactions with families conversational and interactive.

Recognizing Barriers to Communication

Numerous factors can affect the quality of communication between families and professionals. For instance, a family's negative prior experience with a professional may present a barrier to establishing relationships with other professionals (Winton, 1992). Likewise, a professional whose attitude toward dual-language learning is that it is "a problem to be solved" may have a difficult time understanding why parents want to preserve their home language and culture for their children. When professionals work with families who differ from them in their language and/or culture, they must be vigilant to recognize and overcome barriers that hamper communication. These can include not only families' previous experiences in the health care or educational systems but also differences in cultural beliefs, such as those concerning child rearing, disabilities, and parent-child communication.

Making Effective Use of Cultural Mediators, Translators, and Interpreters

Use of a trained cultural mediator, or translator, or interpreter provides a cultural context for all conversations and is an effective tool for establishing trust when a family's culture and/or language is different from the professional's (Moore & Perez-Mendez, 2005a). Families often respond to someone with whom they can easily converse, and they will quickly warm up to others who are able to communicate in the language with which they are most familiar. Use of cultural mediators, who have the added asset of understanding the family's culture, provides additional comfort to parents and family members who may be in a novel situation and unsure of what is expected.

The concept of cultural mediator or cultural broker has been described in early intervention (Maude, Catlett, Moore, Sanchez, & Thorp, 2006) and in special education by several authors (Barrera, 1993; Chen, 1999; Moore, Beatty, & Pérez-Méndez, 1995, 2001). The purpose of involvement of such mediators is to promote respect, understanding, and communication among family members and professionals. The individual must be both bilingual and sensitive to both cultures represented. The cultural mediator also is knowledgeable about community resources and support systems and can promote linkages that increase access to appropriate resources by the family for the early care and education setting. Administrators in El Grupo have worked with the state department of education in developing a meaningful educational program for those bilingual bicultural family members or paraprofessionals who want to develop skills as cultural mediators. El Grupo also supports "veteran parents" to network with other families.

Summary: Importance of Culturally Competent, Relevant, and Meaningful Interactions

Culturally responsive practices demand an understanding of self and culture to build a foundation for meaningful interactions and positive relationships with all families. Programs that recognize and are grounded in the family's experiences and values as a foundation for sharing information may be more successful in attracting diverse families to participate. Consideration of a schedule for meetings that is consistent with family needs and obligations, use of specific rituals or routines that are culturally resonant with the participants' lifeways or beliefs, and other considerations that help clarify expectations for participation may clear the way for successful experiences. As with all families, the opportunity to share stories and experiences with each other often promotes networking, learning from one another, and parent-to-parent connections.

Implementing El Grupo de Familias

As noted, many parents and family members are referred to El Grupo by early intervention providers, health care providers, other parents, or family members. Since its inception, the model has evolved from direct work with children into one that focuses on prevention of later learning challenges though parent education and support. El Grupo uses a model of intervention that is focused on directly enhancing the child's learning of language(s) and building foundations for later conventional literacy in an inclusive environment but, more important, leverages greater change through supporting families to enhance their child's language and preliteracy development at home.

As in any parent education group, the participants of El Grupo de Familias are similar in some ways but diverse in others. The children recruited generally are between the ages of 2 years 6 months and 3 years 6 months, and the families all speak Spanish as their primary or only language in the home. Although the age of the children and the primary language in the homes of the families generally are similar for participating families, the families are diverse in their socioeconomic level, educational experience, years of living in the United States, and knowledge of English. Also, the children vary in their level of knowledge of English and language learning abilities, with some children in every group exhibiting significant difficulties with language acquisition.

El Grupo activities are organized to achieve six primary goals. Descriptions of specific activities that support attainment of each goal are presented next.

Goal 1: Establishing a Culturally and Linguistically Responsive Learning Environment

From the first session of El Grupo, establishing an environment that is culturally and linguistically responsive is a primary consideration. An innovative strategy is used at the very first session to create an environment in which parents feel free to listen to others and to share their own thoughts and experiences.

Getting Started: The "Talking Stick"

There are many strategies used to create a culturally responsive, safe, and comfortable environment in which families can share and learn new information. El Grupo is led by a cultural mediator who is bicultural as well as bilingual. She makes the first contact with each family and introduces families to the group purposes and structure during home visits and telephone calls before the first session. In El Grupo de Familias, the "Talking Stick" is the first activity done as a whole group. The Talking Stick is a powerful traditional tool used by Native Americans as a means of communication. Tribes of different nations have used it for many years. The Talking Stick is a symbol of power. The power lies not with the speaker but with the audience that is listening. The speaker speaks freely and without repercussions. In fact, what is said inside the circle cannot be repeated outside of the circle. The tradition of the Talking Stick is a symbol of power, honor, and integrity among the Native American people and is a respectful way to open dialogue and sharing within any group.

The participants gather in a private room, with chairs arranged in a circle, in which traditional or other suitable music is playing, and an aromatic candle is lighted. The group members hear the story of the Talking Stick and why they are engaging in this ancient Native American practice. They breathe deeply several times, guided by the group's leader. After everyone is relaxed, with eyes closed, the leader holds the Talking Stick and with a gentle voice takes the group on a journey of visualization. The leader asks the group members to visualize their childhood, their native place, their first school, teacher, the road back home to a familiar face, their favorite room in the house, and the smells of favorite foods around them. The leader finishes by bringing the group back to the present and to the current dreams and hopes of the group members for their children now that they live in this country. This is done while the music and aroma of the candle fill the room, along with nostalgia and the very heartfelt feelings that have arisen among the participants.

One by one, without any pressure, the participants then share the story of their visualization while the other group members listen with respect. Members share stories of joy and sorrow, and what they do and do not want for their children. Some share stories about the most important person in their life. This may be someone who has passed along to them positive parenting values and made them who they are now. The stories of other participants are about the difficult and long journey they made to be here and how they work hard to give their children better opportunities. Others remember their school days and remark how different the system is in this country. Emotions and heartfelt feelings overcome them one by one as all listen and share. Even persons who pass the Talking Stick along in silence receive respect for the words that cannot be said, but can be felt among all in the group. At the end of the activity, the participants can look each other in the eyes and feel that they know something very personal that they did not previously know about one another. The leader closes the activity by securing a commitment from the participants as part of El Grupo de Familias and discussing how they will work together to fulfill the dreams and hopes they share for their children.

Sharing of stories is an authentic self-expression that leads to understanding of families' experiences within their sociocultural context, identifying family strengths and resilience, and encouraging the establishment of meaningful relationships. Families and providers recognize that sharing prior experiences with education and schooling associated with diverse backgrounds is often helpful to parents so that they can better clarify their own expectations and desires for their child's education.

Goal 2: Promoting Understanding of Language Acquisition and Options for Preservation of Home Language and Culture

[Educators] should consider the cognitive advantage that can accrue from knowing and using two languages instead of considering only the possibility of the disadvantages, as has been the case traditionally when consulting with parents about the pro's and cons of bilingualism. (Genesee et al., 2004, p. 58)

One of the main goals of El Grupo de Familias is to support families as they make choices about their children's language development within the context of the (dominant) culture and language. Choices about language, such as deciding which language(s) to use in education, determining laws for translating documents and providing legal services, and planning television programming in different languages, are affected by political and economic influences. Such external forces influence personal and family choices. Families who live in the United States and who speak only Spanish are part of a minority ethnolinguistic community. In a minority ethnolinguistic community, the language spoken may receive less institutional support and members of the community may experience lower social status and socioeconomic power (Genesee et al., 2004). Accordingly, it is common for parents to base decisions about their children's linguistic environment on the perceived economic and social advantages, without considering the linguistic implications and best practices for language development. Many immigrant parents encourage their children to speak only English. These parents also may opt to use whatever English they know as the home language, instead of their native Spanish. As previously noted, this creates a "subtractive" bilingual environment, in which the majority language is learned at the expense of the family's native language. When parents with only a rudimentary knowledge of English abandon Spanish in favor of the majority language, they provide their children with an anemic linguistic model. They may not have the vocabulary skills, the syntactical skills, or the articulation skills to provide a rich English language model. Because of these limitations, the danger of language loss is ever present for young children living in the United States who speak Spanish or another minority languages as their first language. Language loss is a phenomenon in which children's rate of forgetting their first language exceeds the rate of learning their second language. The effects of this can be deleterious (Genesee et al., 2004; Goldstein, 2004; Wong Fillmore, 1991). Children can lose the positive effects of their first language development on their second language learning. They may experience the loss of family connections, social-emotional support, family engagement, and family participation in the educational process. Overall, they are at risk for losing their sense of cultural identity, which may have a negative impact on self-esteem.

Preservation of Home Language and Culture Activities

Rather than stressing the possible negative outcomes of abandoning a family's first language, El Grupo de Familias creates an environment that celebrates and highlights the positive outcomes of maintaining the home language while supporting learning the majority language. This is accomplished during a parent session by completing four activities (see Table 2–3) in a session devoted specifically to preservation of home language and culture. These activities include listening to personal stories of bilingual individuals, reviewing a videotape, group sharing, and brainstorming. It is crucial to have candid discussions with families about the research on second language acquisition in general, and about second language acquisition in children with difficulties such as SLI. It often is beneficial to spend extra time after a parent session talking with concerned families and to follow up on their concerns in subsequent sessions.

Goal 3: Providing Culturally Responsive Instruction in Parent-Child Interactions

El Grupo helps parents to learn and apply strategies that they can use across the day to facilitate their children's language and emergent literacy development. Both strategies used in normal conversations and those used in literacy-related activities are introduced. Parents are assisted to integrate new knowledge with their extant values about communication and child-rearing styles. Throughout the El Grupo program, the emphasis is on providing models for parents concerning how they can help their children learn by playing and interacting with them at home throughout the day in culturally relevant ways. They learn about activities (e.g., how to make "la plasticina," or "play dough") they can do at home with rather than for their children. Parents learn and may change their ways of interacting with their children after exposure to effective modeling of interactions, as well as hands-on experience in culturally comfortable contexts that recognize and value their heritage and lifeways.

Table 2–3. Preservation of Home Language and Culture Activities

Activity	Description	Objective
Personal stories	Group leaders (or guest speakers) who were raised bilingually share their stories and feelings about their families' choices	To encourage the families to start thinking and talking to others about the choices they face
Video: *Language and culture: Respecting family choices* (Moore & Perez-Mendez, 2004)	Videotape discusses the importance of family choices and the role of culture in considering children's language development	To provide testimonials from people who went through the same process To celebrate the positive outcomes for those people who chose to maintain their home language
Group sharing	Facilitated by the group leader, families talk to each other about their perspectives of language choices and thoughts about the video	To help create a community of families who can learn from and support each other with these decisions To signal to the group leader where families are in their decision-making process
Brainstorming	Group leaders suggest ways in which parents can support their children's maintenance of their home language in conjunction with learning English and provide some perspectives from the literature	To identify tangible ways in which parents can support their families' language choices To give some context for the choice to maintain the home language while learning the majority language To present local resources for learning English and supporting continued home language development

Talking With Children: Interactive Strategies in Daily Routines, Activities, Places, and Relationships

The work of Hwa-Froelich and Vigil (2004) discusses culturally relevant ways of helping parents use new strategies when talking with their children and emphasizes how caregivers from different cultures interact with their children in different ways. For example, it is reportedly typical for North American, English-speaking mothers to use an attention-following approach with their children, in which the adult comments on the activity or object chosen by the child. People from cultures with a more interdependent value system, however, may tend to direct children's attention. Likewise, in many cultures, caregivers do not participate in play with their children, or they may instruct a child exactly in how to use a toy or object, rather than letting the child explore it himself or herself. In their communication with their children, caregivers from many cultures rely on directives and imperatives, which is different from the communication style that is prevalent among North American middle-socioeconomic- status (SES) parents, who use descriptives while following the child's lead (Hwa-Froelich & Vigil, 2004).

When sharing ideas about language and literacy promotion with families of diverse backgrounds, professionals must be particularly aware of the cultural values and beliefs that they bring to the conversation. A grandmother participant in a recent El Grupo de Familias session supported this notion when she shared this experience with the group:

> I went to a parenting group once. The instructor told me that in the morning I should give my son choices about what he wanted to wear by asking him things like, "Do you want the blue long sleeved shirt or the red and yellow striped T-shirt?" I think it's a nice idea but I never had time for that. I was rushing everywhere so I just told my son, "Here, put that on." I threw him a shirt and maybe helped him pull it over his head as we ran out the door. We were working all the time and didn't have time to spend with our kids.

This transcript provides an example of what can happen when facilitators of parenting groups do not address family and cultural differences. van Kleeck (1994) points out that it is important for leaders of parent education groups to be cautious in making assumptions about the family's lifeways, priorities, and interactions. For example, a professional initially may assume that a family shares her own belief that children learn language best as "equal" participants in conversation, when in fact the family's cultural perspective on this aspect of learning may be the opposite. Because people from different cultures maintain different values regarding communication, with considerable variation even within one culture, facilitators of parenting groups must decide how to integrate such differences in implementing program activities and in group discussions. Parents and family members may choose to preserve home language and specific aspects of their lifeways, or may decide to modify and adapt their interactions with their children as they learn new information about development, language, and literacy.

van Kleeck (1994) suggests that there are three possible options for professionals running parenting groups for diverse families. The professional can either (1) use a parent-training program developed for other families, (2) create a training program to fit the families, or (3) alter a mainstream program to fit the families. This is an important consideration for organizations desiring to develop parent training programs, and with El Grupo, a training program was created specifically to meet the needs of Latino families, although the overall framework of the program allows for variation dependent on the cultural norms and lifeways of the participants, as shown in Table 2–4.

Goal 4: Supporting Emergent Literacy Development

Many of the parents who participate in El Grupo have relatively limited literacy skills and exposure to education beyond the high school level. To facilitate their children's emergent literacy skills and provide children with opportunities to increase their readiness before formal schooling, the program emphasizes the importance of providing children with frequent high-quality literacy experiences at home, particularly shared storybook reading.

Shared Storybook Reading Strategies

At the start of the 10-week El Grupo session, family members complete the At Home Survey (Moore, 2002) in Spanish, a questionnaire that gathers information concerning home activities, including

Table 2–4. Addressing Cultural Norms/Variations in El Grupo de Familias Program

Cultural/Communication Norms	El Grupo Features
Many of the older siblings act as caretakers for the younger children while the parents work.	Invite and actively engage older siblings in reading to younger children and helping in the class.
Other family members may be the primary caregivers of the children.	Aunts, uncles, cousins, and grandparents can attend all or some of the sessions.
At social gatherings, adults interact primarily with one another, not with the children present.	Children participate in a preschool-like environment while parents attend round table conversations, observe the children, and discuss the activities.
Parents do not typically engage in explorative play with their children; rather, they use directive language throughout the day, particularly during household chores.	In providing suggestions for enhancing children's language skills, identify concrete language goals paired with specific activities. For example, rather than telling the parents to engage in play, provide three language elements for the parent to "teach" while involved in daily routines with the child, such as directional concepts: up/down, over/under, below/above.

reading. This questionnaire is presented in Appendix 2-A. If families are not literate in Spanish, it is completed through an interviewing process. As important as this information is to helping El Grupo program leaders guide discussions of literacy, completion of this questionnaire also primes families' awareness of home activities as a mechanism for literacy development. In fact, some family members report that completion of the questionnaire increased their awareness of approaches to use with their children during reading activities.

El Grupo sessions feature provision of information concerning emergent literacy development, as well as direct modeling and practice of interactive reading strategies. Through videotapes, family members can observe staff modeling interactive storybook reading with their children in the classroom; also, parents, grand-parents, and sometimes older siblings are asked to read with the children for staff and others to observe. Key strategies are based on the literature available concerning dialogic reading, print referencing, acting out the story, using open-ended and predictive questions, relating the story to familiar activities or objects, and using prompts and props (Bus, 2001; Ezell & Justice, 2005; Kaderavek & Sulzby, 1998; Justice & Pullen, 2003; Moore & Perez-Mendez, 2005b; Owens & Robinson, 1997; Weitzman & Greenberg, 2002; Whitehurst et al., 1988, 1998). All strategies are emphasized as options through which family members can engage children with books while strengthening their vocabulary knowledge, oral language, and print awareness in both their native language and English. Family members choose the strategies that fit their own style as well as what proves appropriate for the developmental level of the child.

One strategy that has been found to be particularly useful is the "4-squares" technique (see Table 2-5). With this technique, El Grupo facilitators videotape parents reading a favorite story with their children. If parents prefer, they can make the video at home or during the session. Group facilitators and parents observe and discuss the video, during which the facilitator highlights and affirms parents' use of strategies that support their children's learning. The "4 squares" provide a framework for the discussion, including a brainstorming session with parents to identify "next steps" for future reading sessions that will incorporate strategies discussed in El Grupo and that respond to their children's needs and interests. Strategies and suggestions are co-developed with parents, incorporating special circumstances or specific interests, activities, or culturally resonant topics or books that may also support their child's development and progress in early literacy development.

A variety of additional activities are used in El Grupo to emphasize the importance of home literacy activities, including support of the oral tradition associated with many cultures, such as making family albums. Albums developed specifically to document El Grupo activities serve as documentation of children's accomplishments and also include books and ideas for continuing El Grupo

Table 2–5. Reading with Your Child: "4 Squares" Approach

Your Strengths	Your Next Steps
• Talked about the pictures • Asked questions Who? What? • Pointed to familiar letters • Used emotion and sounds as you read the book • Used "wait time" to let child initiate conversation about the story	• Ask what will happen next before you turn the page • Relate the story to child's everyday life. • Ask questions at the end to see if he/she can re-tell part of the story • Continue to respond when he/she recognizes a letter or points to it
Your Child's Strengths	**Your Child's Next Steps**
• Child is engaged and listening • Child turns pages and looks to you to read • Child points at the pictures in the story • Child asks questions: What? Why?	• Let child re-tell the story if interested • Let child finish the sentence or "fill in" the words you know he/she knows • Count with objects, make story interactive • Let child talk about story or what he/she is interested in

activities after meetings have finished. One activity in regular use in the program is creating and decorating "literacy boxes." Families are supported to provide a special box in which their children can keep pens, papers, crayons, scissors, envelopes, recipe cards, name tags, and literacy artifacts, as shown in Figure 2–2.

Goal 5: Increasing Access to Community Resources

An emphasis throughout this chapter has been that a critical focus of El Grupo is facilitating families' self-advocacy and knowledge. Within El Grupo sessions, families learn about community resources that can support their efforts to promote their children's health,

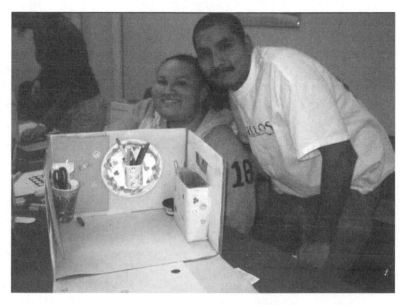

Figure 2–2. Literacy Box.

education, and participation in learning opportunities such as regular use of the library and visits to museums. This includes a focus on how parents can "navigate the system," including understanding of resources and opportunities for their child's education. Parents, especially those with children identified with special needs, also need information regarding quality child care settings, options for preschool programs, recreation center programs, and city and county resources providing human services and or intervention programs.

La biblioteca

A visit to "la biblioteca" (the library) is a favorite El Grupo activity for children, family members, and staff. It involves making connections with the local library, arranging a tour, and obtaining library cards for each child. Sometimes librarians share a story in Spanish with the children and allow children to pick out books with guidance and support so they can use their cards. Family members also are encouraged to check out books themselves and to learn where bilingual books are located, the times for scheduled story times in Spanish and English, how to access computers, and rules about how to check out books and return them. Many family members report that they continue to use this resource after the initial positive and enjoyable experience. Some parents also become aware that their own literacy is important as well and that there are resources in the community to help them strengthen their reading skills in their first language, in addition to learning and becoming literate in English.

Goal 6: Facilitating Parent-to-Parent Connections

Parents and families participating in El Grupo de Familias are encouraged to form enduring, supportive relationships with one another outside of the program sessions.

Support, Friendships, Advocacy, and Participation

Parents in El Grupo typically form friendships and continue to interact with one another long after the last session. Many report that they have developed knowledge and skills that help them advocate for educational options they want for their children as they enter school. Many continue to share celebrations with their El Grupo network. Some parents go on to develop leadership skills by participating in later sessions as "veteran" parents to support others. For example, one El Grupo mother, Jeanette, has developed the knowledge and skills necessary to serve in such an advocacy role. When Jeanette first came to the United States she was passive and fearful of agencies but was desperate for information on how to help her daughter, Matilda, who had a cleft palate and other disabilities. She was determined that Matilda would receive all of the services she needed, including surgery for a poorly repaired cleft palate. Jeanette is now a proactive advocate for other parents experiencing similar challenges and helps parents to gain access to the resources they need through community early intervention services.

Outcomes for Parents and Children

Parents consistently report a variety of benefits from participating in El Grupo de Familias, with benefits reflecting the design principles and goals discussed previously in this chapter. For instance, they report that El Grupo was extremely useful in learning about community resources and accessing appropriate supports for their family. As one parent noted, "We didn't know that our daughter could have her own library card, and now she is very proud."

Parent-to-parent connections were successfully developed throughout El Grupo activities. Parents have reported: "I have never participated in groups like this, where there were other parents." "I learned to read more with my children and to share more with other parents." "The most important thing I learned from El Grupo was how to get involved with other people and teachers."

Parents also report positive outcomes for their children: "My child learned that playing with other children is nice." "My child is using more words, sharing, and following the routine." "My child learned to be more independent and not cry." "My child has more interest in reading and painting." "My child learned to count from 1 to 10 in Spanish from the book *Ten Black Dots*." "My child sings the songs from El Grupo at home. My child now speaks more in Spanish and more in English, before he did not speak in either language." "My kids can't wait to come to El Grupo and they call it their Escuelita (little school)." One mother shared that her daughter waits for her father to come home and as he walks through the door she says, "Daddy, what book do you want me to read to you?"

To illustrate El Grupo impacts, a brief case study—the story of one recently participating El Grupo family—is presented next.

Case Study: Laura's Family

Nine years ago, Laura's family came to El Grupo de Familias. They were referred by an agency that provides "shelter" to families temporarily displaced from their homes. Laura Valle, then 2 years 9 months of age, and her mother attended El Grupo sessions at the University of Colorado in Boulder, Colorado. During an early session, the staff recommended a developmental evaluation with the local school district because Laura demonstrated difficulty with speech intelligibility in Spanish. Laura qualified for speech-language treatment through the Individuals with Disabilities Education Act, Part C, for children birth to 3 years of age. Because her family was monolingual (Spanish), Laura received additional individual services in Spanish.

The family benefited in many ways from participation in El Grupo. Laura's parents reported that they frequently went to the library after receiving a card for Laura through the program. Laura's father reports that between the library and the books received from El Grupo, his wife reads at least three books each night to each of their three children. He notes that the youngest child learns new concepts as his mother reads to the other children. The techniques learned during El Grupo about how to share books with children and engage them in reading in an enjoyable way created an appreciation for reading for the entire family. They believe that because Laura's mother attended El Grupo, the family is now better prepared to handle subsequent challenges with their other children. Through El Grupo, the family learned more about preschool programs and schools available in the community. They learned about the benefits of dual language, bilingualism, ESL programs, and English immersion schools so that they could make informed decisions on the programs they want for their children. They also learned about procedures for families with children with special needs as well as extracurricular programs available in the local school district. In addition, they learned that parent involvement is not only welcome in the schools but also expected. They were given suggestions about what will be expected of their children once they arrive at school.

Perhaps most important, Laura's parents became advocates for their daughter and searched for the best opportunities available to support her educational success. Laura's family moved out of the shelter into their own apartment in a Spanish-speaking area, where they were ready to welcome a baby sister. At that time, two other families in El Grupo were expecting a second child. They, along with the Valle family, held the first "out of the schedule" social event. Since then, the network of parents has been crucial for providing each other support as they continue the journey in the school system and their new culture. The relationships the parents built in El Grupo made them feel that they had become part of the community.

Conclusions

SLPs can provide a wealth of resources and supports to families from diverse backgrounds and their children within a preventive framework. The challenge in working with diverse families is to create a safe environment that respects the family's background and culture, recognizes and incorporates their particular perspectives into planning responsive activities and discussions, and promotes new learning and parent-to-parent connections by building a sense of community that supports their children's growth and development. A program like El Grupo not only supports children in their development of language and literacy in the early years but also leverages long-term change and growth by facilitating access to knowledge and resources by family members. As noted, the activities described in El Grupo de Familias evolved in response to the needs of Spanish-speaking families in the community. The desire of the participating parents to improve their children's growth and development and successful transition into educational placements has driven the process. Of note, the model for El Grupo is readily transferable to any group of families who desire similar outcomes for their children.

References

Adams, M. (1990). *Beginning to read: Thinking and learning about print.* Cambridge, MA: MIT Press.

Artiles, A. J., & Ortiz, A. (Eds). (2002). *English language learners with special education needs.* McHenry, IL: Center for Applied Linguistics and Delta Systems Co.

August, D., & Hakuta, K. (Eds.) (1997). *Improving schools for language minority children: A research agenda.* Washington, DC: National Academy Press.

Barrera, I. (1993). Effective and appropriate instruction for all children: The challenge of cultural, linguistic diversity and young children with special needs. *Topics in Early Childhood Education, 13,* 461–487.

Bateson, M. C. (2000). *Full circles overlapping lives.* New York: Random House.

Bus, A.G. (2001). Joint caregiver-child storybook reading: A route to literacy development. In S. B. Neuman & D. K. Dickinson (Eds.), *Handbook of early literacy research* (pp. 179–191). New York: Guilford Press.

Capps, R., Fix, M., Passel, J. S., Ost, J., & Reardon, A. (2005). *The health and well-being of young children of immigrants.* Center for Law & Policy. Retrieved May 19, 2006, from: http://www.clasp.org.html

Catts, H. W. (1993). The relationship between speech language impairments and reading disabilities. *Journal of Speech and Hearing Research, 36,* 948–958.

Dickinson, D. K., & Tabors, P. O. (Eds.) (2001). *Building literacy with language: Young children learning at home and at school*. Baltimore: Paul H. Brookes.

Dunst, C., Trivette, C., & Deal, A. (1988). *Enabling and empowering families: Principles & guideline for practice*. Cambridge, MA: Brookline Books.

Erikson, E. (1959). Identity and the life cycle: Selected papers. *Psychological Issues, 1*, 50–100.

Erikson, E. (1982). *The life cycle completed*. New York: W. W. Norton.

Ezell, H., & Justice, L. (2005). *Shared storybook reading*. Baltimore: Paul H. Brookes.

Genesee, F., Paradis, J., & Crago, M. (2004). *Dual language development and disorders*. Baltimore: Paul H. Brookes.

Goldstein, B. (2004). *Bilingual language development and disorders*. Baltimore: Paul H. Brookes.

Hakuta, K., & Garcia, E. (1989) Bilingualism and education. *American Psychologist, 44*, 372–379.

Hammer, C., Miccio, A.W., & Wagstaff, D. (2003). Home literacy experiences and their relationship to bilingual preschoolers' developing English literacy abilities: An initial investigation. *Language, Speech, and Hearing Services in Schools, 34*, 20–30.

Hart, B., & Risley, T. R. (1995). *Meaningful differences in the everyday life of young American children*. Baltimore: Paul H. Brookes.

Hwa-Frolich, D. C., & Vigil, D. (2004). Three aspects of cultural influence on communication: A literature review. *Communication Disorders Quarterly, 25*(3), 107–117.

Isbell, E., Sobol , J., Lindauer, L., & Lawrence, A. (2005). The effects of storytelling and story reading on the oral language complexity and story comprehension of young children. *Early Childhood Education Journal, 32*, 157–163.

Justice, L., & Pullen, H. (2003). Promising interventions for promoting emergent literacy skills. *Topics in Early Childhood Special Education, 23*, 99–113.

Kaderavek, J. N., & Sulzby, E. (1998). Parent-child joint book reading: An observational protocol for young children. *American Journal of Speech-Language Pathology, 7*, 33–47.

Kayser, H. (1993). *Bilingual speech language pathology: An Hispanic focus*. San Diego, CA: Singular Publishing Group.

Kessler, C., & Quinn, M. (1987). Language minority children's linguistic and cognitive creativity. *Journal of Multilingual and Multicultural Development, 8*, 173–186.

Krashen, S. C. (1982). *Principles and practices in second language acquisition*. New York: Pergamon Press.

Langdon, H. (1999). Aiding preschool children with communication disorders from Mexican backgrounds. *Bilingual Review, 2*, 30–54.

Lynch, E., & Hanson, M. (1998). *Developing cross-cultural competence* (2nd ed.). Baltimore: Paul H. Brookes

Maude, S., Catlett, C. Moore, S. M., Sanchez, S., & Thorp, E. (2006). Educating and training students to work with culturally, linguistically, and ability-diverse young children and their families. *Zero to Three, 20*, 28–35.

Moore, S. M. (2002). *At home survey*. Ready to Read, Write & Relate program. Denver Great Kids Head Start, Denver, CO.

Moore, S. M., & Perez-Mendez, C. (1998). *Language & culture: Respecting family choice*. CD. Boulder, CO: Landlocked Films. Available at: http://www.landlockedfilms.com

Moore, S. M., & Perez-Mendez, C. (2005a). *Beyond words: Effective use of cultural mediators, translators and interpreters*. Boulder, CO: Landlocked Films. Available at: http://www.landlockedfilms.com

Moore, S., & Perez-Mendez, C. (2005b). *Module 6: Parent and family involvement in English language learners with exceptional needs: ELLEN Toolkit*. Golden, CO: Meta Associates.

Moore, S. M., & Perez-Mendez, C. (2006). *A Story about El Grupo de Familias*. Boulder, CO: Landlocked Films. Available at: http://www.landlockedfilms.com

Moore, S. M., & Perez-Mendez, C. (2006). Working with linguistically diverse families in early intervention: Misconceptions and missed opportunities. *Seminars in Speech & Language, 27*, 187–198.

Moore, S. M., Beatty J., & Pérez-Méndez, C. (1995). *Developing cultural competence in early childhood assessment*. Boulder, CO: University of Colorado.

Moore, S. M., Pérez-Méndez, C., Beatty, J., & Eiserman, W. (1997). *A three-way conversation: Effective use of cultural mediators, interpreters and translators*. Video, VHS. The Spectrum Project. Denver, CO: Western Media Products. Available at: http://www.media-products.com/

Owens & Robinson. (1997). Once upon a time: Use of children's literature in the preschool classroom. *Topics in Language Disorders, 17*, 19–48.

Paradis, J., Crago, M., Genesee, F., & Rice, M. (2003). Bilingual children with SLI: How do they compare to monolingual peers? *Journal of Speech, Language, and Hearing Research, 46*, 113–127.

Restrepo, M. A. (1998). Identifiers of predominantly Spanish-speaking children with language impairment. *Journal of Speech, Language, and Hearing Research, 41*, 1398–1411.

Restrepo, M. A. (2005). The case for bilingual intervention for typical and atypical language learners. *Perspectives on Language Learning & Education, 12*, 13–17.

Roseberry-McKibbin, C. (1995). *Multicultural students with special language needs*. Oceanside, CA: Academic Communication Association.

Sanchez, S. (1999). Learning from the stories of culturally and linguistically diverse families and communities. *Remedial and Special Education*, *20*, 351–359.

Sanchez, S. (2005). Issues of language and culture impacting early care of young Latino children. *Child Care Bulletin*, *24*, 3–4.

Santos, R. M., Corso, R. M., & Fowler, S. A. (2005). *Working with linguistically diverse families*. Longmont, CO: Sopris West.

Schickendanz, J. (1999). *Much more than the ABCs*. Washington, DC: National Association for the Education of Young Children.

Snow C., Griffin, M., & Burns, S. (1998). *Preventing reading difficulties in young children*. Washington, DC: National Research Council.

Stechuk, R., & Burns, S. (2005). Making the difference: A framework for supporting first and second language development in preschool children of migrant farm workers AED. Retrieved January, 16, 2006, from http://www.aed.org/ToolsandPublications/upload/Making_a_Difference.pdf

Tabors, P. O. (1997). *One child, two languages*. Baltimore: Paul H. Brookes.

Thomas, W. P., & Collier, V. P. (1997–1998). Two languages are better than one. *Educational Leadership*, *55*, 23–28.

Thorp, E. K. (1997). Increasing opportunities for partnership with culturally and linguistically diverse families. *Intervention in School and Clinic*, *32*, 261–269.

Turnball, A., & Turnball, R. (2001). *Families, professionals and exceptionality* (4th ed.). Upper Saddle River, NJ: Merrill Prentice Hall.

van Kleek, A. (1994). Potential bias in training parents as conversational partners with their children who have delays in language development. *American Journal of Speech-Language Pathology*, *1*, 67–68.

Weitzman, H., & Greenberg, J. (2002). *Learning language and loving it*.

Westby, C. (1990). Ethnographic interviewing: Asking the right questions to the right people in the right way. *Journal of Children's Communication Development*, *1*, 101–111.

Westby, C. E., Burda, A., & Metha, Z. (2003, April). Asking the right questions in the right ways: Strategies for ethnographic interviewing. *The ASHA Leader*, *8*(8), 4–5.

Whitehurst, G. J., Falco, Lonigan, Fischel, DeBaryshe, M., Valdez-Menchaca, & Caulfield, M. (1988). Accelerating language development through picture book reading. *Developmental Psychology*, *24*, 552–559.

Winton, P. (1992). *Working with families in early intervention: An interdisciplinary preservice curriculum* (2nd ed.). Chapel Hill, NC: Frank Porter Graham Child Development Center.

Wong Filmore (1991). When learning a second language means losing the first. *Early Childhood Research Quarterly*, *6*, 323–346.

APPENDIX 2-A

ENCUESTA EN LA CASA

Nombre del Niño: _____

Nombre de los Padres: _____ **Fecha:** _____ **Lenguaje en Hogar:** _____

Su niño está creciendo y aprendiendo todo el tiempo. Ayúdenos a saber más de los intereses de su hijo, acerca de lo que le gusta hacer en la casa, y acerca de las cosas que hacen ustedes juntos.

A mi niño le gusta … (Marque con una X los cuadros que se aplican)

Garabatear o dibujar figuras ❏ sí ❏ no

¿Qué tanto? ❏ a veces ❏ frecuentemente

El usa ❏ lápices ❏ plumas ❏ crayones ❏ gises ❏ marcadores

El usa ❏ libros de colorear/ otros libros ❏ tijeras ❏ sellos ❏ plastilina ❏ bloques/legos
❏ esténciles (trazar alrededor de formas) ❏ trazar ❏ letras de alfabeto - números
❏ revistas ❏ Otro _____

Juega juegos ❏ emparejar figuras (lotería) ❏ juegos con colores ❏ juegos de contar ❏ juegos con barajas
❏ juegos de palabras (rimas, sonidos y letras) ❏ juegos de computadora (_____)

Habla acerca de lo que está jugando o platica cuentos
acerca de las acciones de figuras (e.g. personas de juguete, animales, autos/camiones) ❏ sí ❏ no

Cocina y juega en la cocina ❏ sí ❏ no

Ve libros o hace que le lean cuentos ❏ sí ❏ no
¿Qué tanto? ❏ a veces ❏ frecuentemente

❏ Pretende leer libros ❏ Recuerda el cuento y platica parte de él
❏ Platica acerca de los dibujos/fotos ❏ Puede repetir todo el cuento
❏ Hace preguntas acerca del cuento

Mi niño…

Conoce las palabras impresas o los letreros en el ambiente (letrero de alto, cajas de cereal)	❏ sí ❏ todavía no
Pide ayuda para aprender los letreros y palabras que ve	❏ sí ❏ todavía no
Reconoce su nombre impreso	❏ sí ❏ todavía no
Sabe algunas de las letras de su nombre	❏ sí ❏ todavía no
Sabe todas las letras de su nombre	❏ sí ❏ todavía no
Pide que le escriban palabras o letras	❏ sí ❏ todavía no
Pretende escribir (haciendo garabatos o escribiendo algunas letras)	❏ sí ❏ todavía no
Escribe su nombre el solo	❏ sí ❏ todavía no

Las cosas favoritas que le gustan hacer a mi niño son:

Las cosas favoritas con las que le gusta jugar a mi niño son:

Creado por Susan Moore para el Proyecto Ready to Read, Write, and Relate (Listos para Leer, Escribir y Relacionarse). Adaptado de *Things We Do At Home Survey por* Moore, McCord, Boudreau (1997) – Child Learning Center, Universidad de Colorado en Boulder

Traducido por Puentes Culturales   PC-V1.0100902

1

continues

A mí me gusta hacer con mi niño…

Hablarle acerca de lo que está jugando	❑ no mucho ❑ a veces ❑ frecuentemente
Hablarle acerca de los planes de la familia y de lo que va a hacer	❑ no mucho ❑ a veces ❑ frecuentemente
Hacer preguntas para ayudarle a pensar en lo que está haciendo	❑ no mucho ❑ a veces ❑ frecuentemente
Jugar a pretender o a las "mentiritas"	❑ no mucho ❑ a veces ❑ frecuentemente
Platicarle historias acerca de nuestra familia y nuestra cultura	❑ no mucho ❑ a veces ❑ frecuentemente
Cantarle canciones, decirle rimas de cuna o jugar juegos de rimar	❑ no mucho ❑ a veces ❑ frecuentemente
Ver libros, leer cuentos o ver videos	❑ no mucho ❑ a veces ❑ frecuentemente
Ir a la biblioteca para oír cuentos o seleccionar libros	❑ no mucho ❑ a veces ❑ frecuentemente
Enseñarle letreros o palabras y decirle que significan	❑ no mucho ❑ a veces ❑ frecuentemente
Decirle los nombres de los colores, letras del alfabeto o números	❑ no mucho ❑ a veces ❑ frecuentemente

Comparto con mi hijo historias acerca de nuestra familia, tradiciones y cultura: ❑ varias veces al día ❑ diario ❑ 2-3 veces por semana ❑ con menos frecuencia
Le leo a mi niño: ❑ varias veces al día ❑ diario ❑ 2-3 veces por semana ❑ con menos frecuencia

Las cosas favoritas que me gustan hacer con mi niño incluyen:

Cuando tengo tiempo me gusta leer … ❑ revistas, ❑ periódicos, ❑ libros y otros materiales.

Ejemplos:

Me gustaría obtener más información acerca de:

Que tipos de cuentos/libros le podrían gustar a mi niño.	❑ sí ❑ no
Recursos e información acerca de cómo aprenden a hablar los niños.	❑ sí ❑ no
Recursos e información acerca de cómo aprenden los niños a leer y escribir.	❑ sí ❑ no
Juguetes, juegos, y otros recursos para ayudarle a mi niño a aprender.	❑ sí ❑ no
Actividades que yo puedo hacer con mi niño para que esté listo para "leer y escribir".	❑ sí ❑ no
Recursos para mejorar mis propias habilidades para leer y escribir.	❑ sí ❑ no
Recursos para apoyar mi propio uso del inglés	❑ sí ❑ no
Estoy interesado en asistir a un taller de trabajo para padres acerca de cómo puedo ayudar a mi niño a aprender más acerca de cómo leer y escribir en la casa.	❑ sí ❑ no

Tengo otras preguntas acerca de…

Creado por Susan Moore para el Proyecto Ready to Read, Write, and Relate (Listos para Leer, Escribir y Relacionarse). Adaptado de *Things We Do At Home Survey por* Moore, McCord, Boudreau (1997) – Child Learning Center, Universidad de Colorado en Boulder

Traducido por Puentes Culturales

2

PC-V1.0100902

Chapter Three

Using Assistive Technology to Support Literacy Development in Young Children with Disabilities

Amelia K. Moody

Overview

Mandates in the Individuals with Disabilities Education Act (IDEA, 2004) require that students with disabilities have access to and participate in the general education curriculum. One way to improve these students' access to important literacy activities is through the use of assistive technology (AT). AT refers to any item, piece of equipment, or product system used to increase, maintain, or improve the functional capabilities of individuals with disabilities, as defined in Public Law 100-407 (U.S. Congress, 1988). AT products relevant to emergent literacy instruction help children by directly enhancing literacy skills, reducing curricular and access barriers, developing independence, and increasing their access to literacy materials. Teachers and clinicians can use technology to allow children better access to literacy experiences as well as increased opportunities for acquiring phonological awareness, print awareness, and comprehension skills, all of which are essential for reading readiness (Carnine, Silbert, Kame'enui, & Tarver, 2004; Snow, Burns, & Griffin, 1998).

This chapter presents an overview of current theory, policy, and research regarding the use of technology to support children'semergent literacy development. AT benefits, limitations, and its uses as a preventive tool for helping struggling learners are addressed as well. Technological adaptations for common emergent literacy activities, such as storybook reading, also are presented. This information can assist clinicians, teachers, and parents to use AT to promote access to important literacy activities at home and in the classroom while enhancing the literacy development of children with special needs.

What Is Assistive Technology?

Assistive technology describes technological tools specifically designed for children who require assistance to access learning. As mandated by law, students with disabilities are required to have access to and participate in the general education curriculum (IDEA, 2004). The use of AT in early intervention is a fundamental part of the educational process for many children with disabilities because it maximizes access to literacy activities and instruction within the classroom.

AT includes "low-tech," "mid-tech," and "high-tech" options. Low-tech devices are low-cost, easy to use support strategies; these include adapted books, picture schedules, highlighting tape, fidget toys, and pencil grips, for instance. One example of a low-tech emergent literacy tool is a puppet. A speech-language pathologist (SLP) can use puppets during storybook-reading sessions to reinforce vocabulary, increase student understanding, and facilitate language exchanges. Mid-tech devices include battery-operated or other inexpensive electronic devices such as speech generation devices (SGDs), books on tape, and talking picture frames. Clinicians can use SGDs, which are recording devices for young children who are nonverbal, to increase verbal expression and participation of young learners. For example, during a storybook-reading activity, a nonverbal child can push a button on the SGD with the recorded message "Turn the page" to elicit an appropriate response from the therapist. High-tech devices encompass higher-cost items such as computers and software devices; these include voice recognition software, text-to-speech software (TTS), digital books, adapted keyboards, and seating or positioning devices. An SLP may use an adapted seat to ensure the proper positioning of a child during a storybook reading session.

Of importance, AT includes a range of different types of tools, many of which are readily accessible and available at very low cost. Although with some tools, application requires more expertise on the part of the therapist or teacher, and costs can be very high, more inexpensive low-tech tools can be readily used to promote children's engagement, participation, and access to important literacy activities.

Assistive Technology and Emergent Literacy Skills

The No Child Left Behind Act of 2001 specifies four areas of emergent literacy development to be promoted in young children (particularly those who are at risk) as indicated by scientifically based reading research (Guidance for the Early Reading First Program, 2003). These four areas are oral language, phonological awareness, print awareness, and alphabet knowledge. Children with developmental disabilities, like many other children, require structured and systematic opportunities to develop skills in each area within the home and the classroom. AT can be used in specific ways to support skills development in each of these four areas.

Oral Language

Oral language development is an important part of the child's emergent literacy foundation and is vital for future reading success (Neuman & Dickinson, 2002). Research has shown that some children have limited exposure to high-quality language input and therefore have fewer opportunities to develop a strong oral language base (Hart & Risley, 1995; van Kleeck, Gillam, Hamilton, & McGrath, 1997). For instance, Hart and Risley (1995) completed a longitudinal study examining the differences among professional, working-class, and poor families' use of language at home and found that children in professional families heard more words per hour (averaging 2,153 words) in comparison with working-class (1,251 words) and poor families (616 words). Differences in language exposure over time were found to relate to children's vocabulary and grammatical growth, with children experiencing less exposure making slower gains.

A study of this magnitude has not been conducted with children with developmental disabilities, but its findings can be generalized to these children to indicate that language input is a critical developmental mechanism for fostering early language achievements. Some experts suggest that children with developmental disabilities may experience less linguistic input than their nondisabled peers and that this input may be relatively more restricted in its grammatical complexity and lexical richness (see Newhoff & West, 1993). A number of language intervention approaches are available to help parents, educators, and SLPs adopt more and improved ways of communicating with children with developmental disabilities (e.g., Bunce, 1995; Weitzman & Greenberg, 2002). Additionally, a variety of AT products also are available to support children's language development, including microcomputers, manipulative books, digital books, and story props. Although research in this area is relatively scarce, the available evidence suggests that these technologies can promote children's language expression and comprehension, as well as their engagement in literacy activities.

McCormick (1987) studied the use of switch-activated toys and computer-play activities for five preschool children with social and language delays who were participating in regular preschool environments. A *switch-activated toy* is one that has been modified to allow a child with a disability to press a switch for its activation, and *computer-play activities* are games and other activities completed on computers. The study examined the extent to which vocalizations, social opportunities, and accessibility options are increased through the use of these types of AT. McCormick found that both forms improved children's oral language production when compared with peers using noncomputerized activities. Research also indicates that social interactions among children increase when children work with computers compared with children participating in non–technology-based activities (Clements, Nastasi, & Swaminathan, 1993).

Kaderavek and Justice (2005) studied the use of manipulative books as a means for improving the language expression of children with language impairment during storybook reading. A *manipulative book* is a book that has some sort of hands-on feature, such as flaps that can be lifted to reveal a picture, for example. These researchers compared language use of children reading nonmanipulative books with their mothers with that of children reading manipulative books with their mothers; the children reading the manipulative book were found to talk more and use more complex language.

In another study involving storybooks used in the context of AT, De Jong and Bus (2002) also found that digital books promoted children's early literacy skills by facilitating interest, discussion, and interactions with the book. *Digital storybooks*—also called CD-ROM storybooks, talking books, interactive books, and computer books—are books in an electronic form that allow children to listen to a recording of the story while viewing related pictures and highlighted text on a computer screen. These books also allow young readers to explore interactive features (Parham, 1993; Trushell, Burrell, & Maitland, 2001). For example, in one digital storybook, using the mouse to click on a picture of a door causes the door to open to another page.

Digital storybooks may be particularly beneficial for children who exhibit low engagement during reading activities; these children may be more likely to choose to read a digital book on the computer with text and interactive graphics than to look at a traditional paper book. AT can enhance children's exposure to words and language by providing them with additional exposure to language and written words while providing interactive pictures and sounds to increase the young reader's interest.

As another example of use of AT to promote language, storybook reading *props* have been found to improve children's vocabulary development. Wasik and Bond (2001) studied 127 4-year-olds from low-income families over a 15-week period of regular storybook reading. The adult readers were trained to use interactive book techniques to promote children's language abilities (i.e., defining vocabulary terms, asking open-ended questions) and also engaged the children with props from "theme boxes" for each book (e.g., small toy rake, shirt, flower). Adults in the control group were given regular storybooks for the read-aloud activity, with no such instructions or props. Results indicated that children in the interactive reading group performed significantly better on vocabulary measures than did children in the control group, indicating that storybook props have a positive effect on vocabulary development for preschoolers who are from low-income families. Although these findings cannot be directly generalized to pupils with significant disabilities, the results are indeed promising that engaging children in storybooks utilizing a range of interactive behaviors and props may enhance their gains from the activity.

Phonological Awareness

Phonological awareness refers to an individual's awareness of the constituent phonological structures of spoken language, such as syllables and phonemes (Stanovich, 1991). Research promoting phonological awareness instruction is prevalent in the field of early literacy (Carnine et al., 2004; Neuman & Dickinson, 2002; Snow et al., 1998), with an increasing number of studies examining the results of instruction on children with disabilities (e.g., O'Connor, Jenkins, Leicester, & Slocum, 1993).

Assistive technology research is increasingly gaining attention as a way to improve phonological awareness and to supplement phonological awareness instruction, particularly the use of computer programs that gradually train children to attend to syllables, rhymes, and phonemes (Kersholt, van Bon, & Schreuder, 1994; Mitchell & Fox, 2001; Torgesen & Barker, 1995; Wise & Olson, 1995; Wise, Olson, Ring, & Johnson, 1997; Wise, Ring, & Olson, 1999).

Mitchell and Fox (2001) investigated two computer programs developed to increase phonological awareness in kindergarten and first grade students whose literacy related skills were below grade level. The programs targeted rhyme identification, segmenting, and blending. Pre- and post-test assessments indicated that children who received computer-based phonological awareness instruction combined with teacher-led phonological awareness instruction showed a significant increase in phonological awareness over that observed for a control group in which the children received instruction only from the phonological awareness computer program. This study indicates that AT should be paired with effective instructional techniques.

Howell, Erickson, Stanger, and Wheaton (2000) studied the effects of computer-based reading instruction that encompassed

15 minutes of instruction supported by an adult followed by 15 minutes of extended practice and found significant improvements in children's phonological awareness. Researchers have suggested that programs that combine decoding instruction with phonological awareness activities are significantly more effective than regular instruction (Wise et al., 1997) or instruction plus computer "free play" (Wise et al. 1997; Wise & Olson, 1995).

Phonological awareness computer programs are effective not only for school-aged children but also for preschoolers. Lonigan, Driscoll, Cantor, Brenlee, Anthony, and Goldstein (2003) evaluated the use of computer-assisted instruction (CAI) for enhancing phonological sensitivity skills in 45 preschool children who were at risk for reading difficulties. Comparison with control subjects, who received instruction without computers, showed use of CAI to significantly improve children's rhyming and expressive vocabulary scores. Taken together, these studies show that AT can effectively support the acquisition of phonological awareness.

Print Awareness and Alphabet Knowledge

Print awareness is the ability to understand the form and function of print, as well as the association between units of written and oral language (Justice & Ezell, 2005). Acquisition of these print concepts during the preschool years promotes reading competence later on (Ehri, 1989). Dimensions of print awareness include print and book reading conventions, concept of word, literacy terms, and alphabet knowledge (Justice & Ezell, 2005). *Print conventions* refer to the basic understanding of textual patterns, such as reading from top to bottom and left to right. *Concept of word* refers to children's knowledge of words as printed units. *Literacy terms* are the explicit metalinguistic terms used to discuss aspects of reading and writing (e.g., word, letter, spell). *Alphabet knowledge* also is a component of print awareness, which represents children's knowledge of the individual letters of the alphabet. Among print awareness skills, alphabet knowledge is the best predictor of later reading achievements in decoding (Adams, 1990).

Children's earliest experiences with books and other literacy activities support developments in print awareness. AT can provide an important supplement to these experiences by giving children the opportunity to manipulate letters and words, learn about print directionality, and explore different print concepts, particularly the use of hypermedia. *Hypermedia* refers to multiple-media presentations including graphics, digital speech, music, or video (Higgins & Boone, 1993). Higgins and Boone (1993) reported that hypermedia-based reading programs can assist children in linking print with meaning by allowing them to select words, hear their pronunciation, and see a picture to obtain the word's meaning. De Jong and Bus (2002) found that children using digital books paid more attention to text than they did when reading regular books.

One additional approach used to teach alphabet knowledge is the *Montessori approach*. Maria Montessori was a physician who developed a concrete and sensory-based teaching approach for working with children with mental retardation using specialized materials (Daoust, 2004). The Montessori teaching philosophy involves carefully structuring interactions among the child, environment, and teacher using manipulative materials that promote sensory-based learning. This approach features a range of activities for teaching literacy skills, including those focused on the alphabet letters, such as sandpaper letters, movable alphabet letters, and letter cutouts for tracing letters (Heddens, 1986). Some research support is provided by a study by Centofanti (2002), who introduced alphabet letters and phonological knowledge to kindergarten children with developmental delays by having them trace letters (e.g., on sandpaper, or in clay). This study found a significant increase in children's ability to recognize and recall letter names. Although some educators believe that manipulatives are useful for assisting children in understanding abstract concepts by introducing concrete materials (Heddens, 1986), the use of manipulatives has been sorely understudied for use with at-risk children.

Text-to-speech (TTS) software is another commonly used support in the promotion of print awareness. TTS refers to computer programs that translate text appearing on the computer screen into digital speech to assist students with disabilities who have decoding difficulties (Lewis, 1998). Although TTS may be used to promote children's early knowledge about print, many of these programs do not outperform traditional instructional approaches (Strangman & Dalton, 2005). Dawson, Venn, and Gunter (2000) found that TTS software was less effective than teacher instruction in improving children's early word recognition.

Storybook Reading Technologies

The beneficial influence of adult-child storybook reading is well established in the literature (e.g., Bryant, Maclean, & Bradley, & Crossland, 1990; Byrne & Fielding-Barnsley, 1989; Stahl & Murray, 1994), and a number of studies have focused specifically on children with disabilities. AT can be used to increase children's exposure to storybooks and results in improvements in all areas of literacy discussed previously. Emergent literacy skills are supported through the use of storybook reading in the following ways: (1) they reinforce concepts and content, (2) they support interactions, (3) they promote scaffolding, (4) they prompt decision making, and (5) they provide explicit instruction (Johnson, 2003; Wepner & Cotter, 2002).

First, storybook reading with AT can reinforce concepts and content (Wepner & Cotter, 2002). Children who repeatedly read storybooks have the opportunity to learn more about the subject matter and the ideas encompassed in the story. Also, exposure to storybooks of different modalities can further reinforce learning. For example, if the child enjoys a storybook reading with an adult and then explores the digital version of the book on the computer, he or she will gain additional exposure to the content of the book.

Second, technological supports can promote interactions between the child and the adult in a reading session (Wepner & Cotter, 2002). Rather than simply listening passively to a story, a child can be provided with a puppet to represent a character in a book and act out the sequence of the book with a clinician, teacher, or peers. Thus, language can be facilitated through the use of low-tech storybook manipulatives.

Third, AT promotes the scaffolding of instruction to allow the clinician or educator to place the book's content within a child's zone of proximal development (Johnson, 2003). For instance, a storybook can be adapted to minimize the wording on the page for children who comprehend only two- and three-word utterances. For example, the original wording "the blue dog ate a big bowl of food" may be condensed to simply "the blue dog." The SLP or a parent can successfully reduce text so that the child understands the story but does not get overwhelmed with language. Once the child understands the story, the SLP can slowly build up the text as child builds his or her vocabulary and comprehension.

Fourth, AT provides increased choices for both clinicians and children in that a number of AT options allow children the opportunity for greater self-initiation and independence as applied to exploring books. For instance, with digital books, children can explore these books on their own and push buttons to hear text, rather than relying on an adult to do the reading. This option allows children to explore books on their own and provides them with ongoing exposure to the vocabulary and concepts of a storybook.

Finally, AT can provide children with more explicit exposure to emergent literacy concepts (Wepner & Cotter, 2002). For instance, a digital storybook may use visual displays to link spoken words with visual depictions of the word in print. Such displays also can link meanings of words to the words themselves. For example, if a book's storyline describes a door slamming, the relevant text may be accompanied by an icon that when clicked expresses the sound of a door slamming with a bang, thereby helping the child to acquire a better understanding of the terminology in the book.

Thus, storybook reading is an important means for developing the emergent literacy skills of children with disabilities. Meta-analyses including those by Scarborough and Dobrich (1994), and Bus, van IJzendoorn, and Pellegrini (1995) indicate that storybook reading promotes long- and short-term literacy achievements. Some commonly used low-tech and mid-tech storybook reading technologies are digital storybooks, manipulative storybooks, adapted storybooks, audio books, and expansions. These technology solutions can increase access and independence for young readers. Of importance, in using these technological options with children with disabilities, it is necessary to consider not only the frequency with which children engage with these technologies but also the quality of the interactions that occur within the technology context (see Chapter 9).

Digital Storybooks

Digital storybooks (also called CD-ROM books, talking books, interactive books, and computer books) commonly are found in schools and homes. They can be read both individually and in small groups to provide children with repeated exposure to text through captions and highlighting (Parham, 1993; Trushell et al., 2001). Digital storybooks facilitate interest, discussions, and interactions that promote literacy (De Jong & Bus, 2002) and also assist with vocabulary development (Lefever-Davis & Pearman, 2005).

Shalom, Akerman, and Levin (2002) investigated how preschoolers and their mothers chose the path the story would follow with use of electronic storybooks versus traditional storybooks and found that parents and children engaged in many of the same behaviors and utterances observed for traditional storybooks. However, some of the features of digital books evoke concern among researchers. Interactive features can serve as a distraction (Trushell et al., 2001), promote passivity in the reading process (Lefever-Davis & Pearman, 2005), and decrease recall abilities (Trushell & Maitland, 2005). Talley, Lancy, and Lee (1997) used CD-ROM storybooks with 73 4-year-old children in an 8-week intervention comparing less "well-read" students to "well-read" students and found that digital storybooks helped bridge the gap between children with extensive exposure to printed storybooks and those with less experience by significantly increasing the intrinsic motivation and usage time for those with less print experience.

Manipulative Storybooks

There are many types of books that provide opportunities for children to explore objects and textures, including touch-and-feel books, interactive books, and books with manipulatives (see Figure 3–1). *Manipulative storybooks* are books with tangible options embedded in the books to extend the story into play, enhance young readers' interest, and provide children with disabilities better access to the book. These books often are used in preschool settings and homes to increase children's active engagement with the text and to expand stories through play and discussion. For example, flap books and character props can allow children to play and interact with the book itself.

Research supports the usefulness of these features. For instance, Glenberg, Gutierrez, Levin, Japuntich, and Kaschak (2004) tested the use of reading manipulatives with first and second graders and found that the manipulation of objects improved children's text

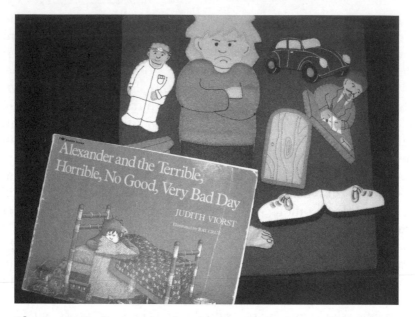

Figure 3–1. A storybook with manipulatives will enhance the child's interest and promote engagement with the story.

memory and comprehension when compared with that achieved by re-reading of the book. As previously discussed, Kaderavek and Justice (2005) investigated the language use of four mothers and their children with language impairment during reading of typical and manipulative storybooks in the home and found that children demonstrated greater mean length of utterance and increased percentage of questions when using manipulative books.

Adapted Storybooks

Storybooks used during reading activities can be easily adapted for children with various physical, sensory, or cognitive needs, and there are many ways to doing so, as shown in Table 3–1. Children with disabilities often have difficulty turning pages and handling storybooks. To prevent frustration by placing the book out of the child's reach, AT can provide low-tech solutions such as laminating

Table 3–1. Book Access Adaptations

Adaptation	Directions	Rationale/Tips for Use
Separate/ strengthen pages	Cut out pages, laminate, and tape the book back together. Scan each book page and print in color.	Promotes focus, attention to the book. Make sure you use a laminate with the appropriate thickness.
Add page protectors	*Floppy pages:* Cut the book apart, slip the pages into page protectors, and put them in a 3-ring binder. *Rigid pages:* Buy two copies of the book. Cut the book apart and insert two copies of each page in the same page protector with a manila folder in between the two pages.	This works well if the child will be "pushing" or "sliding" the pages, rather than lifting pages.
Adapt pages for interaction	Use small pieces of self-adhesive fastening tape to attach laminated pictures, numbers, or words to increase interactions during reading. The child can remove and replace the objects as the book is read. Affix a small plastic bag to the back of the book so loose pieces do not get lost.	Make sure pieces are developmentally appropriate and not a choking hazard.
Simplify text	Rewrite simplified version of the story's text on sticky notes and place over the original text.	Less text allows the child to enjoy the pictures in the books and read text at an appropriate level.

continues

Table 3–1. *continued*

Adaptation	Directions	Rationale/Tips for Use
Individualize adaptation to child's needs	Adapt books for individual enjoyment. Use communication displays and voice output devices with each book that have messages related to the contents so that the child can communicate to others about the story.	Pair with communication books and speech generation devices (SGDs).
Add page fluffers	Page fluffers are anything that separates pages so that they are easier to turn. Materials you can use are jumbo paper clips, bulldog clips, tag board, and buttons of glue in the upper corner of the book.	You can make these thicker by using foam board or multiple layers.
Repeat lines of text	Repeat lines of text to support reading fluency by repetition of words and the added rhythmic element.	
Add sentence strips	Cover the existing text or put an additional strip at the bottom of the page.	Boardmaker, PixWriter (Mac™), and Writing with Symbols (PC) have various symbol and text capabilities.
Highlight text	Use highlighting tape to target specific words or text in the book.	

Source: Adapted with permission from Eichleay, K., Young, E., & DuBuske, S. (2003). *Adapting books access.* Retrieved September 30, 2006, from: http://www.boston.k12.ma.us/teach/technology/emmanuel/GuidelInesBks.pdf

pages and adding page protectors. For instance, page protectors can be used to protect storybooks from damage with repeated touching and turning by children who have difficulties with dexterity. Page fluffers are another option for children with fine motor difficulties, as shown in Figure 3–2. Pages are "fluffed" by placing paper clips, adhesive-backed foam, or buttons of glue from a hot glue gun in the upper corner of the book page to lift and separate pages (Eichleay, Young, & DuBuske, 2003).

Audio Books

Audio books are books on tape or CD that are professionally recorded. These can promote student interest in and access to storybooks and also can improve children's listening and vocabulary skills (Baskin & Harris, 1995). Audio books can be recorded at slower speeds so that children who read at a slower pace can follow along with the text when reading silently or aloud. Although there is limited research on the use of audio books with young children, these provide a viable option for improving engagement with books for children who are easily distracted and for improving

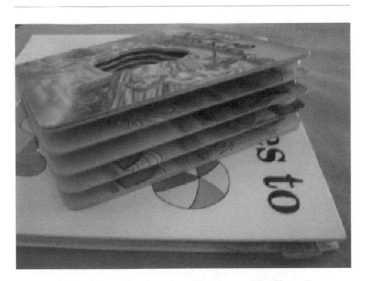

Figure 3–2. Book with page "fluffers."

independent access to books for children who cannot handle books because of physical disabilities.

Expansion Activities

Expansion activities are opportunities to extend literacy experiences beyond simply reading the text, as shown in Table 3–2. Puzzles, props, concept maps, and songs can be used to review book characters and concepts in "fun" and meaningful ways with preschool children. For example, after hearing the story of the three little pigs, children can act out the story by "building houses" and reenacting the story to reinforce vocabulary from the story. Another option is using pictures to discuss concepts in the story, as shown in Figure 3–3. Expansion activities can encourage children's use of new vocabulary and enhance story comprehension (Glenberg et al., 2004). Expansion activities are low-tech examples of how to facilitate language skills and interactions relating to books and can be a valuable way to improve access to storybook content for children with disabilities.

Table 3–2. Expansion Activities

Activity	Description	Tips for Use
Stick props	Laminate paper story props and put on a stick (e.g., tongue depressor or large paint stirrer).	Make sure that pictures coincide with story pictures; e.g., if the hair is red, make it red on the prop.
3D props	Create raised/3D props, backing them with foam, cheap camping mat, foam core, etc. Attach hook Velcro on the back of props for interactive activities. Use stuffed animals to represent characters.	Some students may only be able to play with props as their access to the story; as long as it relates to the story, they are accessing it.

Table 3–2. *continued*

Activity	Description	Tips for Use
Raps or songs	Write a catchy tune or rap with a rhythm.	Tune may help students remember information better, improve motivation.
Graphic organizers	Create graphic organizers related to the story: vocabulary; narrative structure; know/want to know/learn; who, what, where, why, when, etc.	Good for students who need to see the story. Recreate story narrative or relationships graphically.
Kinesthetic/ sensory modalities to support learning	Make letters/words out of clay.	Uses both the visual and kinesthetic/ sensory modalities to support learning.
Puzzles	Create patterns of story characters for students to cut out and assemble.	
Have students make their own published books	Use multimedia programs and word processing software.	
Talking photo album	Place book pages in a talking picture frame and record the text.	The child can explore the book independently.
Digital books	Books are available for purchase online with interactive media features (highlighted text, characters in motion, etc.).	

Source: Adapted with permission from Eichleay, K., Young, E., & DuBuske, S. (2003). *Adapting books access*. Retrieved September 30, 2006, from: http://www.boston.k12.ma.us/teach/technology/emmanuel/Guidel inesBks.pdf

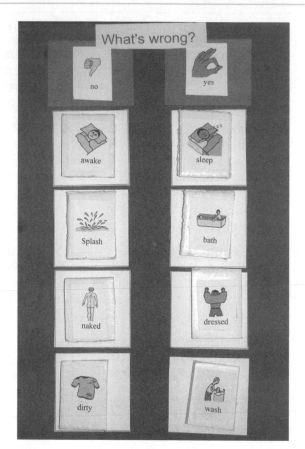

Figure 3–3. Use of pictures relating to concepts in a story to broaden its meaning for children is a low-tech but valuable expansion activity.

Promoting Literacy Access in the Environment

Structuring the Environment

The use of AT devices requires systematic attention to ensuring that the environment in which they are embedded is organized to maximize children's exploration of and exposure to literacy. Roskos and Neuman (2002) recommend three major critical design features for promoting the literacy richness of classroom environments: (1) the presence of and accessibility to print, (2) the proximity of literacy materials, and (3) the portability of literacy objects and activities, in keeping with the well-recognized mobility of the preschooler.

The presence of and accessibility to print refers to how print is placed around the classroom, therapy room, or home. Emergent literacy materials should be diverse in number and type and should be placed in multiple centers around the classroom or therapy room. AT supports such as pictures and props can be used for this purpose. For example, pieces of furniture or supplies within the room, including cabinets, mirrors, puzzles, and easels, can be labeled to promote print awareness. Centers also can incorporate emergent literacy activities, such as a "post office" center for writing, a book area for exploring print, a computer center with digital books, or a blocks area with manipulatives where stories can be acted out.

The proximity of literacy materials refers to children's ease of access to these materials. Literacy materials need to be in locations where they can be readily seen or reached by children. Universal design is recommended to ensure that educational access is provided to all learners in the classroom, particularly those with special needs (George, Schaff, & Jeffs, 2005). Effective instructional environments enable maximum learning to take place by appropriate organization and access of materials and activities (McDonnell, Thorson, McQuivey, & Kiefer-O'Donnell, 1997). Activity centers should allow enough space for children to interact individually or within groups (Roskos & Neuman, 2002). Children who use wheelchairs, walkers, or canes should have enough space to use and store their equipment in each center. Computers and other interactive equipment should be placed on adjustable tables so that children of different sizes are properly positioned. Additionally, children using AT devices for communication (augmentative and alternative communication) should always have access to their devices so that they can properly communicate. For example, for a child who uses pictures to communicate, communication boards relevant to each center can be placed around the room.

Finally, the portability of literacy objects and activities is important, because young children often are highly mobile and can have short attention spans. When materials are attached to a static surface, such as a chalkboard for writing or a tape recorder for listening to books, children cannot take items with them and cannot generalize literacy experiences to other centers or activities in the classroom. For example, if a child is playing in the kitchen in a classroom and decides he needs to run to the store to buy food, it would be helpful if he could take a pad and pencil from the kitchen and move to another center.

Children with disabilities may have particular trouble with their own mobility. By creating literacy activities that are portable, educators and therapists can improve these children's access to literacy across the curriculum. For instance, a laptop or handheld computer is more portable than a desktop computer. Portability of items also makes it easier for clinicians who may be conducting therapy in multiple environments, including the playground, classroom, or therapy room.

Additional Supports

For implementing AT in the classroom to promote children's literacy development and engagement in literacy activities, two additional tools may be useful: activity schedules and video modeling. *Activity schedules* are notebooks or cards that provide information about a child's schedule in a series of pictures or words (Kimball, Kinny, Taylor, & Stromer, 2004). Some children may require activity schedules to learn how to engage and interact appropriately within the environment. Activity schedules and visual rule reminders are common examples of low-tech classroom supports that can assist learners by providing information and structure to children in order for them to gain better access to literacy activities. These supports also help to promote children's functional independence and decrease their disruptive behaviors (Kimball, Kinney, & Taylor, 2003; Kimball et al., 2004).

Video modeling also can be used to demonstrate appropriate literacy behaviors for children. This tool allows children to view videos of other children engaged in particular literacy activities, such as a book reading event. With this form of technology support, children have been found to acquire new language and behaviors at a greater rate than with in vivo modeling (Charlop-Christy, Le, & Freeman, 2000). Watching peers engaged in reading tasks can help children hear what fluent reading sounds like and can help them to learn how to use appropriate voice inflection (Taylor, Hasselbring, & Williams, 2001) and to ask questions about specific aspects of storybooks, such as words and letters (Horner, 2004). Studies of social skills interventions using video modeling suggest that children with disabilities can learn a range of behaviors by observing peers engaged in different tasks (e.g., Maione & Mirenda, 2006), and it seems likely that these results can be generalized to improve children's exposure to the ways in which children engage in various literacy activities, including not only storybook reading but also dramatic play that involves literacy events.

Limitations of Technology

Technology can be a powerful learning tool. Nonetheless, the use of AT is not without its limitations, which include lack of training in its use, lack of research, and existence of cultural barriers. First, the use of AT can be intimidating for professionals and students if they do not know how, when, or why to use it. In a survey of more than 130 early childhood teachers, 95% reported they would like to increase their technology skills, 49% reported being anxious around computers, and 74% feared they might make mistakes when using technology (Specht, Wood, & Willoughby, 2002). Professionals who lack AT training also may require assistance finding, using, and fixing hardware and software problems. Although some SLPs may avoid technology because of these barriers, fear of technology should not be permitted to hinder children's access to it. Rather, it is important for SLPs and other professionals to seek training programs so that they can become informed and stay updated with current technology trends and instructional options. Effective professional development programs should include modeling and peer-coaching methods to help professionals integrate technology into instruction in ways that maximize children's learning (Cunningham, 2003). Once professionals are well trained in the use of AT, they can make educated decisions about which students should be using AT to improve their access to emergent literacy instruction.

A second limitation of AT is its fairly limited research base. Relative to other instructional tools, AT is fairly new; likewise, it typically is used with children exhibiting relatively low-incidence disabilities. For these reasons, the research base concerning effectiveness of AT is relatively small, and studies typically involve only a few children, so that it can be difficult to draw generalizations. As Edyburn states (2003), although technology programs are readily used in schools, they often lack the strong research base required by federal legislation standards. Unfortunately, few studies in traditional literacy journals have historically addressed technology issues. According to Kamil and Lane (1998), when the content of four major reading and writing research journals was examined, only 12 out of 437 research articles focused on technology and literacy. Throughout this chapter, the available evidence concerning the efficacy or effectiveness of different types of AT was cited, although sometimes generalizations were made from findings with typical children and findings from qualitative and case study methodologies. Undoubtedly, as the use of AT increases and becomes more widely accepted as a means to improve the emergent literacy skills of children with disabilities, research will increase and professionals' confidence in the methods they select will be enhanced accordingly.

A final limitation concerning use of AT is that some families, including lower-income families, may have less access to AT resources, particularly high-tech options (e.g., computers), and may require additional instruction before they become comfortable and independent with such technologies (Warren-Sams, 1997). Too often, children with disabilities have access to AT devices at schools but not at home, which significantly limits the extent to which they can generalize their experiences and knowledge to contexts outside of the classroom. Exploring ways to allow children to use AT at home (e.g., a lending library of digital books, allowing parents to borrow laptop computers for computer games at home) is an important consideration for ensuring that children's access to AT encompasses all important learning contexts.

Perhaps the most important limitation concerning AT concerns what it cannot do, and that is to serve as a total substitute for good instruction. Rather, as has been emphasized in this chapter, AT is a supplemental tool that can serve as an important adjunct to high-quality instruction by improving children's access to literacy. AT is most effective when it encourages and enhances instruction, rather than replacing and hindering it. When used in this manner, it can serve as a critical mechanism for unlocking the door to literacy for all children.

References

Adams, M. J. (1990). *Beginning to read: Thinking and learning about print.* Cambridge, MA: MIT Press.

Baskin, B., & Harris, K. (1995). Heard any good books lately? The case for audiobooks in the secondary classroom. *Journal of Reading, 38,* 372–376.

Bryant, P., MacLean, M., Bradley, L., & Crossland, J. (1990). Rhyme and alliteration, phonemic detection, and learning to read. *Developmental Psychology, 26,* 429–438.

Bunce, B. H. (1995). *Building a language-focused curriculum for the preschool classroom: Volume II.* Baltimore: Paul H. Brookes.

Bus, A.G., van IJzendoorn, M. H., & Pellegrini, A.D. (1995). Joint book reading makes for success in learning to read: A meta-analysis on intergenerational transmission of literacy. *Review of Educational Research, 65,* 1–21.

Byrne, B., & Fielding-Barnsley, R. (1989). Phonemic awareness and letter knowledge in the child's acquisition of the alphabetic principle. *Journal of Educational Psychology, 81,* 313–321.

Carnine, D. W., Silbert, J., Kame'enui, E. J., & Tarver, S. G. (2004). *Direct instruction reading.* Upper Saddle River, NJ: Pearson.

Centofanti, J. (2002). *A single subject multiple baseline and feminist intertextual deconstruction of gender differences among kindergarteners in learning the alphabet using clay and tactual/kinesthetic multiple intelligences and Montessori pedagogy.* Doctoral dissertation, Texas Technology University. Retrieved July 8, 2006, from: Proquest database.

Charlop-Christy, M. H., Le, L., & Freeman, K. A. (2000). A comparison of video modeling with in vivo modeling for teaching children with autism. *Journal of Autism & Related Disorders, 30,* 537–552.

Clements, D. H., Nastasi, B. K., & Swaminathan, S. (1993). Young children and computers: Crossroads and directions from research. *Young Children, 48,* 56–64.

Cunningham, J. (2003, July 1). Between technology and teacher effectiveness: Professional development. *Technology & Learning.* Retrieved April 23, 2005, from: http://www.techlearning.com/story/showArticle.jhtml?articleID=10810511

Daoust, C. J. (2004). *An examination of implementation practices in Montessori early childhood education.* Doctoral dissertation, University of California Berkeley. Retrieved July 8, 2006, from: Proquest database.

Dawson, L., Venn, M., & Gunter, P. (2000). The effects of teacher versus computer reading models. *Behavioral Disorders, 25,* 105–113.

De Jong, M. T., & Bus, A. G. (2002). Quality of book reading matters for emergent readers: An experiment with the same book in a regular or electronic format. *Journal of Educational Psychology*, *94*, 145–155.

Edyburn, D. (2003). Research and practice. *Journal of Special Education Technology*, *5*, 16–27.

Ehri, L. C. (1989). The development of spelling knowledge ands its role in reading acquisition and reading disability. *Journal of Learning Disabilities*, *22*, 356–364.

Eichleay, K., Young, E., & DuBuske, S. (2003). *Adapting books access*. Retrieved September 30, 2006, from: http://www.boston.k12.ma.us/teach/technology/emmanuel/GuidelinesBks.pdf

George, C. L., Schaff, J. I., & Jeffs, T. L. (2005). Physical accommodation in today's schools: Empowerment through assistive technology. In D. Edyburn, K. Higgins, & R. Boone (Eds.), *The handbook of special education technology research and practice* (pp. 355–377). Whitefish Bay, WI: Knowledge by Design.

Glenberg, A. M., Gutierrez, T., Levin, J. R., Japuntich, J., & Kaschak, M. P. (2004). Activity and imagined activity can enhance young children's reading comprehension. *Journal of Educational Psychology*, *96*, 424–436.

Hart, B. H., & Risley, T. R. (1995). *Meaningful differences in the everyday experience of young American children*. Baltimore: Paul H. Brookes.

Heddens, J. (1986). Bridging the gap between the concrete and abstract. *Arithmetic Teacher*, *33*, 14–17.

Higgins, K., & Boone, R. (1993). Technology as a tutor, tool, and agent for emergent reading. *Journal of Special Education Technology*, *12*, 29–37.

Horner, S. (2004). Observational learning during shared book reading: The effects on preschoolers' attention to print and letter knowledge. *Reading Psychology*, *25*, 167–188.

Howell, R. D., Erickson, K., Stanger, C., & Wheaton, J. E. (2000). Evaluation of a computer-based program on the reading performance of first grade students with potential reading failure. *Journal of Special Education Technology*, *15*, 5–14.

Individuals with Disabilities Education Improvement Act. (2004). 20 U.S.C.S § 1400.

Johnson, D. (2003). The role of development and social interaction in the selection of children's literature to promote literacy acquisition. *Early Childhood Research and Practice*, *5*. Retrieved July 10, 2006, from: http://ecrp.uiuc.edu/v5n2/johnson.html

Justice, L. M., & Ezell, H. K. (2005). *Shared storybook reading: Building your children's language and emergent literacy skills*. Baltimore: Paul H. Brookes.

Kaderavek, J., & Justice, L. M. (2005). The effect of book genre in the repeated readings of mothers and their children with language impairment: A pilot investigation. *Child Language Teaching and Therapy*, *21*, 75–92.

Kamil, M., & Lane, D. (1998). Researching the relation between technology and literacy: An agenda for the 21st century. In D. Reinking, M.C. McKenna, L. D. Labbo, & R. D. Kieffer (Eds.), *Handbook of literacy and technology: Transformations in a post-typographic world* (pp. 323–341). Mahwah, NJ: Lawrence Erlbaum Associates.

Kersholt, M. T., van Bon, W. J., & Shreuder, R. (1994). Training in phonemic segmentation: The effects of visuals support. *Reading & Writing: An Interdisciplinary Journal*, *6*, 361–385.

Kimball, J. W., Kinney, E. M., & Taylor, B. A. (2003). Lights, camera, action! Using engaging computer-cued activity schedules. *Teaching Exceptional Children*, *36*, 40–45.

Kimball, J. W., Kinney, E. M., Taylor, B. A., & Stromer, R. (2004). Video enhanced activity schedules for children with autism: A promising package for teaching social skills. *Education and Treatment of Children*, *27*, 280–298.

Lefever-Davis, S., & Pearman, C. (2005). Early readers and electronic texts: CD-ROM storybook features that influence reading behaviors. *Reading Teacher*, *58*, 446–454.

Lewis, R. (1998). Assistive technology and learning disabilities: Today's realities and tomorrow's promises. *Journal of Learning Disabilities*, *31*, 16–26.

Lonigan, C., Driscoll, K., Cantor, B., Brenlee, G., Anthony, J., & Goldstein, H. (2003). A computer-assisted instruction phonological sensitivity program for preschool children at-risk for reading problems. *Journal of Early Intervention*, *25*, 248–262.

Maione, L., & Mirenda, P. (2006). Effects of video-modeling and video feedback on peer-directed social language skills of a child with autism. *Journal of Positive Behavior Interventions*, *8*, 106–118.

McCormick, L. (1987). Comparison of the effects of microcomputer activity and toy play on social and communication behaviors of young children. *Journal of the Division for Early Childhood*, *11*, 195–205.

McDonnell, J., Thorson, N., McQuivey, C., & Kiefer-O'Donnell, R. (1997). The academic engaged time of students with low-incidence disabilities in general education classes. *Journal of Mental Retardation*, *35*, 18–26.

Mitchell, M. J., & Fox, B. J. (2001). The effects of computer software for developing phonological awareness in low-progress readers. *Reading Research and Instruction*, *40*, 315–332.

Neuman, S. B., & Dickinson, D. K. (2002). *Handbook of early literacy research*. New York: Guilford.

Newhoff, M., & West, E. A. (1993). Toward an understanding of adult inter-actions with children delayed in communication skills. *Seminars in Speech and Language*, *14*, 253–263.

O'Connor, R. E., Jenkins, J., Leicester, N., & Slocum, T. (1993). Teaching phonological awareness to young children with learning disabilities. *Exceptional Children*, *59*, 532–546.

Parham, C. (1993). CD ROM storybooks: New ways to enjoy children's literature. *Technology and Learning*, *13*, 34–44.

Roskos, K., & Neuman, S. B. (2002). Environment and its influences for early literacy teaching and learning. In S. B. Neuman & D. K. Dickinson (Eds.), *Handbook of early literacy research* (pp. 281–292). New York: Guilford.

Scarborough, H. S., & Dobrich, W. (1994). On the efficacy of reading to preschoolers. *Developmental Review*, *14*, 245–302.

Shalom, F. M., Akerman, J. S., & Levin, G. A. (2002). Reading between the pixels: Parent-child interaction while reading online storybooks. *Early Education and Development*, *13*, 435–451.

Snow, C. E., Burns, M. S. & Griffin, P. (Eds). (1998). *Preventing reading dif-ficulties in young children*. Washington, DC: National Academy.

Specht, J., Wood, E., & Willoughby, T. (2002). What early childhood educa-tors need to know about computers in order to enhance the learning environment. *Canadian Journal of Learning and Technology*, *28*, 31–40.

Stahl, S. A., & Murray, B. A. (1994). Defining phonological awareness and its relationship to early reading. *Journal of Educational Psychology*, *86*, 221–234.

Stanovich, K. E. (1991). Word recognition: Changing perspectives. In R. Barr, M. Kamill, P. Mosenthal, & P. Pearson (Eds.), *Handbook of read-ing research* (pp. 415–482). New York: Longman.

Strangman, N., & Dalton, B. (2005). Using technology to support strug-gling readers: A review of the research. In D. Edyburn, K. Higgins, K., & R. Boone (Eds.), *The handbook of special education technology research and practice* (pp. 355–377). Whitefish Bay, WI: Knowledge by Design.

Talley, S., Lancy, D. F., & Lee, T. R. (1997). Children, storybooks, and com-puters. *Reading Horizons*, *38*, 116–128.

Taylor, R., Hasselbring, T. S., & Williams, R. D. (2001). Reading, writing, and misbehavior. *Principal Leadership*, *2*, 33–38.

Torgesen, J. K., & Barker, T. A. (1995). Computers as aids in the prevention and remediation of reading disabilities. *Learning Disability Quarterly*, *18*, 76–87.

Trushell, J., Burrell, C., & Maitland, A. (2001). Year 5 pupils reading an Interactive Storybook on CD-ROM: Losing the plot? *British Journal of Educational Technology*, *32*, 389–401.

Trushell, J. & Maitland, A. (2005). Primary pupils recall of interactive storybooks on CD-ROM: Inconsiderate interactive features and forgetting. *British Journal of Educational Technology, 36(1)*, 57–66.

Technology-Related Assistance for Individuals with Disabilities Act of 1988, PL 100-407. (August 19, 1988). Title 29, U.S.C. 2201 et seq: U.S. Statutes at Large, 102, 1044–1065.U.

United States Department of Education (2004). *Guidance for the Early Reading First Program, 2003*. Retrieved August 31, 2006 from: http://www.ed.gov/programs/earlyreading/erfguidance.doc

van Kleeck, A., Gillam, R. B., Hamilton, L., & McGrath, C. (1997). The relationship between middle class parents' book sharing discussion and their preschoolers' abstract language development. *Journal of Speech and Hearing Research, 40*, 1261–1271.

Warren-Sams, B. (1997). *Closing the equity gap in technology access and use*. Portland, OR: Center for Origin, Race, and Sex Equity (CNORSE), Northwest Regional Educational Laboratory and the Northwest Educational Technology Consortium. Retrieved March 28, 2005, from: http://www.netc.org/cdrom/equity/html/index.htm

Wasik, B., & Bond, M. A. (2001). Beyond the pages of a book: Interactive book reading and language development in preschool classrooms. *Journal of Educational Psychology, 93*, 243–250.

Weitzman, E. & J. Greenberg, J. (2002). *Learning language and loving it. A guide to promoting children's social, language, and literacy development in early childhood settings* (2nd ed.). Toronto, ON, Canada: Hanen Centre.

Wepner, S. B., & Cotter, M. (2002, February). When do computer graphics contribute to early literacy learning? *Reading Online, 5(6)*. Retrieved from: http://www.readingonline.org/newliteracies/lit_index.asp?HREF=/newliteracies/weper/index.html

Wise, B. W., & Olson, R. K. (1995). Computer-based phonological awareness and reading instruction. *Annals of Dyslexia, 45*, 99–122.

Wise B. K., Olson, R.K., Ring, J., & Johnson, M. C. (1997). Computer-based remedial training in phoneme awareness and phonological decoding: Effects on post-training development of word recognition. *Scientific Studies of Reading, 3*, 235–253.

Wise, B. W., Ring, J., & Olson, R. K. (1999). Training phonological awareness with and without explicit attention to articulation. *Journal of Experimental Child Psychology, 72*, 271–304.

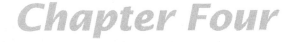

Chapter Four

Clinical Consultation with Teachers for Improved Preschool Literacy Instruction

D. Sarah Hadden
Robert C. Pianta

The Importance of Language and Literacy Development in Young Children

Overview

Recent years have seen a marked increase in the number of children enrolled in early education programs. It is estimated that approximately 70% of all 3- and 4-year-olds in this country currently are enrolled in some type of early education program (Clifford & Maxwell, 2002). Increased attention to ensuring the quality of early education is predicated on the belief that such experiences will improve the child's readiness for formal schooling (Pianta, 2006). Accordingly, early childhood educators are under increasing pressure to make sure that children enter school with the prerequisite skills they

The work on which this chapter is based was supported in part by the Interagency School Readiness Consortium, through a grant from the National Institute of Child Health and Human Development (R01 HD 046061). We extend our appreciation to the teachers and program staff who generously cooperated with this project and who continue to be examples to us of the promise of early childhood education.

need to benefit from academic instruction. This is particularly true in the areas of language and literacy (Pianta, 2006). Studies demonstrating the link between a child's literacy abilities at the beginning of school and such abilities later in life suggest that this focus on early literacy is indeed appropriate (Dickinson & Brady, 2006).

The importance of language and literacy development in young children is well documented. Research not only reveals a link between a child's vocabulary size and his or her early reading skills but also confirms that tests of preschool language abilities are relatively good predictors of a child's reading skills in later years (Snow, Burns, & Griffen, 1998). Learning to speak is a natural process—but learning to read is not. To become competent readers, young children need to have a good grasp of oral language, as well as an understanding of the fundamental aspects of reading such as alphabet knowledge, print concepts, and phonemic awareness (Dickinson, McCabe, Anastasopoulos, Peisner-Feinberg, & Poe, 2003). Children who begin formal reading instruction without these skills are much more likely to struggle than are children who have well-developed skills. A key function of preschool should be to help reduce the number of children who enter school without the fundamental early literacy skills that support their success in formal reading instruction (Snow et al., 1998).

The Potential for Preschool to Reduce Reading Difficulties

Although formal reading instruction in preschool often is not considered to be developmentally appropriate (Breedekamp & Copple, 1997), it is clear that the preschool environment is an ideal place to promote early language and early literacy skills that provide a foundation for later reading ability (Dickinson & Tabors, 2001). A preschool program that explicitly provides children with rich language and literacy experiences can be a significant factor in the prevention of later academic difficulties (National Association for the Education of Young Children, 1998).

Many publicly funded preschool programs were established precisely to ensure that children enter kindergarten with the prerequisite skills that they need to become successful learners. For instance, Head Start, the federal compensatory education program for low-income children, was founded in 1965 to provide such children with skills they would need to be successful when they entered school, as well as to provide health care and nutritional services. More recently, the No Child Left Behind Act of 2001 established the Early Reading First Program with the express purpose of teaching children—particularly low-income children—the skills they will need to become successful learners. In addition, many state and local governments have moved to establish publicly funded preschool programs for at-risk children as an additional means to close the achievement gap (Martinez-Beck & Zaslow, 2006). Unfortunately, publicly funded preschool programs often serve high numbers of children who experience multiple risk factors such as poverty, minority status, or limited English proficiency— risk factors that in and of themselves often interfere with the successful acquisition of the skills that undergird early literacy (e.g., Bowey, 1995; Justice & Ezell, 2001). For example, children who live in poverty are much less likely to have access to a print-rich environment than are children who come from more economically advantaged homes (Snow et al., 1998). Similarly, sheer language exposure for poor children is more limited than for other children. Hart and Risley (1995) found that children who live in poverty hear far fewer words than do children from working class and professional families. Because the acquisition of literacy skills is dependent to a certain extent on a child's prior language experiences, many children in publicly funded early childhood programs are at a disadvantage from the start.

Quality of Preschool Programs

Unfortunately, the extant data on the quality of early education programs in the United States suggest that although most such programs are "socially positive," they also are "instructionally passive" (Pianta, 2006). The National Center for Early Development and Learning's (NCEDL) six-state study of preschool programs reveals that there is considerable variation in the kinds of preschool experiences afforded to children (Bryant, Clifford, Early, Pianta, Howes, Barbarin et al, 2002). NCEDL researchers conducted systematic observations in 250 preschool classrooms in six states and found striking differences in the kinds and amounts of literacy-based instruction delivered to the children. Children in some classrooms were exposed to close to one hour's worth of literacy instruction on a daily basis, but many other children (approximately 30%) received little to no literacy instruction. Furthermore, researchers have found that preschool teachers often lack knowledge of effective strategies for teaching early literacy and language skills (Justice & Ezell, 1999). Thus, although preschool has the potential to be the great equalizer for low-income children, this often is not the case. Children from low-income households, who might benefit the most from high-quality early education experiences, are far less likely to attend preschools that provide a stimulating language environment than are children who come from middle class and upper class households (Karp, 2006; Pianta, 2006; Snow et al., 1998).

Professional Preparation of Early Childhood Teachers

Early education programs stem from different traditions, ranging from enrichment programs for children from middle and upper income families, to compensatory education for children who are at risk for school failure, to child care programs for working families, to special education programs for children with identified disabilities (Welch-Ross, Wolfe, Moorehouse, & Rathgeb, 2006). Although all of these programs serve young children, they may operate in different ways. As a case in point, children who live in a community that provides universal preschool may attend a full-day, state-funded program. Some children from low-income homes may attend a half-day program in a federally funded Head Start classroom, whereas others may be enrolled in a faith-based preschool program funded through a voucher program for low-income families. Children with identified disabilities may attend a segregated early childhood program designed for children with special needs, or they may receive services in an integrated community-based preschool.

The professional preparation of early childhood teachers may vary depending on the type of program in which the teachers work. A majority of teachers (86%) working in publicly funded preschool programs have a bachelor's degree (Martinez-Beck & Zaslow, 2006). By contrast, Head Start requires that at least 50% of its teachers have, at a minimum, an associate's degree in either early childhood education or a related field with experience teaching preschool-aged children (Martinez-Beck & Zaslow, 2006; Welch-Ross et al., 2006). This requirement, however, was mandated in the 1998 reauthorization of the Head Start Act and thus is relatively recent. In general, there is a wide variation in the licensing and credentialing standards for early childhood teachers. Each of the 50 states has different rules and regulations governing the licensure/training requirements for early childhood teachers (Karp, 2006; Pianta, 2006; Welch-Ross et al., 2006). Some states and locales may require that teachers have a 4-year bachelor's degree in early childhood development or education, whereas others may require that teachers obtain only a Child Development Associate (CDA) certificate from a 2-year college program (Welch-Ross et al., 2006). This variation in licensing and credentialing requirements suggests that early childhood teachers enter the profession with widely disparate skill sets for teaching language and early literacy skills. A teacher who has graduated from a 4-year college or university with a degree in early childhood education may have completed a program that includes both a two-course sequence on promoting language and literacy in young children and a course on early reading methods. By contrast, a teacher who has completed a community college program may have received no formal training in methods to promote language and literacy. Although a 4-year degree does not guarantee that a teacher will deliver high-quality language and literacy experiences (Early et al., in press), knowledge of the content increases the odds that the teacher may successfully promote these skills.

The Role of Professional Development

Training and ongoing support of the early education workforce are seen by many experts as key to improving the quality of early education programs, particularly in early language and literacy (Karp, 2006; Pew Charitable Trusts, 2005; Pianta, 2006). However, just as the requirements for educator licensure/certification vary with locale and type of program, what passes for professional development also varies widely. For example, Head Start programs are required to spend a portion of their annual funds on training and technical assistance activities designed to improve program quality. However, programs have wide latitude in how they spend these funds (Welch-Ross et al., 2006).

At the federal level, the No Child Left Behind Act of 2001 (NCLB) requires that states ensure that teachers have access to "high-quality" professional development activities (Borko, 2004). Guidelines for this piece of legislation specifically state that one-day inservices and workshops are not considered to be acceptable professional development opportunities. Rather, the regulations call for programs that are "sustained, intensive, classroom-focused . . . and are not one-day or short-term workshops or conferences." Similarly, regulatory guidelines interpreting the 2001 reauthorization of Title I–funded preschool programs support the use of ongoing mentoring and coaching programs (Welch-Ross et al., 2006).

Although traditional models of professional development (e.g., one-day workshops) have been widely criticized (Birman, Desimone, Porter, & Garet, 2000), most professional development offerings for early childhood professionals currently focus on quick and "fun" activities that teachers can implement with their students (Dickinson & Brady, 2006). Thus, although early childhood educators may indeed participate in ongoing professional development, it is unlikely that they will have access to opportunities that directly relate to their day-to-day practice. It is even less likely that they will have access to ongoing professional development explicitly designed to increase their ability to promote language and early literacy skills.

Summary

Preschool is an ideal place to promote language and early literacy skills. Unfortunately, many early childhood educators lack either the formal training or the ongoing professional support needed to ensure that they are delivering appropriate instruction in these areas. The rest of this chapter outlines an approach to professional development that speech-language pathologists (SLPs) can use to support the teacher's ability to provide high-quality language and early literacy instruction in the preschool classroom.

A Consultative Model for Supporting Early Education Teachers

Overview

Many publicly funded early childhood programs such as Head Start or Early Reading First Programs are served by a speech-language pathologist (SLP) who works directly with children with identified communication impairments to promote their language and literacy skills. SLPs who work within these inclusive models may conduct language circles, book-reading activities, and explicit lessons that specifically target the foundational skills that children will need to become successful readers. However, these SLPs typically are itinerant personnel who serve multiple classrooms or programs at the same time, which means that their time in any given classroom is limited. Therefore, it is important that SLPs work consultatively with classroom teachers to help them improve the quality of their language and literacy instruction across the day, which will facilitate language and literacy development not only for children with identified disabilities but, undoubtedly, for all of the children in the classroom.

The consultative model presented in this section can be used by SLPs to help teachers increase their ability to deliver high-quality language and literacy-rich instruction to support both typical children and children with identified special needs. The model is based on MyTeachingPartner (MTP), an innovative professional development project housed in the Center for Advanced Study of Teaching and Learning (CASTL) at the University of Virginia.

MyTeachingPartner

The MTP program provides professional development to teachers in a wide range of publicly funded preschool programs. Participating teachers receive Web-based support to help them implement instructional activities that improve children's language and literacy skills. The Web-based support includes a comprehensive curriculum comprising a scope and sequence for classroom language and literacy instruction, as well as videos demonstrating high-quality implementation of curricular activities. In addition, teachers receive consultative services from an MTP consultant who has expertise in early childhood education. The primary aim of the MTP consultancy is to provide intensive, sustained, practice-focused support and feedback for teachers through an ongoing professional consultation relationship. Consultants and teachers work together over a 2-year period consisting of regular cycles of observation, reflective analysis, and feedback delivered remotely through electronic journaling and videoconferencing via the Internet. The consultancy cycle process, which is explicitly nonevaluative, is focused on providing individualized feedback based on observations of teacher classroom instruction, with the goal of improving the teacher's processes of self-observation, problem-solving, and reflection. An illustration of the cyclical process is presented in Figure 4–1.

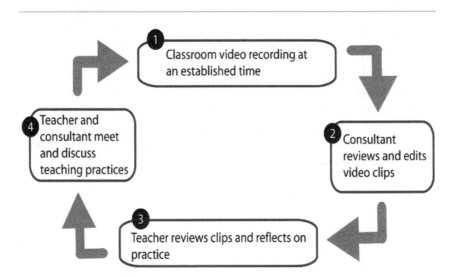

Figure 4–1. Sample MTP consultancy cycle. (Reprinted with permission from Pianta, R. C., Hall, A. P., Dudding, C., Whitaker, S., Kraft-Sayre, M., & Downer, J. [2004]. *MTP procedural manual for teachers.* Center for Advanced Study of Teaching and Learning, University of Virginia.)

MTP Consultancy Cycle

The starting point for an MTP consultancy cycle is videotaping, by the teachers themselves, of a segment of their classroom teaching at regular intervals. Teachers then send their videotapes to their MTP consultant, who edits that tape using a set of prescribed guidelines that focus on indicators of quality teaching identified by the Classroom Assessment Scoring System (CLASS) (Pianta, La Paro, & Hamre, 2006), a validated observational tool that focuses on teacher-child interactions, including the quality of language and literacy instruction. The CLASS describes dimensions of social and emotional interactions in a classroom, such as the climate in the classroom and a teacher's sensitivity to the needs of the children. The CLASS also describes instructional dimensions, such as the level of productivity in a classroom or the extent to which teachers provide instruction that promotes concept development. Prior research shows that the CLASS is predictive of children's social and emotional growth (Pianta, 2006). Table 4–1 presents an overview of the CLASS dimensions.

Once the videotape is edited, the MTP consultant posts the edited video, along with written questions designed to promote reflection, to a password-protected Web site for later review by the teacher. The teacher then views the video online and responds in writing to the consultant's questions. This process provides teachers with the opportunity to objectively view their practice and to reflect on their teaching. The final step in the consultancy occurs when the teacher and the consultant participate in an Internet-mediated videoconference to discuss the edited video and issues related to classroom performance.

Guiding Principles of Consultancy

In clinical practice, SLPs can use a variation of the MTP consultancy model to maximize the quality of language and literacy instruction within preschool classrooms. In this model, the SLP serves as the teacher's consultant, and interactions between the teacher and the SLP occur face to face instead of over the Internet. The model assumes that the SLP is assigned to work with the teacher

Table 4–1. Dimensions of Classroom Instruction Observed in the Classroom Assessment Scoring System (CLASS)

Emotional Support

Positive Climate	The overall emotional tone of the classroom and the connection between the teacher and the students
Negative Climate	The level of expressed negativity such as anger, hostility, or aggression exhibited by teachers and/or students
Teacher Sensitivity	Teacher's responsivity to students' academic and emotional needs
Regard for Student Perspectives	The degree to which teacher's interactions with students and classroom activities place an emphasis on students' interests, motivations, and points of view and promote student autonomy

Classroom Organization

Behavior Management	The teacher's ability to prevent and redirect misbehavior
Productivity	How well the teacher manages instructional time and routines so that students have the opportunity to learn
Instructional Learning Formats	How teachers engage students in activities and facilitate activities to maximize learning opportunities

Instructional Support

Concept Development	How teachers promote higher-order thinking and problem solving
Quality of Feedback	How teachers use feedback to extend students' learning and understanding
Language Modeling	How teachers facilitate and encourage children's language
Literacy Focus	How teachers expose children to precursory knowledge of written and oral language

Table 4–1. *continued*

Student Outcomes

Student Engagement	How well students are focused and participating

Source: Reprinted with permission from Pianta, R. C., La Paro, K. M., & Hamre, B. K. (2006). *Classroom Assessment Scoring System [CLASS].* Unpublished measure, University of Virginia, Charlottesville.

across an extended period of time, such as an academic year. The SLP and the teacher will participate in regularly scheduled cycles of videotaped observations of classroom practice, reflective analysis, and conferencing, with the express goal of increasing the teacher's ability to observe, reflect on, problem-solve, and, ultimately, improve his or her practice.

A fundamental aspect of the consultative relationship is its nonevaluative nature. The SLP and the teacher are viewed as collaborative partners. The SLP, using his or her training in language and early literacy, essentially mentors or coaches the teacher to implement higher quality instruction. The SLP serves as a resource person who can provide information, feedback, and support. Through the give and take of the consultative relationship, the teacher experiences a safe environment in which to try new skills.

Steps in the Consultative Model

Establishing a Relationship

As discussed previously, the nature of the consultancy relationship is collaborative and supportive. Participants should recognize that the consultancy relationship builds over time. In the initial stages of the relationship, the SLP should attend to the need to build a relationship and focus on providing positive support to the teacher. It is in this stage of the relationship that the SLP should make a concerted effort to point out things that the teacher does well. For example, the SLP may comment: "The transition activity you use to dismiss the children by the first letter in their name is a great way to encourage letter recognition." The SLP can then make the transition to providing feedback, framed as constructive criticism, as it becomes clear that the teacher is ready to receive this kind of feedback. Because different teachers will enter the consultative relationship with various skills, one of the challenges the SLP will face is identifying appropriate interventions for different teachers.

Observing Practice

Although it is certainly possible for the SLP to conduct both formal and informal observations during the time spent in the classroom, this modified consultative model depends on the teacher's having the opportunity to observe his or her own practice. To facilitate this self-observation, the teacher videotapes him- or herself teaching on a regular basis (e.g., every 2 to 3 weeks). The videotape is shared with the SLP and becomes a starting point for discussing the teacher's practice. In some cases, the SLP may view the videotape first and then ask the teacher to independently review specific clips before meeting to discuss them. In other instances, the teacher and the SLP may engage in shared viewing of selected segments. Shared viewing provides teachers with practice in developing their observation skills, because it allows the SLP to point out discrete interactions that the teacher has with the children. For example, the SLP may point out that the teacher's instructional practices consistently include the beneficial technique of repeating and extending what the children say, as a means of clarifying that the point of the review is to promote evidence-based practice for increasing children's language skills. As the teacher's observational skills improve, the SLP may ask the teacher to view the tape in advance and identify a portion of the tape in which things seemed to go well and then identify a portion of the tape in which things seemed more challenging. The SLP and the teacher can then view these segments together and present their thoughts about the lesson.

Many teachers are not used to being videotaped and may feel self-conscious about having a video camera in the room. The SLP can ease this concern by assuring the teacher that the tapes will be used as a vehicle for discussing practice and not as a tool for criticizing the teacher. It also may be important for the SLP to remind the teacher that his or her role is to support, not evaluate, the teacher.

Providing a Lens for Observing

Both novice and experienced teachers can benefit from watching themselves teach. However, many teachers may need assistance in learning how to objectively observe their practice. It is not unusual for some teachers to watch footage of themselves teaching and then declare: "That lesson was a disaster!" or "That lesson went really well!"—without being able to articulate what they saw that led them to make that pronouncement. It also is not unusual for teachers to fail to see things that they are doing well. The shared viewing discussed in the previous section may help the teacher learn to objectively view his or her practice. It also allows the SLP to model neutral observational statements, such as the following: "In this segment, you introduce the children to word 'slither.' You demonstrate what slither means by getting down on your stomach and moving across the floor. You then encourage the children to get down on the floor and move in the same way." With repeated practice, the teacher should be able to make similar observational statements. Asking a teacher to watch a video and keep running notes of what she sees on the tape is another good strategy to help build powers of self-observation.

It is critical that the SLP and the teacher have a shared and valid lens for talking about instructional practice. As discussed earlier, the CLASS can serve as vehicle for guiding the observation and feedback that are central to the consultancy model. As noted, the CLASS looks at both emotional and instructional dimensions of high-quality teaching. Of greatest relevance for this chapter, the SLP and the teacher should focus on two specific CLASS dimensions: language modeling and literacy focus. The CLASS Language Modeling and Literacy Focus scales identify specific, observable indicators of instructional practices that are related to the growth of children's language and literacy skills. The **Language Modeling** scale comprises six different indicators that examine the extent to which the teacher uses language stimulation and language facilitation techniques during individual, small group, and large group activities in the classroom. The **Literacy Focus** scale is composed of three indicators of the extent to which the teacher provides explicit and purposeful instruction of literacy concepts (Pianta et al., 2006). Tables 4-2 and 4-3 present descriptions of the indicators of these two important dimensions, as well as scoring ranges for each

Table 4-2. CLASS Language Modeling Scale: Quality Indicators and Scoring

Language Modeling

Captures the quality and amount of teachers' use of language stimulation and language facilitation techniques during individual, small group, and large group interactions with students. Components of high-quality language modeling include self-talk and parallel talk, open-ended questions, repetition, expansion/extension, and use of advanced language.

Indicator	Score Ranges		
	Low (1, 2)	Mid (3, 4, 5)	High (6, 7)
Frequent Conversation	Teacher rarely converses with students.	Teacher sometimes converses with students.	Teacher often converses with students.
Student-Initiated Language	When conversations occur, they are teacher-controlled.	Conversations between teachers and students are sometimes teacher-controlled and sometimes more student-initiated.	Although there is a mix of teacher and student talk, there is a clear and intentional effort by the teacher to promote students' language use.

Score Ranges

Indicator	Low (1, 2)	Mid (3, 4, 5)	High (6, 7)
Open-Ended Questions	The majority of the teacher's questions are close-ended.	Teacher asks a mix of close-ended and open-ended questions.	The teacher asks many open-ended questions.
Repetition and Extension	Teacher rarely, if ever, repeats or extends students' responses.	Teacher sometimes repeats or extends students' responses.	Teacher often repeats or extends students' responses.
Self-Talk, Parallel Talk	Teacher rarely maps his/her own actions and the students' actions through language and description.	Teacher occasionally maps his/her own actions and the students' actions through language and description.	Teacher consistently maps his/her own actions and the students' actions through language and description.
Advanced Language	Teacher does not frequently use advanced language with students.	Teacher sometimes uses advanced language with students.	Teacher often uses advanced language with students.

Source: Reprinted with permission from Pianta, R. C., La Paro, K. M., & Hamre, B. K. (2006). *Classroom Assessment Scoring System [CLASS].* Unpublished measure, University of Virginia, Charlotteville.

Table 4–3. CLASS Literacy Focus Scale: Quality Indicators and Scoring

Literacy Focus

Captures the *frequency* and *quality* of students' exposure to precursory knowledge of *written and oral language*—print units, alphabet letters, and phonological units (syllables, onset/rime, phonemes). Exposure to oral and written language is a component of the score, but even high exposure is not sufficient for a teacher to receive a mid-range or high score. High-quality literacy instruction is explicit, purposeful, and systematic.

Scoring Ranges

Indicator	Low (1, 2)	Mid (3, 4, 5)	High (6, 7)
Explicit	Teacher rarely exposes children to phonological units of oral language or the printed units of written language. There is little evidence of explicit teaching of literacy concepts.	Teacher inconsistently uses terms to describe literacy or language units and/or sometimes clearly identifies the purpose of the activity.	The teacher uses words that relate to oral or written language, its components, and how it works to focus children's interest specifically on the elements of code and to make explicit the purpose of the activity.

Scoring Ranges

Indicator	Low (1, 2)	Mid (3, 4, 5)	High (6, 7)
Purposeful	Teacher does not make clear the connection between code-based activities and written or spoken language.	Teacher occasionally relates code-based activities and written or spoken language.	Teachers link the code-based activities (learning to read and write letters, knowing which words rhyme, knowing how many syllables are in a word) to the broader purpose of written or spoken communication.
Systematic	Activities are not well planned nor engage children in letters, words, or phonemes.	Activities are sometimes planned and organized in a way that engages children in letters, words, or phonemes.	Activities are well planned and sequenced so that they engage children in the code units (letters, words, phonemes) of oral and written language.
Exposure	Teacher rarely, if ever, exposes children to literacy and language units.	Teacher sometimes exposes children to literacy and language units.	Teacher consistently exposes children to literacy and language units, such as letters and numbers.

Source: Reprinted with permission from Pianta, R. C., La Paro, K. M., & Hamre, B. K. (2006). *Classroom Assessment Scoring System [CLASS].* Unpublished measure, University of Virginia, Charlotteville.

indicator. The CLASS is a high-inference coding system, and SLPs who wish to implement this type of consultancy model will benefit from formal training on this measure. After completion of training, the SLP should familiarize the teacher with each of the language modeling and literacy focus indicators. Basing the observation on these indicators will help the teacher and the SLP to focus on similar aspects of high-quality language and literacy instruction.

Relating observations to these two CLASS dimensions not only gives the teacher and the SLP a common language for discussion of instructional practices but also helps each of them narrow the focus to a specific aspect of instruction. Rather than having to think about all of the skills that make up effective literacy instruction, they can talk about, for example, how the teacher draws the children's attention to print in their environment. A teacher who has never taught literacy skills initially may find the task to be overwhelming. Deciding to concentrate on print concepts or alphabet knowledge may make the idea of teaching literacy seem more manageable.

Initial observations of teaching practice may not necessarily focus explicitly on either of these CLASS dimensions. Some teachers are still honing their observation skills, so if a teacher is not feeling confident about his or her ability to promote language and literacy, it may be counterproductive to focus on the CLASS dimensions early on. Over time, the SLP should gradually introduce these two CLASS dimensions using specific indicators to guide the observation, feedback, and subsequent discussions.

Setting Up a Schedule for Observation and Feedback

The teacher and the SLP should engage in a regularly scheduled cycle of videotaped observation and feedback (e.g., every 2 to 3 weeks), reflective analysis, and dialogue about instructional practices. After the teacher videotapes segments of his or her teaching sessions, he or she gives the tape to the SLP for review. The SLP reviews the tape before the feedback session, because the meeting between the teacher and the SLP will be more productive if the SLP has previously identified areas of strength and areas in which the teacher may consider modifying practice.

Conducting Feedback Sessions

Each consultative cycle represents an opportunity for the teacher to receive individualized feedback and support from the SLP. The teacher, in return, offers insight and feedback related to her skills and ideas about teaching. This feedback is based on observation of the teacher's classroom practice and the quality and type of interactions she has with the children. This type of feedback is particularly salient for teachers, because it directly relates to what they are doing in the classroom. Early in the relationship, the SLP may lead the conference discussions, focusing on relationship building and learning about the teacher's classroom routines. As the relationship between the teacher and the SLP develops, the teacher may take a more active role in leading the meeting and identifying topics of conversation.

The SLP needs to strike a balance between identifying positive examples of the teacher's practice and helping the teacher focus on more challenging aspects of his or her teaching. Focusing on things that a teacher is doing well may feel counterintuitive if the SLP feels that the teacher has a lot of work to do to increase his or her skills. Nonetheless, it is important to identify areas of strength as a means of building a consultative relationship, because it will be easier for a teacher to accept feedback that may be construed as being negative if the teacher has a solid relationship with the SLP. Identifying things that the teacher does well also is a good way to increase the teacher's feelings of efficacy. The focus on the positive does not mean that the SLP will never give the teacher constructive criticism. However, focusing on the positive in the beginning increases the chance that later critical feedback will be received within the context of a supportive relationship.

It is critical that the SLP prepares for a feedback session by viewing the teacher's videotape and identifying segments for discussion. It may be helpful for the SLP to prepare some specific statements and questions in advance. For example, the SLP may show the teacher a segment in which he or she is successfully mapping her actions for the children and then comment: "Here you are showing the children how to do the cutting and gluing activity that is available in the art area. You clearly explain the steps involved in finding the paper, cutting out the shapes, picking out glitter and feathers, and then gluing things together." This positive statement allows the teacher to understand that mapping actions to words helps promote the children's language skills. The SLP may pull out another segment of tape designed to promote teacher reflection. For example, the SLP may say, "In this clip, you ask Joanna to describe how her snack tastes. As you can see, Joanna smiles at you and shrugs her shoulders, suggesting that she isn't sure how to answer your question. How could you have either rephrased your question or supported Joanna so she could answer your question?"

Setting Goals

Setting specific goals for the teacher to work on is a key component of the consultancy relationship. In keeping with the principles of the consultative relationship, these goals are not imposed on the teacher by the SLP; rather, they are developed collaboratively. The CLASS scales can be a helpful tool for doing this. Together the SLP and the teacher identify a specific area of language or literacy instruction to focus on, such as alphabet knowledge or phonological awareness, and then identify indicators to target. In the beginning, the SLP should encourage the teacher to focus on skills that he or she already has. This helps to build the teacher's self-confidence and also helps to build the consultative relationship. Once the teacher and the SLP identify a specific area to address, the SLP can identify smaller objectives that the teacher can work on over time. For example, a teacher may decide to focus her efforts on increasing the children's phonological awareness. The SLP can help the teacher understand that phonological awareness consists of a broad range of skills, ranging from basic skills such as identifying common letter sounds and identifying the first sound in a word to more complex skills such as tapping out and blending syllables.

Benefits of a Consultative Model

In view of the concerns about traditional models of professional development, there is growing interest in the use of consultation as a means of supporting educators in the field. Through the consultative process, SLPs can help teachers become more knowledgeable about strategies to encourage language and early literacy. The model described here is designed specifically to address teachers' needs for ongoing, individualized feedback based on their own practice. Unlike the traditional model of professional development, in which teachers attend one-day workshops or inservice training sessions on topics that have been predetermined by an administrator, the consultative model links professional development to the actual experiences of the teachers and children in the classrooms. In doing so, the consultative model meets the guidelines established by the NCLB Act for sustained professional development initiatives, while addressing many of the criticisms that have been levied against traditional models of professional development.

Case Study

Meg is a preschool teacher working in an early childhood center. Meg, who has a bachelor's degree in psychology, has always enjoyed working with children; this is her first teaching position. She has had no experience or training related to promoting language and literacy skills. She is taking courses toward certification but has yet to take a class that includes information on ways to support these skills. When the center director told the staff that she wanted them to focus more explicitly on language and literacy, and that an SLP would be working individually with each teacher, Meg's initial response was neither positive nor enthusiastic. Meg equated literacy instruction with the kinds of worksheet-driven activities she had been given when she had learned to read in kindergarten and first grade. She had often expressed her belief that literacy instruction did not belong in the preschool classroom. Now she was concerned about the children: "I'm not sure the kids will be having much fun anymore." She also expressed misgivings about the effect on her teaching role: "I don't think I want an SLP to come in and tell me how to teach my class!"

Mark, the SLP who worked in Meg's center, knew that Meg was reluctant to engage in the consultative process. Thus, he worked hard to establish a positive relationship with her. He did not want to be seen as a supervisor who was going to come in, observe, and criticize. Thus, Mark and Meg spent their first few meetings simply talking about their ideas about teaching and children. In doing so, they learned that even though they came from different disciplines, that they had very similar goals for the children: Both were invested in establishing a safe and secure environment where the children were able to learn and grow.

Once they started to view videotapes together to examine Meg's language and literacy instruction in the classroom, Mark made certain that he did not give the impression of performing a formal evaluation. He pointed out that the language and literacy activities that Meg already was using in her teaching had specific value. For example, he noted that Meg's practice of having the children act out nursery rhymes and storybooks was a creative and effective way to develop the children's narrative skills while simultaneously promoting phonological awareness.

As they watched videotapes together, Mark narrated what he saw and then began to ask Meg to talk about her observations of her own teaching practices. By using the language modeling and literacy focus CLASS indicators as a guide, they were able to focus their discussions on specific, observable aspects of Meg's instruction. For example, Mark showed Meg that pointing out the letters in the children's names when they signed in each morning would increase their knowledge of letter names. Similarly, after watching herself teach, Meg realized that she asked far more closed-ended questions than she had thought. As a result, she made a concerted effort to increase her use of open-ended questions.

As time progressed, Mark made certain that he continued to focus on the positive aspects of Meg's instruction. However, he also felt that Meg was ready to receive more constructive feedback about her teaching. In one particular session, Mark asked Meg to watch footage that showed her engaged in an animated conversation with the children. He talked about how these kinds of interactions promote the children's language capabilities. He followed this with another videotaped segment from the same day that showed Meg reading a book to the children. He noted that the children seemed anxious to share their ideas with Meg, but that she often ignored their bids to communicate. This led to a discussion about how the children's desire to contribute conflicted with her own need as the teacher to finish a story or activity. Meg acknowledged that she found this to be a difficult balance. On the one hand, she recognized that it was important for her be responsive to the children. On the other hand, she felt some pressure to get through her lessons. As a result of their conversation, Meg was able to think about how she felt about interruptions during a lesson. She also learned some effective strategies to acknowledge the children's ideas without completely losing focus on the task at hand. For example, she learned to say, "You all seem to have some really good ideas about this. We need to finish this book right now, but I will ask you to share your ideas with me at lunch."

Over time, Meg came to see the importance of intentionally paying attention to how she addressed children's language and literacy skills within her classroom instruction. With Mark's assistance, she learned the importance of explicitly focusing on aspects of language and literacy instruction identified in the CLASS, such as using advanced language to increase the children's vocabularies or pointing out environmental print. She also learned that language and literacy instruction did not need to be boring, because Mark showed her ways to incorporate language and literacy activities that were fun for the children. Meg set up a writing center in her classroom and was amazed to see how often the children chose to write letters on the marker boards. She was similarly surprised when she looked over at the dramatic play area one day and overheard the children spontaneously playing rhyming games.

As the year of consultation came to an end, Meg reported a high level of satisfaction with the experience. She said that although initially she was skeptical, she had come to value having the opportunity to have someone else help her think about her professional practice. Watching herself teach and examining her practice in relation to specific indicators of high-quality language and literacy instruction allowed her to see what she was doing well, as well as reflecting on ways to improve her instruction. She noted that "Mark pushed me to try things that I never would have considered in the past." She was pleased to see that the children were doing things that she never thought they were capable of doing. All in all, Meg felt that it was a positive learning experience.

For his part, Mark also reported satisfaction with the consultative process. He had been aware of Meg's reluctance to participate and had some concerns at the onset about how well the process would work. However, he felt that providing objective feedback within the context of an ongoing relationship allowed Meg to view her practice in a nonthreatening way and to develop new skills. Indeed, his observations of her practice across the year showed considerable growth in her ability to teach language and literacy skills.

Conclusion

Professional preparation and ongoing professional development activities are ideal mechanisms for teaching early childhood educators the skills they need to provide children with appropriate language and literacy-rich experiences. Professional development should be driven by teachers' needs for information, support, and feedback centered on classroom interactions with children; therefore, it must be a process that (a) actively involves teachers; (b) allows for flexibility to meet the individualized needs of teachers in their own classrooms; and (c) encourages problem solving and reflection (Birman, Desimone, Porter, & Garet, 2000; Burbank & Kauchak 2003). The consultative model described in this chapter begins with the skill, knowledge, and interest level of the teacher and encourages professional growth through guided observation of practice, reflection, and individual conversations with the SLP. The use of the CLASS as a framework for the consultative process provides the participants with a common metric that allows them to measure professional growth and evaluate the quality of the language and literacy instruction in the classrooom.

References

Birman, B. F., Desimone, L., Porter, A. C., & Garet, M. S. (2000). Designing professional development that works. *Educational Leadership, 57*(8), 1–8.

Borko, H. (2004). Professional development and teacher learning: Mapping the terrain. *Educational Researcher, 33*(8), 3–15.

Bowey, J. A. (1995). Socioeconomic status differences in preschool phonological sensitivity and first-grade reading achievement. *Journal of Educational Psychology, 87,* 476–487.

Bredekamp, S., & Copple, C. (Eds.) (1997). *Developmentally appropriate practice in early childhood programs.* Washington, DC: National Association for the Education of Young Children.

Bryant, D., Clifford, R., Early, D., Pianta, R., Howes, C., Barbarin, O., et al. (2002, November). *Findings from the NCEDL multi-state pre-kindergarten study.* Annual meeting of the National Association for the Education of Young Children, New York.

Burbank, M. D., & Kauchak, D. (2003). An alternative model for professional development: Investigations into effective collaboration. *Teacher and Teacher Education, 19*(5), 499–514.

Clifford, R. M., & Maxwell, K. (2002, April). *The need for highly qualified prekindergarten teachers.* Preparing Highly Qualified Prekindergarten Teachers Symposium, Frank Porter Graham Child Development Institute, University of North Carolina, Chapel Hill, NC.

Dickinson, D. K., & Brady, J. (2006). Toward effective support for language and literacy through professional development. In M. Zaslow & I. Martinez-Beck (Eds.), *Critical issues in early childhood professional development* (pp. 141–170). Baltimore: Paul H. Brookes.

Dickinson, D. K, McCabe, A., Anastasopoulos, L., Peisner-Feinberg, E. S., & Poe, M. D. (2003). The comprehensive language approach to early literacy: The interrelationships among vocabulary, phonological sensitivity, and print knowledge among preschool-aged children. *Journal of Educational Psychology, 95*(3), 465–481.

Dickinson, D. K., & Tabors, P. O. (Eds.). (2001). *Beginning literacy with language: Young children learning at home and school.* Baltimore: Paul H. Brookes.

Early, D. M., Maxwell, K. L., Burchinal, M., Alva, S., Bender, R., Bryant, D., et al. (in press). Teachers' education, classroom quality, and young children's academic skills: Results from seven studies of preschool programs. *Child Development.*

Hart, B., & Risley, T. R. (1995). *Meaningful differences in the everyday experience of young American children.* Baltimore: Paul H. Brookes.

Justice, L. M., & Ezell, H. K. (1999). Knowledge of syntactic structures: A comparison of speech-language pathology graduate students to those in related disciplines. *Contemporary Issues in Communication Science and Disorders, 26,* 119–127.

Justice, L. M., & Ezell, H. K. (2001). Descriptive analysis of written language awareness in children from low income households. *Communication Disorders Quarterly, 22,* 123–134.

Karp, N. (2006). Designing models of professional development at the local, state, and national levels. In M. Zaslow & I. Martinez-Beck (Eds.), *Critical issues in early childhood professional development* (pp. 225–229). Baltimore: Paul H. Brookes.

Martinez-Beck, I., & Zaslow, M. (Eds.) (2006). *Critical issues in early childhood professional development.* Baltimore: Paul H. Brookes.

National Association for the Education of Young Children. (1998). *Learning to read and write: Developmentally appropriate practices for young children.* Washington, DC: Author.

Pew Charitable Trusts. (2005). *National Early Childhood Accountability Task Force briefing.* Philadelphia: Author.

Pianta, R. C. (2006). Standardized observation and professional development: A focus on individualized implementation and practices. In M. Zaslow & I. Martinez-Beck (Eds.), *Critical issues in early childhood professional development* (pp. 231–254). Baltimore: Paul H. Brookes.

Pianta, R. C., Hall, A. P., Dudding, C., Whitaker, S., Kraft-Sayre, M., & Downer, J. (2004). *MTP procedural manual for teachers.* Center for Advanced Study of Teaching and Learning, Unpublished manual, University of Virginia, Charlottesville.

Pianta, R. C., La Paro, K. M., & Hamre, B. K. (2006). *Classroom Assessment Scoring System [CLASS].* Unpublished measure, University of Virginia, Charlottesville.

Snow, C., Burns, S., & Griffen, P. (Eds.), (1998). *Preventing reading difficulties in young children.* Washington, DC: National Academy Press.

Welch-Ross, M., Wolf, A., Moorehouse, M., & Rathgeb, C. (2006). Improving connections between professional development and early childhood policies. In M. Zaslow & I. Martinez-Beck (Eds.), *Critical issues in early childhood professional development* (pp. 369–393). Baltimore: Paul H. Brookes.

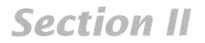

Section II

Clinical Approaches

Chapter Five

Adult Responsiveness as a Critical Intervention Mechanism for Emergent Literacy: Strategies for Preschool Educators

Elaine Weitzman
Luigi Girolametto
Janice Greenberg

Overview

The development of emergent literacy skills begins long before children enter school, and oral language ability, one of the most important emergent literacy skills, is a powerful predictor of a child's success in learning to read and spell (Catts, Fey, & Proctor-Williams, 2001; Catts, Fey, Zhang, & Tomblin, 2001; Roth, Speece, & Cooper, 2002). It is widely accepted that children's oral language skills develop within the context of reciprocal social interactions with mature users of the child's language community (Bohannon & Bonvillian, 1997). The quality and quantity of these early linguistic interactions predict children's developmental outcomes in both language ability and reading success (Snow, 1988, 1994). For the millions of young children participating in early education, these important language-learning interactions occur with a variety of nonparental adults in large-group interactions. In today's society, 80% of children younger than 6 years of age in the United States

(Marshall, 2004) and 54% of children younger than 5 in Canada (Bushnik, 2006) spend considerable time in some form of non-parental care. Consequently, monitoring the quality and quantity of educator-child interactions in early education settings is vitally important to ensuring the optimal development of oral language and emergent literacy skills of preschool children.

This chapter addresses the role of early childhood educators in facilitating the development of oral language and emergent literacy skills in preschool children. The specific focus is on the importance of *linguistic responsiveness* as a critical intervention mechanism for facilitating developmental progress in the oral language and emergent literacy skills of 3- to 5-year-old children. Also emphasized is the role of the speech-language pathologist (SLP) in enhancing educators' use of linguistic responsiveness within educator-child interactions in child care centers and preschools. Many of the principles and practices described in this chapter are drawn from Learning Language and Loving It™—The Hanen Program® for Early Childhood Educators and Preschool Teachers (Weitzman & Greenberg, 2002).

Theoretical Framework

Early education settings provide a naturalistic context for educators to facilitate children's oral language and emergent literacy skills because multiple opportunities exist for high-quality educator-child conversational interactions (Girolametto, Weitzman, Lefebvre, & Greenberg, in press). Many of these interactions take place within daily routines that involve written language (e.g.,reading story-books, writing children's names on artwork, making wall charts), providing excellent opportunities for facilitating not only vocabulary and grammatical skills but also children's knowledge of print concepts and story comprehension (e.g., Dickinson & Tabors, 2001). Unfortunately, children's experiences in child care and other early education environments are highly variable, and many educators lack adequate knowledge of how to promote oral language and emergent literacy development in preschoolers (Dickinson & Tabors, 2001). Consequently, not all children in these settings are regularly included in high-quality conversational exchanges and literacy-related interactions (Dickinson & Smith, 1994; Flowers, Girolametto, Weitzman, & Greenberg, in press).

SLPs are in an excellent position to support early childhood professionals' efforts to promote children's language and emergent literacy skills within early education settings, and to ensure that all children have frequent exposure to high-quality conversational and literacy-related interactions. As described throughout this chapter, supporting early childhood professionals to be more responsive in their language- and literacy-focused interactions with children is an effective approach to achieving these ends. SLPs' knowledge of developmental language and literacy milestones and their expertise in facilitating the attainment of these milestones through linguistically responsive interactions with children equip them to provide appropriate support, consultation, and professional development opportunities to early childhood educators. These functions are consistent with the American Speech-Language-Hearing Association (ASHA) guidelines on the roles and responsibilities of SLPs with respect to the facilitation of reading and writing skills (ASHA, 2001), and with the legislated regulations in the Individuals with Disabilities Education Act (IDEA) Amendments of 2004 to provide prevention and intervention programs in the child's natural environment (Paul-Brown & Caperton, 2001).

The premise that educators can influence children's acquisition of language and literacy through linguistic responsiveness finds support in Vygotskian theory, which asserts that adult-child interactions provide cultural and social guidance that mediates children's development of thinking, learning, and problem-solving skills (Rogoff, 1990; Vygotsky, 1978). Learning is viewed as a process of gradual mastery achieved through mediated practice and social interaction with adults, after which concepts become internalized and consolidated. Promoting children's oral language and emergent literacy skills within the context of naturalistic conversations reflects the social nature of learning. Vygotsky (1981) suggested that the social interactions that occur between children and more capable adults provide the context for a shared construction of knowledge and understanding. Thus, learning is a dynamic, interpersonal process, in which the educator constantly assesses the child's level of understanding in order to decide how best to provide responsive linguistic input.

Linguistic responsiveness is a form of verbal scaffolding in which the educator helps the child learn various types of discourse and linguistic concepts through supported and responsive linguistic interactions (Triplett, 2002). Educators adjust the amount of support they provide in response to children's existing skill levels, decreasing support so that the children are challenged to perform at a higher level, but providing more support when children appear to be having difficulty (Bowman, Donovan, & Burns, 2001). Thus, the process of learning is facilitated without direct instruction but through ongoing mediation and scaffolding (Jarvis & Robinson, 1997). Integral to the concept of scaffolding is the notion of teaching within the child's "zone of proximal development," which refers to a level of performance that is between independence and frustration (Vygotsky, 1978). According to Vygotsky, children learn best when educators target concepts within this zone (i.e., above independent performance) and progressively model and scaffold knowledge to higher levels within the individual child's zone of proximal development.

When this theoretical perspective is applied to the development of oral language and emergent literacy, interactions occurring in everyday activities in child care and preschool (e.g., sensory activities, motor play, lunch and snack time, storybook reading) provide multiple opportunities for educators to model language focused on present events as well as decontextualized language focused on past and future events, emotions, and hypothetical or imaginary situations. Such interactions also provide opportunities to model language focused on aspects of written language, such as print and phonological concepts. As children's language and literacy skills develop, educators can scaffold children's engagement in these interactions to higher levels within the zone of proximal development. For example, during educator-child conversations, the educator may follow the child's lead with questions that help the child link the "here and now" to past experiences. As children begin to make these links on their own, educators may follow up a conversational topic by introducing other examples of decontextualized language, such as making a prediction or providing an explanation. When applied successfully, responsive teaching "awakens and rouses to life those functions which are in the process of maturing . . . " (Vygotsky, 1956, p. 278).

The Mechanism of Responsiveness

"Sensitivity and responsiveness have been identified as key features of caregiving behavior related to positive health and development outcomes in young children" (Richter, 2004, p. 1). Studies in neuroscience suggest that children's neurological development occurs in response to social and interpersonal processes (Nelson & Bloom, 1997) and that the brain's development is dependent upon supportive experiences with adults (Richter, 2004). Blair (2002) suggests that synchronous interactions involving frequent, extended sequences of contingent interactions between very young children and adults lead to the development of neurological links, thereby promoting neurological growth. Responsive caregiving also leads to secure attachments between child and adult, thereby laying the foundations for positive social adjustment and optimal cognitive and language development (Richter, 2004).

Although it is clear that optimal brain development is tied to the quality of caregiving children receive, it is less clear how responsive input promotes children's language and emergent literacy development. The social interactionist perspective of language acquisition, which is compatible with Vytotskian theories of development, suggests that the nature of responsive input matches the child's cognitive processes, which in turn mediate language learning (Bohannon & Bonvillian, 1997). This perspective maintains that responsive language input that is contingent upon the child's focus or topic is more easily processed and permits the child to redirect more cognitive resources for language learning (Girolametto & Weitzman, 2006).

A consideration of the mechanism by which responsiveness facilitates the processing of linguistic input must include the potential contribution of intrinsic motivation, which is "the life force or energy for the activity and development of internal structure . . . " (Deci & Ryan, 1985, p. 8). Intrinsic motivation fulfills three psychological needs: the need for autonomy (being the originator or agent of the action); the need for competence (feelings of satisfaction as a result of mastery); and the need for relatedness (the experience of warmth and positive regard). When these three needs are fulfilled, children's active engagement with the environment can flourish, fueled by their intrinsic motivation (Grolnick, Deci, & Ryan, 1997;

Ryan & Deci, 2000). Therefore, the adults' use of responsive language may concurrently promote the children's sense of autonomy, competence, and the experience of relatedness, thereby increasing children's intrinsic motivation to interact and learn.

Linguistic Responsiveness and the Quality of Early Education

Empirical support for the role of linguistic responsiveness in oral language and emergent literacy acquisition is derived from numerous studies that have examined the relationship between linguistic responsiveness and children's developmental outcomes. These studies have shown positive short- and long-term outcomes from children's participation in high-quality early childhood programs that feature supportive and stimulating interactions with adults, positive interactions with peers, and opportunities for cognitively challenging play experiences (Burchinal, 1999; Phillips, McCartney, & Scarr, 1987; Vandell, 2004; Vandell & Wolfe, 2000). High-quality child care experiences featuring these characteristics provide a protective mechanism for children from disadvantaged home environments, resulting in higher scores on tests of language development and cognitive functioning in comparison with similar children without such child care experiences (Burchinal, Campbell, Bryant, Wasik, & Ramey, 1997; Burchinal, Lee, & Ramey, 1989; McCartney, Dearing, & Taylor, 2003). The most important characteristic of high-quality child care in terms of fostering children's improved developmental outcomes is "the quality of instructional interactions and emotional relationships formed between educators and children" (Mashburn & Pianta, 2006, p. 152).

The quality of early education is not universally high in the United States and Canada. In the National Institute of Child Health and Human Development (NICHD) study of early child care (NICHD Early Child Care Research Network, 2000), which analyzed the early education experiences of more than 1,000 children, only 10% of early child care settings were found to be excellent, and 60% were rated low on this dimension (Vandell, 2004). Similarly, the You Bet I Care Study of child care in Canada (Doherty, Lero, Goelman, Tougas, & LaGrange, 2000) showed that only about one third of early education settings provided experiences that supported and encouraged children's social, language and cognitive development. The implications of these studies clearly compel administrators, supervisors, consultants, and educators to dedicate considerable resources to the creation of high-quality early childhood programs that involve responsive interactions between educators and children and provide cognitively stimulating play environments. In addition, these findings confirm the critical importance of professional development for educators in order for them to support children's optimal development of language and emergent literacy skills. When working with early childhood educators to promote the quality of early education environments, SLPs need to recognize how various features of these environments influence educators' linguistic responsiveness and interactions with children. These features include process and structural quality; educators' formal education and involvement in professional development; use of classroom time; and child characteristics.

Process and Structural Quality in Early Education Settings

In operationalizing the concept of quality in relation to early education settings, researchers have identified two basic dimensions: process quality and structural quality (Hayes, Palmer, & Zaslow, 1990). *Process quality* refers to the nature of educator-child interactions, including the variety, complexity, and emotional and cognitive content of the language the educator uses, the frequency of interactions, and the degree of engagement/detachment and nurturance/harshness communicated during these interactions (Katz, 2004). There are numerous terms for the types of educator behavior that reflect high levels of process quality, such as warmth, sensitivity, and richness of language, and these all reflect high levels of linguistic responsiveness. Process features of the early education environment are dynamic and fluid, changing over time and even across contexts. For instance, a caregiver may be highly responsive in one type of activity (e.g., dramatic play) and less responsive in other types of activities (e.g., mealtime).

Structural quality, by contrast, describes aspects of the early education environment that are tangible and regulable, and these are typically governed by standards that specify acceptable levels of these features to ensure minimal levels of caregiving (Katz, 2004). Structural features include child-adult ratio and group size, both of which have been related to child care quality and to responsiveness in particular (Vandell & Wolfe, 2000). Lower child-to-adult ratios result in increased educator-child interaction and more stimulating and responsive care (Clarke-Stewart, Gruber, & Fitzgerald, 1994; NICHD Early Child Care Research Network, 1996, 2000; Phillipsen, Burchinal, Howes, & Cryer, 1997; Ruopp, Travers, Glantz, & Coelen, 1979). Favorable ratios allow educators to give children more individualized attention, resulting in more responsive and less controlling educator behavior (Shim, Hestenes, & Cassidy, 2004). Children whose classrooms meet recommended guidelines for child-to-educator ratios exhibit better receptive language and functional communication skills over time than do children in classrooms that do not meet recommended ratio guidelines (Vandell, 2004).

The size of the group also predicts educators' behavior, with educators who care for smaller groups of children showing more responsive and less restrictive caregiving, and with three to four children appearing to be an ideal group size (NICHD Early Child Care Research Network, 1996, 2000; Palmerus, 1996; Ruopp et al., 1979; Whitebook, Howes, & Phillips, 1989). When group size approaches or exceeds seven children, educators' responsiveness is reduced and directiveness increases (Pellegrino & Scopesi, 1990). Structural quality has a considerable impact on process quality, as shown by children's increased participation in language-rich interactions with their educators in child care centers with better-quality structural features, compared with children in poorer-quality environments (Goelman, 2003).

Educators' Formal Education and Professional Development

Educators' level of education and participation in professional development have been consistently tied to responsive behavior. For example, educators with a college degree are more likely to be responsive to children, to encourage them, and to promote their verbal skills than those without a degree (Berk, 1985; Connor, Son, Hindman, & Morrison, 2005). Level of formal schooling has been significantly and positively associated with adult sensitivity and responsive involvement with children and negatively related to detachment (Kontos & Wilcox-Herzog, 2002; Ruopp et al., 1979). When SLPs work with early childhood educators with less formal training or educational backgrounds, they can draw on research showing that specialized professional development can increase educator-child interaction and responsivity (Howes, 1983; Kontos, Howes, Shinn, & Galinsky, 1995), as discussed later in this chapter.

Use of Classroom Time

The way educators structure children's daily activities can affect program quality and the potential for high-quality educator-child interaction. A report on the quality of pre-kindergarten classrooms conducted by the National Center for Early Development and Learning (NCEDL) Pre-Kindergarten Study (Bryant, Clifford, Early, & Little, 2005) revealed that children spent relatively large amounts of time (about 30%) unengaged and waiting during daily routines like hand washing or toileting or engaged in large-group activities like circle time, with minimal direct interaction with their educators. Despite the fact that the programs studied by NCEDL met standards of quality for child-to-adult ratios, class size, and educator education (a majority had a bachelor's degree), the organization of classroom activities precluded the educators' engagement with children in extended conversations (Bryant et al., 2005).

As the NCEDL study has shown, early childhood classrooms vary significantly in the number of opportunities children have to engage in small-group activity centers, which in turn provide opportunities for increased teacher-child interaction. Smith (2001) found that although preschool educators report spending time with children in small groups, actual observations of classrooms do not support the teacher reports. Dickinson and Tabors (2001) also found that educators spent very little time in small group activities, and in one third of the classrooms they studied, no small groups were observed at all. When SLPs work with early childhood educators, they need to consider how the use of time and structure of activities within the classroom may be affecting linguistic educators' responsiveness.

Child Characteristics

Children's characteristics also play a role in the frequency and quality of responsive interactions in early education settings. According to the bidirectional model of influence (Bell, 1979), the amount of responsive feedback children receive is, in large part, determined by the frequency of their initiations toward the adults in their environments. As a result, children who initiate for social purposes and who interact more frequently within adult-child interactions may elicit greater responsive feedback from adults than those who do not. Thus, sociable children with typically developing language skills are at an advantage in relation to children who are less sociable (Bohannon & Bonvillian, 1997; Girolametto & Weitzman, 2002). In part, sociability may explain differences in language growth between boys and girls: Girls develop language skills at faster rates than those observed for boys during the preschool years in classrooms where educators met recommendations regarding educator education (Burchinal et al., 2000). Educators' responsive input also appears to be influenced by the presence of a language delay or disability. Children with language disabilities may initiate communication with adults less often than typical children, thus eliciting fewer opportunities for high-quality conversations with adults. Also, educators may ignore nonverbal initiations of young children with disabilities, invite them to interact infrequently, and use language to direct their behavior more frequently than with children without disabilities (Girolametto, Hoaken, van Lieshout, & Weitzman, 2000a; Pecyna Rhyner, Lehr, & Pudlas, 1990).

Consequences of Limited Educator Responsiveness

Much of the research that has studied characteristics of adult-child interaction within early education settings has found educators' talk to children to be directive and unresponsive (Cicognani & Zani, 1992; Girolametto et al., 2000a; Pellegrino & Scopesi, 1990; Polyzoi, 1997; Schaffer & Liddell, 1984; Tizard & Hughes, 1984).

The consequences of unresponsive interactions are far-reaching. Extant research shows that children whose educators are more detached and intrusive have lower vocabulary scores on average than those with educators who demonstrate greater warmth and responsiveness (Connor et al., 2005). In addition, the less verbally stimulating and responsive the child care environment and the more conflict children experience in relationships with educators, the less engaged they are in their classroom, the more poorly they perform on measures of language development, and the greater the risk of poor academic achievement (Ladd, Birch, & Buhs, 1999; Ladd & Burgess, 2001; Pianta & Stuhlman, 2004).

A disturbing finding from the research on the influence of early education environments is that children from families of lower socioeconomic status (SES) are more likely to be placed in lower-quality classrooms than children from higher SES families. In lower-quality classrooms, educators demonstrate less warmth and responsiveness and typically have fewer years of education. Thus, children raised in poverty experience a socially inequitable system in that they are less likely to experience rich learning environments either at home or in child care. This combination of disadvantageous circumstances predicts lower language and literacy skills, which in turn predicts lower Grade 1 language and literacy outcomes for lower SES children. This is known as the "Matthew effect" (Stanovich, 1986), which describes how, in reading, the "rich get richer and the poor get poorer." In this context, the Matthew effect refers to the progressive decline of children who are slow starters in the areas of language and literacy development due to environmental disadvantage and the widening gap between slow starters and fast starters, with most students who fall behind in reading skills never catching up with their peers.

Children with developmental disabilities are significantly disadvantaged by a lack of responsiveness in their educators. Ensuring educator sensitivity and responsiveness has not typically been a focus of early childhood special education; rather, the emphasis is placed on fostering children's development in specific domains through directive, systematic instruction in a structured environment (for a review, see the article by Rimm-Kaufman, Voorhees, Snell, & La Paro, 2003). A consistent finding in studies of educators' communication with children with disabilities is that educators often are nonresponsive or minimally responsive to children's efforts to initiate interactions and provide few opportunities for children to continue to interact around child-initiated topics (Pecyna Rhyner et al., 1990). Supporting educators to improve the quality and quantity of their responsive interactions with children with disabilities and those from low SES households represents an important consultative and collaborative service of the SLP.

Responsive Strategies for Early Childhood Educators: Rationale and Description

SLPs who consult with and support educators in early education settings need to be familiar with strategies that constitute responsive interaction and their impact on children. Learning Language and Loving It™—The Hanen Program® for Early Childhood Educators and Preschool Teachers (Weitzman & Greenberg, 2002) is a well-known model of in-service education for early childhood professionals designed for use by SLPs who consult in early childhood settings. The objectives of this program are to facilitate language and emergent literacy development through naturalistic interactions between educators and preschool-aged children. Educators learn to use responsive strategies to promote children's oral language development in everyday activities and to facilitate emergent literacy skills within print-focused activities, such as book reading and writing activities. Investigations of the efficacy of this in-service program indicate that it effectively improves educators' language and emergent literacy facilitation strategies (Girolametto, Weitzman, & Greenberg, 2003, 2004; Girolametto et al., in press). Moreover, these studies indicate that typically developing children whose educators attended the Learning Language and Loving It program show increased talkativeness, use more diverse vocabulary, and increase their peer interactions in comparison to control peers. For a complete description of this program and a review of its efficacy, see the recent article by Girolametto, Weitzman, and Greenberg (2006).

Learning Language and Loving It ascribes to a social-interactive perspective of language development, which is compatible with the Vygotskian theory of social learning discussed earlier in this chapter (Vygotsky, 1978). The responsive interaction strategies that educators use to promote children's language and emergent literacy development are grouped into three categories (Girolametto et al., 2006):

1. *Child-oriented strategies* are designed to encourage children to initiate conversations and to foster frequent episodes of joint interaction around children's interests.
2. *Interaction-promoting strategies* are designed to foster balanced turn-taking and extended conversations between adults and children that last more than a three-turn exchange, countering typical patterns of classroom interaction such as the question-answer-evaluation pattern.
3. *Language-modeling strategies* are designed to expand children's oral language skills (both contextualized and decontextualized), as well as model emergent literacy skills and concepts.

Child-Oriented Strategies

Educators use child-oriented strategies to encourage children to initiate conversations so that educators can then provide responsive input that is contingent upon the children's initiations. An important point here is that language and emergent literacy skills are learned within the context of conversational interactions, in which children are full and active participants; thus, "conversational interaction" comes before "information." Therefore, educators desiring to build children's language and literacy skills should first focus on encouraging children to initiate and become engaged in conversational interactions before trying to provide specific information that they think will enrich the children's knowledge. By doing so, educators create opportunities for children to hear responsive input on a topic of interest, thereby setting up a situation in which "children who lead get the language they need" (Weitzman & Greenberg, 2002, p. 66). Table 5–1 outlines the child-oriented strategies included in Learning Language and Loving It.

The successful application of child-oriented strategies helps educators to be responsive to children's topics of conversation. When used appropriately, they increase children's motivation to attend, interact, and converse. The following examples illustrate the impact child-oriented strategies may have on an educator-child interaction, with the first example illustrating a *lack* of responsiveness and the second illustrating a *high degree* of responsiveness.

Table 5–1. Child-Oriented Strategies to Promote Conversational Interactions

Child-Oriented Strategies

These strategies encourage children to initiate and engage in conversational interactions. Educators' responses are contingent upon the children's topics and plan-of-the-moment.

Strategy	How Educators Apply Strategy	Outcomes for Children
Observe, wait, and listen	▪ Pay close attention to children to observe exactly what they are interested in or are communicating. ▪ Wait expectantly for initiations (e.g., educator looks directly at children, leans forward, looks expectant). ▪ Use a slow pace that allows time for children to initiate, respond, and complete their messages.	▪ Internalize conversational principle that both initiations and responses are expected during interactions ▪ Initiate or respond verbally or nonverbally
Be face to face	▪ Adjust physical level so educator looks directly at children (e.g., educator sits on the floor or in a child-sized chair, leans forward, bends down).	▪ Feel engaged, connected ▪ Demonstrate more interest in interacting ▪ Communicate more frequently

Strategy	How Educators Apply Strategy	Outcomes for Children
Follow the children's lead	▪ Respond immediately with warmth and enthusiasm.	▪ Feel acknowledged and understood
		▪ Are encouraged to take another turn
	▪ **Imitate** what children say (useful in engaging shy children or if educator does not understand a child's communication).	▪ May repeat previous word or utterance, add more information, or take another turn
	▪ **Interpret:** Put words to children's gestural/nonverbal communication (i.e., say it as they would if they could).	▪ Benefit from the scaffolding effects of a more advanced language model
	▪ **Comment:** Provide information related to the child's initiation or response.	
Join in and play	▪ Actively join in the play or ongoing activity as an equal partner.	▪ Become interested in educator as a conversational and play partner
	▪ Build on the children's topics.	▪ Are encouraged to continue in the activity
	▪ Converse and play without dominating.	▪ May initiate and respond more often

Source: From Weitzman, E., & Greenberg, J. (2002). *Learning language and loving it: A guide to promoting children's social, language, and literacy development in early childhood settings* (2nd ed.). Toronto: The Hanen Centre. Copyright 2002, Hanen Early Language Program. Reprinted with permission.

In both examples, an educator is sitting at a table with several pre-school-aged children who are drawing pictures on the topic of a book they have just read. One child in the group, Luis, is drawing a picture that resembles an animal.

Example 1: Lack of child-oriented strategies

Luis appears to be finished with his picture . . .

Educator: What else are you going to draw? Do you want to draw the little girl? *(does not wait for child to initiate; asks questions the child may not be interested in answering)*

Luis: I'm making a monster.

Educator: But what about the little girl in our story? James, can you tell Luis what the girl in our story did to her fingers and toes? *(redirects the children's attention to her focus, which is not in tune with children's plan-of-the-moment)*

James: She painted her fingernails and toenails silver and purple. Yuck!

Educator: That's right, silver and purple. What else did she do? *(directs the activity and does not give children an opportunity to initiate conversation)*

Example 2: Appropriate use of child-oriented strategies

Luis appears to be nearly finished with his picture. The educator watches in silence, looking interested in what Luis is doing. She waits to see what he says . . .

Luis: I'm making a scary monster. Here's his head and legs. *(child initiates after educator waits in silence, looks expectant, and smiles)*

Educator: Your monster looks a bit like the big moose in our story. *(follows the child's lead with a comment)*

James: Yeah, the girl thought the moose was going to come and eat her up.

Educator: So the girl thought that the big moose in our story was a monster. How did she feel about that? *(follows the child's lead with a comment and a question and waits for child to respond)*

Luis: She was afraid but the babysitter didn't let the moose in the house.

Educator: Yes, she was very frightened, but she didn't need to be because the moose never came into the house. *(follows the child's lead with a comment)*

James: I'm gonna make a monster too.

Educator: Wow, we're going to have two monsters. I wonder if they are friendly monsters. *(follows child's lead with a comment, which encourages children to respond)*

As is evident from these two examples, an educator's use of child-oriented strategies can vastly change the dynamics of an interaction, and increases the likelihood that children will initiate and sustain conversations. One might wonder why the educator in Example 1 differed so much from the educator in Example 2. In part, educators' use of child-oriented strategies may be influenced by their beliefs about how children learn and about the role of educators in facilitating children's learning. If educators espouse a didactic view of learning, they will adopt an adult-centered approach to interactions with children, guided by predetermined views of what children should learn and the need to transmit this information to the children. Educators who adhere to a constructivist or sociocultural theory of learning may have more success at adopting child-oriented strategies because of their belief that children actively construct knowledge as they engage with their environment (Bowman et al., 2001).

Because educators' own beliefs may influence their openness to or ease in adopting more child-oriented strategies in the classroom, SLPs may need to facilitate educators' self-examination of their beliefs and attitudes in relation to how children learn and the educator's role in this process. Learning Language and Loving It provides a summary of different roles that educators play in the classroom and describes how these roles may affect children's opportunities to initiate and interact (Weitzman & Greenberg, 2002). These roles include:

1. The *Director* role—the educator is always in control, giving directions, asking questions
2. The *Entertainer* role—the educator is playful and fun but dominates the interaction

3. The *Timekeeper* role—the educator focuses on staying on schedule, limiting potential for interaction

4. The *Too-Quiet Teacher* role—the educator sits with the children but hardly interacts with them

5. The *Helper* role—the educator answers for children or provides assistance before the children have indicated a need for it

6. The *Cheerleader* role—the educator provides a lot of praise and positive reinforcement but usually terminates the interaction thereafter

7. The *Responsive Partner* role—the educator is attuned to child's abilities, interests and needs and responds with warmth and interest

Although educators need to play each of these roles at times throughout the day, the Responsive Partner role is the ideal role and the one that provides the greatest benefit to children's language and literacy development. Often, educators are not aware of the dominant roles they play (e.g., a Director role) or of the impact these roles have on children's interactions and development. Although directive interaction behaviors do not preclude the use of responsive interaction behaviors (de Kruif, McWilliam, Ridley, & Wakely, 2000), program quality depends on educators' predominant use of the Responsive Partner role (Weitzman & Greenberg, 2002). A Responsive Partner joins in and plays with the children as an equal play partner, supporting and elaborating on the play, thereby facilitating the children's cognitive and language skills, particularly when engaged in pretend play (Bowman et al., 2001; Saracho, 2004).

Educators seeking to become more responsive may also need some help in evaluating how children's conversational styles (Weitzman & Greenberg, 2002) can affect their interactions in the classrooms. Identifying which of the four prevalent conversational styles fits a given child helps educators appreciate which children are likely to need more encouragement to initiate and interact:

1. The *Sociable Child*—initiates and responds with ease

2. The *Reluctant Child*—seldom initiates but responds when he or she "warms up" and feels comfortable

3. The *Child with His/Her Own Agenda*—plays alone, initiates only when he or she needs something (if this style is persistent, it may be indicative of a social-pragmatic disorder)

4. The *Passive Child*—seldom responds or initiates (persistent passivity can be indicative of a developmental delay)

Highlighting the interplay between educators' roles and children's conversational styles helps educators identify potential mismatches between the two. For example, during interactions with an educator in the Director or Entertainer role, the reluctant child is unlikely to initiate and interact (Weitzman & Greenberg, 2002). By contrast, taking on a role that is more responsive will be more efficacious for engaging the reluctant child.

Interaction-Promoting Strategies

The goal of interaction-promoting strategies is to encourage children to maintain conversations so that educators can continue to model progressively more complex language and literacy concepts relevant to the children's topic. These strategies are presented in Table 5–2. When providing information to educators about interaction-promoting strategies, SLPs need to emphasize the value of (1) responsive one-to-one educator-child interactions, during which the dyad explores and elaborates on a single topic, and (2) small-group conversations, in which the educator and several children collaboratively contribute to a topic and elaborate it further, sharing the turn-taking across all group members. The former may occur as children arrive at or prepare to leave the child care center or during incidentally occurring exchanges during the day. Small-group interactions typically occur at focused activity centers (e.g., water table, creative activities); during activities involving constructive, sensory, or dramatic play; or at mealtimes, when educators can sit and interact with children for extended periods, giving some undivided attention to each child (Cote, 2001; Girolametto & Weitzman, 2002; Kontos, 1999). Groups larger than four children may provide significantly reduced opportunities for involving children in extended conversations.

The first focus of interaction-promoting strategies is to involve all children in activities and conversations. Educators can use a variety of strategies designed to foster children's conversational engagement, as shown in Table 5–2. These strategies include actively scanning the group, observing each child, and noticing his or her

Table 5-2. Key Interaction-Promoting Strategies for Fostering Extended Conversations

Interaction-Promoting Strategies

Educators' use of these strategies facilitates children's participation in extended conversations and results in more turns on topic.

Strategy	How Educators Apply Strategy	Outcomes for Children

Use a variety of questions to encourage conversation	▪ Use a variety of open-ended "Wh" questions (e.g., who, what, where, why, when, how, what if).
	 ▪ Wait silently and expectantly for a response—give the child time to think!
	 ▪ Use questions that:
	   – respond to the children's topics
	   – verify the children's messages
	   – request unknown information
	   – stimulate the children's creative thinking (e.g., "What would happen if . . . ?" "Why do you think . . . ?")
		▪ Become engaged in the conversation
		 ▪ Learn how to answer a variety of questions
		 ▪ Learn how to maintain a topic over more turns
		 ▪ Learn new information and vocabulary
		 ▪ Develop decontextualized language skills when asked questions that require use of abstract language, such as reasoning, projecting, imagining, etc.

Strategy	How Educators Apply Strategy	Outcomes for Children

Encourage turn taking	■ Use comments to:
	  – show interest
	  – acknowledge the child's message
	  – provide contingent information
	■ Link a comment and a question.
	■ Balance the number and length of adult-to-child turns.
	■ Wait silently and expectantly for a response—give the child time to take a turn!
		■ Become engaged in the conversation
		■ Learn how to answer a variety of questions
		■ Learn how to maintain a topic over more turns
		■ Learn new information and vocabulary
		■ Develop decontextualized language skills when asked questions that require use of abstract language, such as reasoning, projecting, imagining, etc.

Scan in groups	■ Carefully observe each child in small group activities to:
	  – adapt responses to encourage the attention, participation and interaction of all children
	  – ensure that no one child is uninvolved or dominates the interaction
		■ All children have equal opportunities to:
		  – use the materials and become involved in an activity
		  – initiate to the educator and other children
		  – take turns in extended interactions

Source: From Weitzman, E., & Greenberg, J. (2002). *Learning language and loving it: A guide to promoting children's social, language, and literacy development in early childhood settings* (2nd ed.). Toronto: The Hanen Centre. Copyright 2002, Hanen Early Language Program. Reprinted with permission.

level of participation and interaction. On the basis of these observations, the educator can take appropriate steps to facilitate the child's engagement. Too often, children with reluctant or passive conversational styles are overlooked in a group, unless educators make a conscious effort to observe and include them (Weitzman & Greenberg, 2002).

The use of interaction-promoting strategies usually results in a more equal ratio of adult-to-child talk, in which the educator listens to the children, tailors comments and questions to their interests, and does not dominate the conversation. In this type of conversation, there are short periods of time when the educator is seen to be listening closely to the children without interrupting them, followed by responses that are clearly contingent upon what the children have said. Dickinson (2001) reported that a lower ratio of teacher-to-child talk, as measured during free play, was linked to better child performance in narrative production, decontextualized language, emergent literacy, and receptive vocabulary, underscoring the importance of interaction-promoting strategies and shared turn-taking.

A second focus of interaction-promoting strategies is on giving children opportunities to remain engaged in conversations that are longer than typical Question-Response-Evaluation formats, applicable to both individual and small-group contexts. Conversations in which educators and children discuss ongoing activities, recall past events, tell stories, provide explanations, and describe imaginary situations have been shown to be highly beneficial to the development of children's oral language and emergent literacy skills (Goelman, 2003; Snow, 1988). The following two examples contrast a lack of interaction-promoting strategy use (Example 1) with exemplary use of such strategies (Example 2). In both examples, the educator is reading a storybook with several preschoolers.

Example 1: Lack of Interaction-Promoting Strategies

Jessica: They're not sharing. *(while looking at a picture of a cat and dog in the book)*

Educator: What aren't they sharing? *(asks question to which answer is already known)*

Jessica: The chair.

Educator: That's right. They're not sharing the chair. *(typical Question-Response-Evaluation format does not result in educator's pursuing further information on topic; resumes reading)*

Example 2: Appropriate Use of Interaction-Promoting Strategies

Jessica: They're not sharing. *(while looking at a picture of a cat and dog in the book)*

Educator: Yes, they're not being very nice to one another. What's happening here? *(points to picture; encourages turn-taking by linking a comment with an open-ended question, and waits expectantly)*

Samuel: He pushed him.

Educator: Who pushed who? *(scaffolds, asking child for more explicit information)*

Samuel: Ginger Cat pushed the Yellow Dog onto the floor.

Educator: Yes, and Yellow Dog looks very upset. *(scans the group, looking at all the children and pauses, waits expectantly)*

Jessica: They need to share.

Educator: Yes, they need to find a way to share the chair. What could they do? *(encourages turn-taking by linking a comment with an open-ended question requiring children to problem-solve; waits expectantly)*

Jessica: They could take turns.

Educator: Just like all of you take turns when you share a toy. Jamal, what do you think they should do? *(scans the group and notices that Jamal is uninvolved; directs an open-ended question to Jamal, requiring him to provide an opinion, and waits)*

Jamal: The Yellow Dog got there first.

Educator: Do you think he should have the chair all to himself because he got there first? *(encourages turn-taking*

by asking a question requiring child to explain his opinion)

Jamal: If he gets there first, he can have the chair.

Educator: Who thinks that the Yellow Dog should have the chair because he got there first? *(encourages turn-taking by asking a question and waits expectantly to elicit a turn from another child)*

Laura: I think he should get the chair 'cuz he was there first, but now he's on the floor!

Educator: Yes, and he's very surprised to find himself on the floor. What do you think he's going to do now? *(encourages turn-taking by linking a comment with an open-ended question requiring children to predict; waits expectantly)*

Educators may successfully scaffold children's participation in extended conversations by using interaction-promoting strategies, as illustrated by the conversation in Example 2. These strategies provide opportunities for educators to facilitate oral language as well as important aspects of emergent literacy, such as decontextualized language (see page 149 for a description of decontextualized discourse). Whitehurst and Lonigan (1998) suggest that 2- and 3-year-old children may be able to answer questions only about concrete objects, actions, and events on the page of the storybook, whereas 4- and 5-year-old children are able to answer more decontextualized questions, as shown in Example 2. Furthermore, although younger children may respond equally to open-ended and closed questions, 4-year-old children often use longer utterances in response to open-ended questions, confirming the value of this type of question for promoting interaction and eliciting language (de Rivera, Weitzman, Greenberg, & Girolametto, 2005). Therefore, SLPs consulting with early childhood educators may need to help educators match the level of their interaction-promoting questions to the diverse ages and abilities of the children in their groups and provide regular follow-up in the classroom to help educators fine-tune this strategy as children develop their skills.

Engagement in extended conversational exchanges also helps children learn to assume the perspective of the listener and provide the specific, explicit types of information the listener needs.

These exchanges help young children take another person's perspective and escape from their own egocentricity (Tough, 1985). When children are exposed to responsive input that is just above their level of competence (but still within their zone of proximal development), they experience models of how adults think and how to add new information that is contingent upon a listener's perspective. These sorts of extended exchanges provide an appropriately challenging language learning environment, facilitating the internalization of what has been negotiated and learned in the social context (Berk & Winsler, 1995). The most important aspect of these interactions is that the emphasis is on the interactive process between the educator and children so that the educator does not dominate, instruct, or correct the children; rather, learning takes place as the interaction unfolds.

Language-Modeling Strategies

Language-modeling strategies build children's oral language skills and may also be used to model important emergent literacy concepts, including decontextualized language, print concepts, and letter names. Table 5–3 outlines the language-modeling strategies included in Learning Language and Loving It. To facilitate educators' understanding of the type of language models that best support oral language and emergent literacy development, SLPs should ensure that the difference between contextualized and decontextualized discourse is understood. *Contextualized* discourse is tied to the immediate environment and is used when knowledge or context is shared by conversation partners so that the speaker need not be highly explicit. A child may say, "I don't want it so I'll leave it here" and be understood perfectly well from the immediate context. Young children's early language development involves the contextualized use of language, because most of their talk revolves around the "here and now."

Decontextualized discourse occurs when meaning is conveyed primarily through language, with minimal reliance on context or shared understanding. This type of discourse focuses on past, future, abstract, and imaginary situations and requires more precise and specific vocabulary as well as formal syntactic markers to clarify the temporal and causal nature of events (Curenton & Justice, 2004).

Table 5–3. Key Language-Modeling Strategies for Developing Oral Language Skills

Language-Modeling Strategies

Educators' use of language-modeling strategies includes utterances that expand or extend the syntactic and semantic content of the children's utterances and provide a model of more advanced oral language skills and emergent literacy knowledge.

Strategy	How Educators Apply Strategy	Outcomes for Children
Use a variety of labels	• Use a variety of vocabulary (nouns, verbs, adjectives; include unfamiliar or rare words). • Emphasize key words. • Repeat words, especially unfamiliar vocabulary. • Use specific vocabulary rather than nonspecific words (e.g., "it," "this," "that," "there," "thank you"). • Clarify word meanings during conversations.	• Pay attention to new vocabulary • Begin to connect new vocabulary with their meaning • Use new vocabulary • Expand vocabulary
Expand on what the child says	• Respond, repeating the child's words and adding one or two more words to model more complex forms. • Respond, using the child's words and adding some new ideas.	• Hear a more mature language model • Hear new vocabulary • May use new vocabulary • May use more complex morphology and syntax

Strategy	How Educators Apply Strategy	Outcomes for Children

Extend the topic	■ Model the "language of learning"/ decontextualized language by using comments or questions to:
	
	  – ask for/give information about the past or present
	
	  – ask for/give reasons for what is happening
	
	  – talk about feelings and opinions
	
	  – project into other people's lives, experiences, and feelings
	
	  – predict/hypothesize about what will happen
	
	  – talk about imaginary things or play a pretend role
		■ Begins to understand more concepts and ideas
		
		■ Learns to use the "language of learning"/ decontextualized language to go beyond the here-and-now to analyze and understand the world

Source: From Weitzman, E., & Greenberg, J. (2002). *Learning language and loving it: A guide to promoting children's social, language, and literacy development in early childhood settings* (2nd ed.). Toronto: The Hanen Centre. Copyright 2002, Hanen Early Language Program. Reprinted with permission.

It should not be assumed that children who have developed contextualized language skills will automatically develop the ability to use decontextualized language. Children can be effective conversationalists when there is no need for use of decontextualized language, but may have limited ability to engage in extended discourse during which they must reflect on language and communicate novel information (Dickinson & Beals, 1994). When implementing language-modeling strategies, early childhood educators may need specific guidance on how to provide models that extend children's comprehension of decontextualized language.

The following two examples illustrate use of language-modeling strategies by contrasting an educator who neglects use of these strategies (Example 1) with one who shows exemplary use of these strategies (Example 2). In both, an educator is sitting with children at a small table while they drink water and have a snack. The first example shows how an educator misses an opportunity to engage children in an extended conversation that would provide rich language models.

Example 1: Lack of Language-Modeling Strategies

Jamal: My T-shirt's wet. *(he just spilled water on his shirt)*

Educator: It's okay. It will dry when we go outside. *(turns to another child)*

Example 2: Appropriate Use of Language-Modeling Strategies

Jamal: My T-shirt's wet. *(he just spilled water on his shirt)*

Educator: It's okay. We're going outside soon. Do you know what will happen to the water on your T-shirt when we go outside? *(extends topic—invites Jamal to predict, using decontextualized language)*

Jamal: It's gonna get dry?

Educator: Yes, it will get dry. *(expands on child's utterance)*. How will it get dry? *(extends the topic—invites children to explain, using decontextualized language)*

Jackson: The sun's gonna dry it.

Educator: Yes, the sun is so hot today. *(expands on child's utterance)* It will suck up the drops of water from your T-shirt. *(extends the topic)*

Maria: Where will the drops go?

Educator: Where do you think the drops will go? *(extends the topic—sees if children can develop a theory of their own, hypothesize, and use decontextualized language)*

Jamal: All the way up to the sun? Then the sun's gonna suck them up.

Educator: Well, the sun is so far away, the water won't go all that way—that's millions of miles. But yes, the drops of water will be sucked up into the air by the heat of the sun *(extends the topic, builds on children's rudimentary understanding of the sun's capacity to absorb water into the air)*.

Jackson: But we can't see them.

Educator: That's right. We won't be able to see the drops of water *(expands on child's utterance)*.

Maria: 'Cuz they go far away? Then we can't see them?

Educator: We can't see the drops of water because they evaporate into the air and they are so tiny, that we can't see them. Do you know what evaporate means? *(labels—introduces a "rare" word: "evaporate")*

Jamal: No.

Educator: It means the drops of water get sucked into the warm air. They evaporate and we can't see them because they are so tiny, but they are still there in the air. *(extends the topic—explains meaning of rare word)*

Jackson: Can I try to make water evaporate in a cup?

Educator: That's a good idea. How will you do that? *(extends the topic—sees if child can explain, which requires use of decontextualized language)*

Jackson: I'll put water in a cup and leave it outside in the sun.

Jamal: Then we'll see how long it takes to 'vaporate.

Educator: That's a great idea. We can see how long it takes for all the water to evaporate. *(expands on child's utterance)* How about we make a line on the cup to mark the water level? Then when we put the cup outside we can track the level as the water evaporates. *(extends the topic)*

Jamal: Yeah!

Example 2 illustrates how an educator uses not only language-modeling strategies (e.g., use a variety of labels, expand on what the child says, extend the topic) but integrates these with child-oriented strategies to follow the children's lead, and with interaction-promoting strategies to extend the conversation. This conversation has the potential to be the first of many conversations that slowly build on the children's interest in and understanding of evaporation. Future conversations may include exploration with sponges and water, other examples of evaporation, and discussions about clouds and rain.

Linguistic Responsiveness and Emergent Literacy

Children's participation in high-quality interactions that feature adults' frequent use of child-oriented, interaction-promoting, and language-modeling strategies serves an important role in promoting their language development within the early education setting. As supported by our own research, educator use of these strategies promotes children's verbal productivity in terms of number of utterances used, multiword combinations, and peer-directed utterances (Girolametto et al., 2003). Use of these strategies, however, also can serve to enhance children's emergent literacy skills, as discussed next.

Responsiveness in Shared Book Reading

One of the most important language and literacy experiences for preschool children is storybook reading. This context provides an opportunity for educators to expose children to high-quality literature and to the kind of decontextualized language that is fundamental to the acquisition of literacy. When reading stories to children, educators can help them gain meaning from the text by ensuring their active participation, which improves their story comprehension and language development, especially when they hear the same story several times (Morrow, 1988, 1989). Although frequent, regular exposure to storybook reading is critical to children's development of language and emergent literacy, it is not always an integral part of the routines in early education settings. At least in some early education classrooms, children may spend more time each day in transition between activities than listening to storybooks (Dickinson, McCabe, & Anastasopoulos, 2002).

SLPs need to support educators in their program planning so that storybook reading is a regular part of the daily scheduled activities for the class as a whole, as well as being a regular part of informal, small-group activities. Beyond ensuring the frequency of this activity, SLPs also can help educators to integrate the use of child-oriented, interaction-promoting, and language-modeling strategies into the shared reading routine, with language-modeling strategies focused specifically on the use of decontextualized language.

Educators may have difficulty extrapolating the use of interaction-promoting strategies from general interactions with children to the context of storybook reading, because for some educators, book reading is characteristically an adult-directed activity. The SLP can help educators who typically share books with children in a directive fashion to understand the rationale for making storybook reading a highly interactive activity that need not adhere to any particular script, or to reading the text exactly as written. It may also be helpful for educators to think of book reading as consisting of three stages: *before reading*, *while reading*, and *after reading*; the SLP can work with educators to build responsive strategies into all three stages, as outlined in Table 5–4.

Linguistic Responsiveness and Verbal Print References

Within storybook reading and writing activities, language-modeling strategies, particularly labels and expansions, constitute an ideal vehicle for making references to print that model higher-level literacy concepts for children. As with all language models, print references should ideally follow children's lead in terms of topic and help to focus children's attention on the form of written language.

Table 5–4. Key Strategies for Responsive Storybook Reading

Responsive Book Reading Strategies

Educators' use of child-oriented, interaction-promoting, and language-modeling strategies enable children to gain meaning from the book, to participate in the conversations about the book, and to gain exposure to and experience with decontextualized language.

When to Use Strategy	How Educators Apply Strategy	Outcomes for Children
Before reading	▪ Prepare children to read the book: – Read and point to the title. – Show the cover. – Introduce author and illustrator. – Ask children to predict what the story is about based on title and cover. – Ask a question that creates a purpose for reading the book.	▪ Activate their background knowledge ▪ Become familiar with literacy concepts such as "author," "illustrator," and "title" ▪ Gain exposure to meaningful print ▪ Approach book reading with a purpose
While reading	▪ Observe, wait, and listen: – Read at an unhurried pace, giving the children time to look at and discuss each page. – Pause and wait expectantly at key points to encourage initiations. – Observe the children to pick up verbal and nonverbal initiations.	▪ Initiate by making comments or asking questions ▪ Gain meaning from the book and relate it to what they already know

When to Use Strategy	How Educators Apply Strategy	Outcomes for Children
While reading continued	▪ Follow the children's lead by responding to their initiations by labeling, interpreting, expanding, and commenting or asking a question.	▪ Feel acknowledged ▪ More likely to continue to take turns in the conversation ▪ Are actively engaged in the book reading process

	▪ Encourage turn taking: Use a variety of labels, expand on children's utterances, and extend the topic. Use a variety of questions, labels, and comments for the purpose of:
	– teaching new vocabulary
	– relating the book to the children's own knowledge and experiences
	– encouraging children to use decontextualized language to:
	  ○ talk about characters' feelings
	  ○ project themselves into the story and describe how they would feel or behave in that situation
		▪ Are supported to make sense of the book and relate it to what they already know
		▪ Are exposed to new vocabulary, concepts, and ideas
		▪ Understand the book at a higher level and gain exposure to decontextualized language
		▪ Participate in the conversation using decontextualized language

continues

Table 5-4. *continued*

When to Use Strategy	How Educators Apply Strategy	Outcomes for Children
While reading continued	○ explain why something happened or why one of the characters said or did something ○ predict what will happen next ○ imagine a different ending or what happened beyond the ending of the story	
After reading	▪ Ask questions to encourage children to express their opinions about the book, to link ideas with other books they have read. ▪ Offer interesting follow-up activities, such as role playing the story or creating a piece of artwork about the story.	▪ Feel opinions about the book are valued ▪ Make connections between books read ▪ Language and concepts learned in the story are reinforced through a related follow-up activity

Source: From Weitzman, E., & Greenberg, J. (2002). *Learning language and loving it: A guide to promoting children's social, language, and literacy development in early childhood settings* (2nd ed.). Toronto: The Hanen Centre. Copyright 2002, Hanen Early Language Program. Reprinted with permission.

When adults make explicit print references, preschoolers learn that letters can be named, are associated with sounds, and can be combined in different ways to produce words that have meaning (Justice & Ezell, 2004). For example, adults may point out alphabet letters (e.g., "That's an S"), draw attention to the sound of a letter (e.g., "This letter makes the sound /s/"), or refer to a specific word (e.g., "Let's write the word 'sun'"). By integrating interaction-promoting strategies within these exchanges, educators can engage children in extended conversations that scaffold children's understanding of these abstract but highly important concepts.

There are many opportunities for educators to make print references during storybook reading, craft, writing, activities, and other daily routines. It appears, however, that they rarely do so without instruction (Dickinson & Tabors, 2001; Flowers et al., in press; Justice & Ezell, 2000). SLPs can help educators increase the frequency of print references within the context of activities that follow the children's lead, extend conversational turn-taking, and model language (Weitzman & Greenberg, 2002). By adhering to these principles, educators learn to integrate print only when appropriate to the topic (e.g., writing short stories that the children dictate, writing names and descriptions on artwork, writing messages on sign-up sheets, journals, or daily records) and explicitly promoting emergent literacy skills by pointing out letters, words, print conventions, and sound patterns (e.g., sounds of letters, rhymes).

Some activities may be more amenable to print referencing than others. Girolametto, Weitzman, Lefebvre, and Greenberg (in press) examined educators' use of print references in two contexts: during storybook reading and during a post-story craft activity in which educators encouraged children to dictate messages about pictures they drew. Educators used fewer than 2 print references in 15 minutes of storybook reading but used approximately 36 print references in a post-story craft activity of similar duration. Extant guidelines recommend that adults should use no more than three to five print references per storybook to prevent the children from being distracted from the storyline (Justice & Ezell, 2004) but can use more during other activities, such as writing-enriched craft activities, depending on the children's interest and motivation. Thus, SLPs offering in-service education on print referencing may want to explore storybook reading and pre- and post-story activities (e.g., print-related activity centers, role playing with shopping lists) that provide naturalistic and focused opportunities for educators to use verbal print references.

Promoting Educators' Use of Responsive Strategies

Assessing Educators' Use of Responsive Strategies

The emphasis throughout this chapter has been not only on the importance of linguistic responsiveness to facilitating children's language and literacy skills within early education settings but also on the important roles that SLPs can play in promoting educators' responsiveness. To facilitate improvements in early childhood educators' frequency and quality of responsive behaviors, SLPs may wish to utilize a formal instrument for both formative and summative purposes. Specifically, the Teacher Interaction and Language Rating Scale (Girolametto, Weitzman, & Greenberg, 2000b) was developed to evaluate educators' implementation of child-oriented, interaction-promoting, and language-modeling strategies before, during, and after in-service education. This scale can be a valuable tool for SLPs when working with educators to increase their linguistic responsiveness. It can be used to identify specific targets for educators to work on during an in-service program (formative assessment) and to characterize the overall effectiveness of in-service (summative assessment). Appendix 5–A presents an abbreviated version of the scale items (for a complete copy of the scale, contact The Hanen Centre at www.hanen.org). This instrument has been used in several studies to document educators' use of responsive strategies (Girolametto & Weitzman, 2002; Girolametto, Weitzman, & van Lieshout, 2000c) and to monitor progress during in-service programs (Girolametto et al., 2003).

The first four items on the scale—Wait and Listen, Follow the Children's Lead, Join in and Play, Be Face-to-Face—are child-oriented strategies. If educators receive a rating of 4 or below ("Needs Fine-Tuning") on any of these items, these specific items may be the first objectives of training or consultation. For example, if the SLP observes that an educator waits, follows the children's lead by commenting, and is face to face but does not join in the children's play as a play partner, he or she can provide guidance to the educator on how to increase and improve use of this strategy. By joining in the children's play as a partner, the educator takes advantage of opportunities to engage the children in a pleasurable interaction that, in turn, will provide multiple opportunities for using responsive strategies and modeling more advanced play skills. The Join in and Play strategy may be especially important for building comprehension skills in children with language disabilities and children learning English as a second language.

The next three items—Use Appropriate Questions, Encourage Turn-Taking, Scan—assess the educators' use of interaction-promoting strategies. Early childhood educators appear to have particular difficulty keeping children involved in conversations that extend beyond three turns, and all of these items are designed to monitor use of strategies that can increase children's participation in extended conversations. Two of these items deserve special attention. First, Girolametto and Weitzman (2002) reported that educators rarely achieved a rating of 4 or above for the item evaluating the use of questions (i.e., Use a Variety of Questions). Second, in a subsequent study (Girolametto et al., 2003), educators received uniformly low ratings (i.e., below 3) for conversational turn-taking (i.e., Encourage Turn-Taking). These results indicate that both strategies may require additional emphasis during an in-service program or during individual consultation sessions. Educators need to learn how to ask open-ended questions to engage children in decontextualized conversations that are within their zone of proximal development. Implementing turn-taking within a small group situation requires the educator to monitor the ongoing topic and use comments and questions skillfully to maintain the children's interest. In addition, the educator may need to learn how to balance following children's initiations with maintaining the topic when one child in the group makes an initiation that is tangential or off-topic.

The remaining four items are language-modeling strategies: Imitate, Label, Expand, Extend. Two of these items also may require special emphasis during in-service programs. In a study investigating educators' interactions in book reading and "play dough" activities, educators received consistently low ratings (i.e., a rating of

4 or lower) for Expand and Extend (Girolametto & Weitzman, 2002). Use of these two strategies requires educators to listen carefully to children's utterances in order to incorporate them into their subsequent turns and flexibly scaffold the topic by adding new information. Educators may need ongoing supports in using expansions and extensions in one-on-one, small-group, and large-group interactions throughout the day.

When SLPs utilize the rating scale as a professional development tool, the scale should be used and scored within at least two different classroom activities before objectives for in-service training or consultation are established. Sampling multiple contexts of educator-child interaction is important because a strategy that is not used in one activity may be observed in another. For example, in a "play dough" activity (a child-focused activity), an educator may receive high ratings for child-oriented strategies and interaction-promoting strategies. By contrast, during book reading, these strategies are seldom used effectively (Girolametto & Weitzman, 2002). Once an educator can successfully implement a strategy in one context, it makes it easier to (1) highlight the educator's awareness of his or her ability to apply the strategy effectively in one context and (2) facilitate the transfer of the skill to a different context.

Training Educators to Become More Responsive Conversational Partners

A considerable body of research has demonstrated that the quality of early education and child care in the United States and Canada generally is mediocre in terms of the kinds of interactions and stimulation known to result in developmental gains for children (Pianta, 2006). In light of this finding, SLPs have the opportunity to play a major role in providing high-quality in-service education to early childhood educators on the facilitation of language and emergent literacy skills. This in-service education can help educators become more responsive conversational partners with children, one of the most salient characteristics of high-quality early education settings.

In general, the goal of in-service education is to facilitate educators' acquisition of knowledge and skills so that they are able to change their classroom practice, with a consequent positive impact on the children's developmental outcomes. In focusing on responsiveness, the goal is to promote educators' use of child-oriented, interaction-promoting, and language-modeling strategies, all of which may require sustained, intensive support by the SLP. Unfortunately, the most common type of in-service education or professional development offered to early childhood professionals is a workshop, which frequently involves a "one-shot" event from a leader with special expertise. Such workshops have been widely criticized as being ineffective because their brief format does not foster meaningful changes in educators' classroom practices (Garet, Porter, Desimone, Birman, & Yoon, 2001).

Learning Language and Loving It™: A Professional Development Approach

The professional development approach presented next, developed at The Hanen Centre in Toronto, Ontario, goes well beyond a "one-shot" approach and emphasizes the need for ongoing intensive support for educators to enhance their use of responsive strategies. Specifically, Learning Language and Loving It™—The Hanen Program® for Early Childhood Educators and Preschool Teachers aims to help educators (1) understand the rationale for adopting responsive strategies, (2) understand the critical role they play in promoting children's developmental progress, (3) understand that children construct knowledge when they are actively engaged with the people and objects in their environments, and (4) apply responsive strategies flexibly within their everyday interactions with children in their classrooms.

Learning Language and Loving It is a group training program that fulfills the following requirements for effective in-service education, as described by Bowman, Donovan, and Burns (2001) and Garet et al. (2001). First, effective in-service education programs offer a continuous program of study, sustained over time. Accordingly, Learning Language and Loving It is an intensive program that usually consists of a series of eight 150-minute group sessions for up to 20 educators as well as six individual videotaping and feedback sessions. The total time commitment expected from the early childhood educators who attend the in-service education program is approximately 25 hours over a 15-week period.

The second requirement of effective in-service education programs is active participation of learners in the learning process. The format of Learning Language and Loving It is guided by principles of adult education, which espouse active involvement as an essential prerequisite for positive learning outcomes. The Learning Language and Loving It group sessions, which include a variety of media such as PowerPoint slide presentations and videotaped examples of educator-child interactions, are structured so that educators' learning is facilitated through interactive, experiential activities such as small-group discussions, group brainstorming, videotape analysis, and simulated practice activities.

Third, effective in-service education programs include opportunities to apply knowledge in simulated and real-life situations. The strategies learned by educators during the group sessions of Learning Language and Loving It are therefore practiced during group sessions, usually in simulated activities representing frequently occurring classroom situations. These simulations are following by debriefings that encourage educators to ask questions or express concerns and to enable the group leader to highlight issues related to application of the strategy in question.

Fourth, effective in-service education involves the provision of expert mentoring or coaching in real-life situations. In Learning Language and Loving It, each educator is observed and videotaped on site in his or her early education setting by the group leader six times over the course of the 15-week program. On-line coaching is provided to the educator to facilitate his or her application of newly learned strategies to interactions with children during routine classroom activities.

Fifth, effective in-service education provides immediate feedback on learners' application of newly-learned behavior. Using the videotapes filmed in the early education setting, each educator is excused from the classroom so that the videotaped interaction can be viewed together with the group leader of the Learning Language and Loving It program. This provides educators with powerful images of the positive impact they have on children when they use responsive strategies. It also facilitates the development of the educators' self-awareness regarding specific aspects of interactive behavior that need to be modified to increase responsiveness. In addition, the feedback process increases educators' ability to self-monitor the application of program strategies, which is critical to generalized use of program strategies across a variety of activities and children.

Finally, the collective participation of educators from the same setting is essential for effective in-service education. Learning Language and Loving It usually is offered to the entire staff at a child care center or preschool program in order to promote systemic changes in practice over time. By developing a shared understanding of the goals of interacting with children and discussing ideas and concerns with colleagues on a day-to-day basis, educators are more likely to implement the strategies they have learned.

The efficacy of Learning Language and Loving It has been supported in a series of studies showing positive changes for educators and children. Specifically, in comparison with a control group, educators who participated in the 15-week program increased their use of responsive interaction strategies during routine activities (play dough, book reading) with small groups of children (Girolametto et al., 2003). The children in this study also benefited from their educators' positive changes, as they spoke more often during small group interactions and used a more diverse vocabulary and longer utterances than children in the control classrooms. A second study used a shortened version of the program (i.e., 6 weeks of instruction) and focused expressly on educators' role in facilitating peer interaction (Girolametto et al., 2004). In this study, educators learned to use a variety of peer support strategies to invite children to interact with one another. In comparison with a control group, the children in this study interacted with their peers more often and kept the peer-directed conversations going for longer turns.

Two additional studies have examined educators' ability to adopt emergent literacy strategies after participation in the Learning Language and Loving It in-service program (Flowers et al., in press; Girolametto et al., in press). In the first study (using the 15-week program in which emergent literacy was a 1-week topic), educators increased their use of decontextualized language during storybook reading to invite children to share their experiences and comment on emotions of the storybook characters. Furthermore, the children in this study used more decontextualized responses to the educators' comments or questions, in comparison with a control group. A follow-up study (Girolametto et al., in press) focused exclusively on facilitating educators' use of decontextualized language and print referencing strategies when interacting with children; educators in this study participated in 2 weeks of instruction on these topics. In addition to increasing their use of decontextualized language, the educators increased their use of print references during a post-story craft activity to highlight letters, sound-letter correspondences, and word concepts (Girolametto et al., in press). The children in this study also increased their use of decontextualized utterances and references to print. These initial studies point to the positive benefits of in-service programs for promoting systematic changes in educators' responsive interactions; importantly, these changes in educator behaviors appear to result in short-term benefits to children's language and emergent literacy skills. Because the designs of these studies included control groups that did not receive the target program, it is possible to conclude that the educators' involvement in in-service education was the significant factor in producing the observed changes in children's performance.

Conclusion

Early education settings constitute a vitally important environment for promoting children's developmental progress. When educators are responsive and use "a language of caregiving that communicates to children at semantic, syntactic, pragmatic and social-emotional levels" (Goelman, 2003, p. 2.8), they create environments that provide the intellectual, language, and social-emotional nurturing needed to promote children's language and emergent literacy development. The SLP's role in consulting and collaborating with early childhood educators, including use of sustained and intensive in-service programs, is a key mechanism for enhancing the quality of child care, particularly in the area of language and literacy. Learning Language and Loving It™—The Hanen Program® for Early Childhood Educators and Preschool Teachers, which has been field tested and rigorously examined using stringent randomized control trials, provides one example of an effective vehicle through which SLPs can provide educators with efficacious in-service. Moreover, the program adheres to current philosophical guidelines for how best to promote educators' knowledge and skills. In supporting educators' efforts to create responsive, high-quality environments, SLPs are building educators' capacity to reach thousands of children and to promote their learning in the key areas of language and emergent literacy, setting them on the path to optimal academic achievement.

References

American Speech-Language-Hearing Association (ASHA). (2001). *Roles and responsibilities of speech-language pathologists with respect to reading and writing in children and adolescents*. Rockville, MD: Author.

Bell, R. (1979). Parent, child, and reciprocal influences. *American Psychologist, 34*, 821–826.

Berk, L. (1985). Relationship of caregiver education to child-oriented attitudes, job satisfaction, and behavior toward children. *Child Care Quarterly, 14*, 103–129.

Berk, L., & Winsler, A. (1995). *Scaffolding children's learning: Vygotsky and early childhood education*. Washington, DC: National Association for Education of Young Children.

Blair, C. (2002). School readiness: Integrating cognition and emotion in a neurobiological conceptualization of child functioning at school entry. *American Psychologist, 57*, 111–127.

Bohannon, J., & Bonvillian, J. (1997). Theoretical approaches to language acquisition. In J. Berko Gleason (Ed.), *The development of language* (4th ed., pp. 259–316). Needham Heights, MA: Allyn & Bacon.

Bowman, B., Donovan, M., & Burns, M. (2001). *Eager to learn: Educating our preschoolers*. Washington, DC: National Academy Press.

Bryant, D., Clifford, D., Early, D., & Little, L. (2005). How is the pre-K day spent? *Early Developments* (p. 22–28). Published by the Frank Porter Graham Child Development Institute. Retrieved on May 3, 2006 from http://www.fpg.unc.edu/~NCEDL/PDFs/ED9_1.pdf

Burchinal, M. (1999). Child care experiences and developmental outcomes. *The Annals of the American Academy of Political and Social Sciences, 563*, 73–97.

Burchinal, M., Campbell, F., Bryant, D., Wasik, B., & Ramey, C. (1997). Early intervention and mediating processes in cognitive performance of children of low-income African-American families. *Child Development, 68*, 935–954.

Burchinal, M., Lee, M., & Ramey, C. (1989). Type of day care and preschool intellectual development in disadvantaged children. *Child Development, 60*, 128–137.

Burchinal, M., Roberts, J., Riggins, R., Zeisel, S., Neebe, E., & Bryant, M. (2000). Relating quality of center child care to early cognitive and language development longitudinally. *Child Development, 71*, 339–357.

Bushnik, T. (2006). *Child care in Canada*. Children and Youth Research Paper series. Retrieved April 25, 2006, from http://www.statcan.ca/english/research/89-599-MIE/89-599-MIE2006003.pdf

Catts, H., Fey, M., & Proctor-Williams, K. (2001). The relationship between language and reading: Preliminary results from a longitudinal investigation. *Logopedics Phoniatrics Vocology, 25*, 3–11.

Catts, H., Fey, M., Zhang, X., & Tomblin, J. (2001). Estimating the risk of future reading difficulties in kindergarten children: A research-based model and its clinical implementation. *Language, Speech, and Hearing Services in Schools, 32*, 38–50.

Cicognani, E., & Zani, B. (1992). Teacher-children interactions in a nursery school: An exploratory study. *Language and Education, 6*, 1–11.

Clarke-Stewart, K., Gruber, C., & Fitzgerald, L. (1994). *Children at home and in day care*. Hillsdale, NJ: Lawrence Erlbaum Associates.

Connor, M., Son, S., Hindman, A., & Morrison, F. (2005). Teacher qualifications, classroom practices, family characteristics, and preschool experience: Complex effects on first graders' vocabulary and early reading outcomes. *Journal of School Psychology, 43*, 343–375.

Cote, L. (2001). Language opportunities during mealtimes in preschool classrooms. In D. Dickinson & P. Tabors (Eds.), *Literacy begins with language* (pp. 205–221). Baltimore: Paul H. Brookes.

Curenton, S., & Justice, L. (2004). African American and Caucasian preschoolers' use of decontextualized language. *Language, Speech, and Hearing Services in Schools, 35*, 240–253.

de Kruif, R., McWilliam, R., Ridley, S., & Wakely, M. (2000). Classification of teachers' interactive behaviors in early childhood classrooms. *Early Childhood Research Quarterly, 15*, 247–268.

de Rivera, C., Weitzman, E., Greenberg, J., & Girolametto, L. (2005). Children's responses to educators' questions in day care playgroups. *American Journal of Speech-Language Pathology, 14*, 14–26.

Deci, E., & Ryan, R. (1985). *Intrinsic motivation and self-determination in human behavior*. New York: Plenum Press.

Dickinson, D. (2001). Large-group and free-play times: Conversational settings supporting language and literacy development. In D. Dickinson & P. Tabors (Eds.), *Beginning literacy with language* (pp. 235–255). Baltimore: Paul H. Brookes.

Dickinson, D., & Beals, D. (1994). Not by print alone: Oral language supports for early literacy development. In D. Lancy (Ed.), *Children's emergent literacy: From research to practice* (pp. 29–40). Westport, CT: Praeger Press.

Dickinson, D., McCabe, A., & Anastasopoulos, L. (2002). *A framework for examining book reading in early childhood classrooms* (No. 1-014). CIERA Report.

Dickinson, D., & Smith, M. (1994). Long-term effects of preschool teachers' book reading on low-income children's vocabulary and story comprehension. *Reading Research Quarterly, 29,* 105–122.

Dickinson, D., & Tabors, P. (2001). *Beginning literacy with language.* Baltimore: Paul H. Brookes.

Doherty, G., Lero, D., Goelman, H., Tougas, J., & LaGrange, A. (2000). *You bet I care: Key findings and their implications.* Guelph, ON: The Centre for Families, Work and Well-Being.

Flowers, H., Girolametto, L., Weitzman, E., & Greenberg, J. (in press). The effects of in-service education on the promotion of story comprehension and early literacy skills. *Journal of Speech-Language Pathology and Audiology.*

Garet, M., Porter, A., Desimone, L., Birman, B., & Yoon, K. (2001). What makes professional development effective? Results from a national sample of teachers. *American Educational Research Journal, 38,* 915–945.

Girolametto, L., Hoaken, L., van Lieshout, R., & Weitzman, E. (2000a). Patterns of adult-child linguistic interaction in integrated day care groups. *Language, Speech, and Hearing Services in Schools, 31,* 154–167.

Girolametto, L., & Weitzman, E. (2002). Responsiveness of child care providers in interactions with toddlers and preschoolers. *Language, Speech, and Hearing Services in Schools, 33,* 268–282.

Girolametto, L., & Weitzman, E. (2006). It takes two to talk—the Hanen Program for parents: Early language intervention through caregiver training. In R. McCauley & M. Fey (Eds.), *Treatment of language disorders in children* (pp. 77–103). Baltimore: Paul H. Brookes.

Girolametto, L., Weitzman, E., & Greenberg, J. (2000b). *Teacher interaction and language rating scale.* Toronto: The Hanen Centre.

Girolametto, L., Weitzman, E., & Greenberg, J. (2003). Training day care staff to facilitate children's language. *American Journal of Speech-Language Pathology, 12,* 299–311.

Girolametto, L., Weitzman, E., & Greenberg, J. (2004). The effects of verbal support strategies on small group peer interactions. *Language, Speech, and Hearing Services in Schools, 35,* 256–270.

Girolametto, L., Weitzman, E., & Greenberg, J. (2006). Facilitating language skills: In-service education for early childhood educators and preschool teachers. *Infants and Young Children, 19,* 36–48.

Girolametto, L., Weitzman, E., Lefebvre, P., & Greenberg, J. (in press). The effects of in-service education to promote emergent literacy in child care centers: A feasibility study. *Language, Speech, and Hearing Services in Schools.*

Girolametto, L., Weitzman, E., & van Lieshout, R. (2000c). Directiveness in teachers' language input to toddlers and preschoolers in day care. *Journal of Speech, Language, and Hearing Research, 43*, 1101–1114.

Goelman, H. (2003). The language of caregiving and caretaking in child care settings. In L. Girolametto & E. Weitzman (Eds.), *Enhancing caregiver language facilitation in child care settings* (pp. 2.1–2.14). Toronto: The Hanen Centre.

Grolnick, W., Deci, E., & Ryan, R. (1997). Internalization within the family: The self-determination theory perspective. In J. Grusec & L. Kuczynski (Eds.), *Parenting and children's internalization of values: A handbook of contemporary theory* (pp. 135–161). New York: Wiley & Sons.

Hayes, C., Palmer, J., & Zaslow, M. (1990). *Who cares for America's children? Child care policy for the 1990's.* Washington, DC: National Academy Press.

Howes, C. (1983). Caregiver behavior in center and family day care. *Journal of Applied Developmental Psychology, 4*, 99–107.

Jarvis, J., & Robinson, M. (1997). Analyzing educational discourse: An exploratory study of teacher response and support to pupils' learning. *Applied Psycholinguistics, 18*, 212–228.

Justice, L., & Ezell, H. (2000). Enhancing children's print and word awareness through home-based parent intervention. *American Journal of Speech-Language Pathology, 9*, 257–269.

Justice, L., & Ezell, H. (2004). Print referencing: An emergent literacy enhancement strategy and its clinical applications. *Language, Speech, and Hearing Services in Schools, 35*, 185–193.

Katz, J. (2004). *The relationship between early childhood caregivers' belief about child-rearing and young children's development: A secondary analysis of data from the NICHD Study of Early Child Care and Youth Development.* Boston: Harvard University.

Kontos, S. (1999). Preschool teachers' talk, roles, and activity settings during free play. *Early Childhood Research Quarterly, 14*, 363–382.

Kontos, S., Howes, C., Shinn, M., & Galinsky, E. (1995). *Quality in family child care and relative care.* New York: Teachers College Press.

Kontos, S., & Wilcox-Herzog, A. (2002). *Teacher preparation and teacher-child interaction in preschools* (No. EDO-PS-02-11). ERIC Digest.

Ladd, G., Birch, S., & Buhs, E. (1999). Children's social and scholastic lives in kindergarten: Related spheres of influence? *Child Development, 70*, 1373–1400.

Ladd, G., & Burgess, K. (2001). Do relational risk and protective factors moderate the links between childhood aggression and early psychological and school adjustment? *Child Development, 72*, 1579–1601.

Marshall, N. (2004). The quality of early child care and children's development. *Current Directions in Psychological Science, 13*, 165–168.

Mashburn, A., & Pianta, R. (2006). Social relationships and school readiness. *Early Education and Development, 17*, 151–176.

McCartney, K., Dearing, E., & Taylor, B. (2003). *Quality child care supports the achievement of low-income children: Direct and indirect effects via caregiving and the home environment.* Tampa, FL: Society for Research in Child Development.

Morrow, L. (1988). Young children's responses to one-to-one story readings in school settings. *Reading Research Quarterly, 23*, 89–107.

Morrow, L. (1989). The effect of small group story reading on children's questions and comments. In S. McCormick & J. Zutell (Eds.), *Cognition and social perspectives for literacy research and instruction* (Vol. 38th Yearbook of the National Reading Conference, pp. 77–86). Chicago: National Reading Conference.

Nelson, C., & Bloom, F. (1997). Child development and neuroscience. *Child Development, 68*, 970–987.

NICHD Early Child Care Research Network. (1996). Characteristics of infant child care: Factors contributing to positive caregiving. *Early Childhood Research Quarterly, 11*, 269–306.

NICHD Early Child Care Research Network. (2000). Characteristics and quality of child care for toddlers and preschoolers. *Applied Developmental Science, 4*, 116–135.

Palmerus, K. (1996). Child-caregiver ratios in day care centre groups: Impact on verbal interactions. *Early Child Development and Care, 118*, 45–57.

Paul-Brown, D., & Caperton, C. (2001). Inclusive practices for preschool-age children with specific language impairment. In M. Guralnick (Ed.), *Early childhood inclusion: Focus on change* (pp. 433–464). Baltimore: Paul H. Brookes.

Pecyna Rhyner, P., Lehr, D., & Pudlas, K. (1990). An analysis of teacher responsiveness to communicative initiations of preschool children with handicaps. *Language, Speech, and Hearing Services in Schools, 21*, 91–97.

Pellegrino, M., & Scopesi, A. (1990). Structure and function of baby talk in a day-care centre. *Journal of Child Language, 17*, 101–113.

Phillips, D., McCartney, K., & Scarr, S. (1987). Child care quality and children's social development. *Developmental Psychology, 23*, 537–543.

Phillipsen, L., Burchinal, M., Howes, C., & Cryer, D. (1997). The prediction of process quality from structural features of child care. *Early Childhood Research Quarterly, 12*, 281–303.

Pianta, R. (2006). Standardized observation and professional development: A focus on individualized implementation and practices. In M. Zaslow & I. Martinez-Beck (Eds.), *Critical issues in early childhood professional development* (pp. 231–254). Baltimore: Paul H. Brookes.

Pianta, R., & Stuhlman, M. (2004). Teacher-child relationships and children's success in the first years of school. *School Psychology Review, 33,* 444-458.

Polyzoi, E. (1997). Quality of young children's talk with adult caregivers and peers during play interactions in the day care setting. *Canadian Journal of Research in Early Childhood Education, 6,* 21-30.

Richter, L. (2004). *The importance of caregiver-child interactions for the survival and healthy development of young children.* Geneva: World Health Organization.

Rimm-Kaufman, S., Voorhees, M., Snell, M., & La Paro, K. (2003). Improving the sensitivity and responsivity of preservice teachers toward young children with disabilities. *Topics in Early Childhood Special Education, 23,* 151-163.

Rogoff, B. (1990). *Apprenticeship in thinking: Cognitive development in social context.* Oxford, England: Oxford University Press.

Roth, F., Speece, D., & Cooper, D. (2002). A longitudinal analysis of the connection between oral language and early reading. *Journal of Educational Research, 95,* 259-272.

Ruopp, R., Travers, J., Glantz, F., & Coelen, C. (1979). *Children at the center: Final report of the National Day Care Study.* Cambridge, MA: ABT Associates.

Ryan, R., & Deci, E. (2000). Intrinsic and extrinsic motivations: Classic definitions and new directions. *Contemporary Educational Psychology, 25,* 54-67.

Saracho, O. (2004). Supporting literacy-related play: Roles for teachers of young children. *Early Childhood Education Journal, 31,* 201-206.

Schaffer, H., & Liddell, C. (1984). Adult-child interaction under dyadic and polyadic conditions. *British Journal of Developmental Psychology, 2,* 33-41.

Shim, J., Hestenes, L., & Cassidy, D. (2004). Teacher structure and child care quality in preschool classrooms. *Journal of Research in Childhood Education, 19,* 143-157.

Smith, M. (2001). Children's experiences in preschool. In D. Dickinson & P. Tabors (Eds.), *Literacy begins with language* (pp. 149-174). Baltimore: Paul H. Brookes.

Snow, C. (1988). Literacy and language: Relationships during the preschool years. *Harvard Educational Review, 53,* 165-189.

Snow, C. (1994). Beginning from baby talk: Twenty years of research on input in interaction. In C. Gallaway & B. J. Richards (Eds.), *Input and interaction in language acquisition* (pp. 1-12). Cambridge, UK: Cambridge University Press.

Stanovich, K. (1986). Matthew effects in reading: Some consequences of individual differences in the acquisition of literacy. *Reading Research Quarterly, 21,* 360-406.

Tizard, B., & Hughes, M. (1984). *Young children learning*. London: Fontana Paperbacks.

Tough, J. (1985). *Talking and learning: A guide to fostering communication skills in nursery and infant schools*. London: Ward Lock Educational.

Triplett, C. (2002). Dialogic responsiveness: Toward synthesis, complexity, and holism in our response to young literacy learners. *Journal of Literacy Research, 34*, 119-158.

Vandell, D. (2004). Early child care: The known and unknown. *Merrill-Palmer Quarterly, 50*, 387-414.

Vandell, D., & Wolfe, B. (2000). *Child care quality: Does it matter and does it need to be improved?* (No. 78). Madison, WI: Institute for Research on Poverty.

Vygotsky, L. (1956). *Selected psychological investigations*. Moscow: Izdstel'sto Akademii Pedagogicheskikh Nauk SSSR.

Vygotsky, L. (1978). *Mind in society*. Cambridge, MA: Harvard University Press.

Vygotsky, L. (1981). The genesis of higher mental functions. In J. Wertsch (Ed.), *The concept of activity in Soviet psychology* (pp. 144-188). Armink, NY: Sharpe.

Weitzman, E., & Greenberg, J. (2002). *Learning Language and Loving It: A guide to promoting children's social, language, and literacy development in early childhood settings* (2nd ed.). Toronto: The Hanen Centre.

Whitebook, M., Howes, C., & Phillips, D. (1989). *Who cares? Child care teachers and the quality of care in America*. Oakland, CA: Child Care Employee Project.

Whitehurst, G., & Lonigan, C. (1998). Child development and emergent literacy. *Child Development, 69*, 848-872.

APPENDIX 5–A

Teacher Interaction and Language Rating Scale

NEEDS IMPROVEMENT: GOAL FOR PROGRAM	NEEDS FINE-TUNING	DOES NOT NEED IMPROVEMENT		

Almost Never		Sometimes		Frequently		Consistently	
1	2	3	4	5	6	7	N/A

1. **Wait and Listen:** encourages most of the children in the group to initiate verbally and/or nonverbally.

Almost Never		Sometimes		Frequently		Consistently	
1	2	3	4	5	6	7	N/A

2. **Follow the Children's Lead:** when the children initiate verbally or nonverbally.

Almost Never		Sometimes		Frequently		Consistently	
1	2	3	4	5	6	7	N/A

3. **Join in and Play:** as a partner.

Almost Never		Sometimes		Frequently		Consistently	
1	2	3	4	5	6	7	N/A

4. **Be Face to Face:** teacher adjusts her physical level.

Almost Never		Sometimes		Frequently		Consistently	
1	2	3	4	5	6	7	N/A

5. **Use Appropriate Questions:** encourages conversation with most of the children in the group.

Almost Never		Sometimes		Frequently		Consistently	
1	2	3	4	5	6	7	N/A

6. **Encourage Turn Taking:** must achieve 4 or more turns on a topic with one or more children for a score of 5.

Almost Never		Sometimes		Frequently		Consistently	
1	2	3	4	5	6	7	N/A

7. **Scan:** facilitates the participation and interaction of all children in group activities.

Almost Never		Sometimes		Frequently		Consistently	
1	2	3	4	5	6	7	N/A

8. **Imitate:** evaluate only if children are preverbal or at one-word stage.

APPENDIX 5–A. *continued*

Almost Never		Sometimes		Frequently		Consistently	
1	2	3	4	5	6	7	N/A

9. **Use a Variety of Labels:** uses a variety of vocabulary (nouns, verbs, adjectives, adverbs).

Almost Never		Sometimes		Frequently		Consistently	
1	2	3	4	5	6	7	N/A

10. **Expand:** repeats the children's words and corrects the grammar or adds another idea.

Almost Never		Sometimes		Frequently		Consistently	
1	2	3	4	5	6	7	N/A

11. **Extend:** to obtain a rating of 5, the teacher must extend frequently and include at least two functions other than informing (e.g., project, pretend/imagine, explain, talk about the future, talk about feelings).

Chapter Six

Phonological Awareness Instruction in Early Childhood Settings

Barbara Culatta
Kendra M. Hall

Overview

Preschool and kindergarten-age children with poor emergent or early literacy skills, including limited phonological awareness, are at risk for subsequent reading difficulties (Catts, Fey, Zhang, & Tomblin, 2001; Cunningham & Stanovich, 1998; Scarborough, 2001; Torgesen, Al Otaiba, & Grek, 2005). Many children who struggle in acquiring critical early literacy skills have language delays, differences, or deficits and are served by speech-language pathologists (SLPs) (Bird, Bishop, & Freeman, 1995; Bishop & Adams, 1990; Catts & Kamhi, 2005). These SLPs need effective interventions that promote emergent and early literacy skills for the children with whom they work.

Current research suggests that emergent and early literacy interventions should focus on facilitating both meaning (comprehension, vocabulary, print awareness) and skills (letter knowledge, letter-sound associations, phonological awareness, phonics) (Dickinson, McCabe, Anastasopoulos, Peisner-Feinberg, & Poe, 2003; McCardle, Scarborough, & Catts, 2001; National Reading Panel, 2000; Storch & Whitehurst, 2002) while also stimulating children's interest and motivation (Baker, Dreher, & Guthrie, 2000; Guthrie, Wigfield, & VonSecker, 2000; Gutierrez-Clellen, 1999; McKenna, 2001). Both meaning and skills should be taught through systematic, explicit exposure to critical literacy concepts in contexts that are language-rich and highly motivating and engaging for all children, particularly those with linguistic deficits and differences (Center for Research on Education, Diversity and Excellence, 2005; Dickinson & Sprague, 2001; Gutierrez-Clellen, 1999; McGee & Richgels, 2000).

Systematic and Engaging Early Literacy Instruction (SEEL) is an early literacy intervention model that integrates attention to both meaning and skill. SEEL explicitly teaches phonological aware-ness in varied, interactive, playful social contexts (Culatta, Aslett, Fife, & Setzer, 2004; Culatta, Kovarsky, Theadore, Franklin, & Timler, 2003; Culatta, Setzer, Wilson, & Aslett, 2004), providing an effective framework for organizing early literacy interventions. This chapter illustrates how SLPs and teachers together can implement SEEL instruction to develop phonological awareness skills that are a nec-essary foundation for later reading success. Although SEEL also includes explicit attention to facilitating children's print skills (see Figure 6–1), this chapter emphasizes the phonological awareness components of the curriculum. Approaches to facilitating print skills are discussed elsewhere in this book (see Chapter 10). The remainder of the chapter provides (1) a summary of how the cur-riculum addresses phonological awareness skills in an appropriate developmental sequence leading toward reading, (2) a discussion of explicit instructional strategies presented in interactive, mean-ingful contexts and activities, and (3) use of specific examples of instructional activities addressing each of the components of phonological awareness.

SEEL Curriculum: A Developmental Sequence

Phonological awareness refers to an individual's understanding that words can be segmented into sounds and that sounds can be blended to make words. Early achievements in phonological aware-ness include rhyming and alliteration, whereas later achievements include isolating and substituting phonemes in words, known as *phonemic awareness*. Performance on phonological and phone-mic awareness tasks is predictive of later reading success (Bishop & Adams, 1990; Catts et al., 2001; Scarborough, 1990; Wagner & Torgesen, 1987; Whitehurst & Lonigan, 1998), because these skills

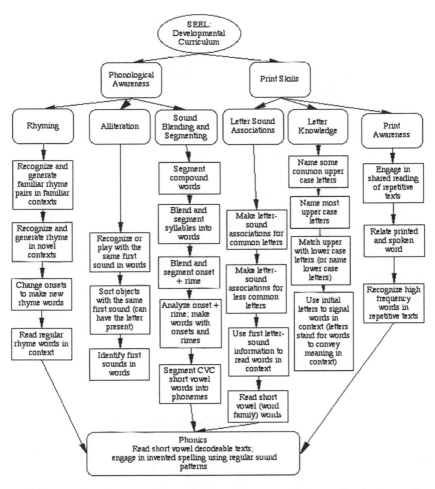

Note: The map represents development within each of the component areas (rhyming, alliteration, sound blending, letter sound associations, letter knowledge, and print awareness) but, does not represent the overlap in development across areas. Skills in one area will influence skills in another (e.g., skills in rhyming support the blending of onset + rime endings).

Figure 6–1. Systematic and Engaging Early Literacy Instruction (SEEL) developmental curriculum.

help children to achieve the *alphabetic principle* (the ability to represent sounds with letters and combine sounds to read and write words).

Most experts agree that phonological awareness skills should be taught in a systematic sequence, with connections between sounds and print being strategically made at appropriate points

(Adams, 1990). Figure 6–1 illustrates how the SEEL curricular progression for phonological awareness follows a developmental sequence of instruction in three areas: rhyming, alliteration, and sound blending and segmenting. Development of these skills enables children to progress from phonological awareness to phonic attainments, including reading regular short vowel family words (i.e., words with the same rime ending such as *bag, tag, rag, drag, flag,* and *wag* or *bet, set, get, pet, wet,* and *net*).

In developing phonological awareness and phonics skills, children progress in a pattern from identifying larger (word and syllable) to smaller (phoneme) units, moving from implicit to explicit awareness, engaging in simple and then more complex tasks, and recognizing sounds in familiar to less familiar words (Adams, 2001; Gillon, 2004; Goswami, 2001; Troia, 2004; Whitehurst & Lonigan, 2001). This chapter explains the development and progressive sequence of these skills.

Rhyming

Children begin the SEEL rhyme curriculum by learning a core of familiar rhyme pairs. Initially, SLPs and teachers present a variety of supported activities targeting children's attention to familiar rime units (a rime unit is the part of a syllable that includes the medial vowel and its final consonant or consonant cluster)—for example, *ug, ip, at, ag, op,* or *et.* Then they transition to novel rhyme pairs and more complex contexts, including play scripts or rhyme stories; eventually children are able to generate multiple examples of novel rhymes in novel contexts without support.

Rhyming connects to reading as phonetically regular rhymed words are attached to print (Gillon, 2004; Goswami, 2001; Goswami & Bryant, 1992; Torgesen et al., 2005; Treiman, 1992). The onset of the rhyming words (initial consonant or consonant cluster) and their rime ending can be designated with different colored markers or spaces (e.g., *b-ug, t-ug, j-ug*). Children segment and blend rhymed words into their onsets and rimes (e.g., "What am I saying? *t-ug*") and change the onset to make new words (e.g., making *sip* or *ip* into *dip, tip, zip, ship, lip,* or *chip*) (Gillon, 2004; Goswami & Bryant, 1990). By noticing similarities in printed and spoken words and analyzing words into their onsets and rimes, children move toward reading by analogy (Torgesen et al., 2005). For instance, the child who recognizes the rime unit *og* in *hog* may use an analogy strategy to read *dog*.

Alliteration

Alliteration, which refers to identifying the same first sound across words, is introduced in SEEL after children are able to generate some familiar rhymed word pairs. Children begin by identifying words in a series that have the same first sound, which the SLP or teacher can highlight by continuing continuants (e.g., "sssssoft"), softly repeating plosives ("a b-b-b-big burly b-b-b-black bear that b-b-bumbles, and bumps into bushes"), and producing words rapidly with sing-song intonation. SLPs can also produce same-first-sound phrases in a "tongue twister" fashion, placing stress on the first part of each word without segmenting the first sound or by segmenting the first sound from the rest of the word and re-blending it. Alliteration activities within the SEEL curriculum then move to sorting words on the basis of their beginning sounds (e.g., identifying a word in a series that does not begin with a target sound), first with high levels of support and then less support. Eventually, children are asked to identify or generate the initial sound in words: "Does *sun* start with /s/?" "Think of a word that starts with /s/" "Which of these words starts with /s/?"

After children can engage in a variety of alliteration tasks, they move into explicit letter-sound associations, represented within the "print skills" strand of the SEEL curriculum. Work on letter-sound associations typically does not begin until children have reasonably well-developed phonological awareness skills, as represented in their ability to sort words on the basis of beginning sounds. Letter-sound association activities help children to link beginning sounds in words with beginning letters. For instance, children may be asked to recall words used in a sort activity (e.g., items placed in the "*S* store"), which the SLP or teacher can write on a white board for the class to use in a shared reading activity: The children give the sound for the initial letter (/s/), the SLP or teacher reads the rest of the word (*oup*), and together they blend the sounds to form the word ("/s/ . . . *oup*. We bought *soup*).

Sound Blending and Segmenting

In its blending and segmenting activities, the SEEL curriculum begins with words and then moves to smaller linguistic units (syllables, onset/rimes). Children clap and march as they segment sentences and compound words into word parts; then they separate words into their syllables (*bas* + *ket*), onsets and rimes (*t* + *op*), and finally phonemes. Initial blending and segmenting activities use tokens, such as bottle caps, to move while chanting the sound parts (Ball & Blachman, 1991) or word wheels to make word-family words by changing the onset while keeping the rime constant (e.g., make *ug* into b-ug, m-ug, j-ug).

Blending and segmenting activities focused on a variety of phonological units (e.g., syllables, onset/rimes) ultimately lead children to blending and segmenting the individual phonemes in words and toward reading predictable words (Gillon, 2004; Goswami & Bryant, 1992; Torgesen et al., 2005). SLPs or teachers can complement blending and segmenting activities involving only sound structures with use of printed letters so that children can strengthen their understanding of the way sounds blend in words during real reading. For instance, children can move tiles with letters on them, with each tile representing a letter-sound of a word, to identify the sequence of sounds in words.

Letter-Sound Associations

SEEL SLPs or teachers begin explicit instruction in letter-sound associations after children can name some common letters, use printed letters or words to stand for objects or events, sort words that begin with the same first sound, and blend onsets and rimes into words (Gillon, 2004; Torgesen et al, 2005). In the SEEL program, teaching letter-sound associations follows this pattern. First, children are taught the letter-sound associations for the most common letters whose names incorporate their sounds (*B, M, T, S*), followed by other frequently occurring letters that also say their names (*R, F, K, D, N, P, L*). Then, children are taught those consonant letters that don't say their names (*C, G, H*) and vowels (*A, E, O, I, U*). Last, less frequent letters (*J, Q, V, X, Y, Z*) and diagraphs (*SH, CH, TH*) are taught. The order for introducing letter-sounds can be varied slightly. When moving through this sequence, SLPs or teachers intersperse new associations with familiar ones, constantly reviewing previously learned concepts to develop automaticity.

To facilitate early reading, connections between the letters and their sounds are formed through activities that emphasize the meaning-related aspects of reading. The following sequence is suggested:

1. SLPs or teachers highlight letter-sound associations in words that carry meaning in specific contexts. (The foregoing alliteration section presents ways to highlight sounds.)
2. Letters themselves are manipulated using action words that begin with the sound the letter makes (e.g., *P*s are poked, patted, punched, pinched, picked, and pasted)
3. Children use the first letter in a key word (a) to "read" in context, (b) to request or earn actions, turns, or objects (e.g., a chance to *wag* a *rag* like a *flag* if they can point to the word that starts with *R*), or (c) to reject or accept (e.g., the letter *N* can stand for "no, not, never," or the letter *P* can stand for "please pass").
4. Children write letters that stand for words to indicate choices or opinions. They can write *F*s if they want a "few free fun fake fish food flakes to flick to and feed to four fat, fussy, frisky, flitting flip-flopping, flapping [paper] fish."

Phonics

Though not a component of phonological awareness, phonics is heavily influenced by phonological awareness (Blachman, 1994; Brady & Fowler, 1988; Ehri et al., 2001; Wagner, Torgesen, & Rashotte, 1994). Researchers suggest that instruction in the two should be integrated (Cunningham, 1990; Gillon, 2004; Goswami, 2001). Thus, in SEEL, a phonological pattern is learned auditorily and subsequently represented with letters. The process of initial phoneme identification, rhyming, and blending of onsets and rimes moves into analyzing and reading word-family words and then into analyzing regularly spelled consonant-vowel-consonant (CVC) words into phonemes. Phonological awareness becomes a bridge to explicit analysis and manipulation of letters and their sounds to create words.

In the SEEL phonics curriculum, children in late preschool and early kindergarten play with sound patterns and notice similarities between written and spoken words (e.g., how *ip* words look and sound). They use graphemes to represent key words from classroom events and activities. Children first blend sounds without print and then add letters written on manipulatives (blocks, chips, or tokens) to create the same words in print. Using skills in rhyming, they create printed word-family words to signal meanings in context, adding onsets to rime endings to change meanings—for example, changing the initial consonant on the word *sip* to make *lip*, *dip*, *tip*, *rip* as they mix a drink from a packet that they rip, tip, snip, and dip; the finished drink they sip with their lip.

By mid-kindergarten, children select letters from alternatives to go with sounds to compose simple words (e.g., "This says *og*—pick the letter for /d/ to go here at the front to make 'dog'"). They read words in meaningful contexts by recognizing the first consonant letter and a familiar single rime ending (e.g., a text with *wag*, *bag*, *tag*, *rag*, *drag*, *flag*). In later kindergarten, they progress to reading of a variety of short-vowel CVC word-family words in decodable texts, first experienced as scripts in oral language. Decodable language experience texts are constructed based on an activity in which children have actually participated (e.g., taking a pretend trip on a ship, getting stuck in the muck) (Perfetti, 1985; Tierney & Readence, 2000).

Thus, kindergarten literacy instruction is designed to develop a strong phonological awareness base so that reading can be functional as letters are mapped onto the understanding of words (Adams, 1990; Cunningham, 1990; Gillon, 2004; Troia, 2004). Students need to realize that (1) letters correspond to sounds, (2) two letters may combine to represent one sound (/sh/, /ch/, or/ ck/) and (3) two sounds can be represented with one letter (/ks/ in "box") (Torgesen & Mathes, 1999). In late kindergarten, children participate in *invented spelling*: spelling words using their knowledge of letter-sound relationships, rather than memorizing conventional spellings (Richgels, 2001).

Implementing SEEL Instruction

To provide high-quality instruction to address the targets specified in the SEEL curriculum, SEEL organizes units around themes, applying the skills in engaging activities in multiple contexts throughout the day. Thus, SEEL instruction is both meaningful and explicit.

Unit Planning

SEEL focuses on two basic unit planning strategies to ensure that instruction is meaningful, intense, and frequent. First, instruction is embedded in activities centered on relevant and engaging content or themes related to children's prior knowledge, such as shopping, taking trips, caring for pets, making friends, or collecting bugs (Blank & White, 1992; Culturally and Linguistically Appropriate Services, 2001; Dickinson, McCabe, & Clark-Chiarelli, 2004; Neuman, Copple, & Bredekamp, 2000; Rand, 1993). Second, SEEL instruction is incorporated in multiple classroom contexts: Skills are introduced in large- and small-group contexts and then reinforced and practiced during free play, centers, classroom routines, and transitions (Gillon, 2004; McGee & Richgels, 2000), providing frequent, varied and salient exposures to literacy targets recommended for early literacy practice (Adams, 2001; Justice & Kaderavek, 2004; Kaderavek & Justice, 2004; Pellegrini, 2001; Richgels, 2001; Snow, Burns, & Griffin, 1998; Verhoeven & Snow, 2001).

Theme-Based Instruction

The SLP and the teacher can jointly develop thematic instruction by identifying the target skill or objective, selecting a theme, choosing a story or stories to fit the theme, identifying key vocabulary to illustrate the phonological pattern and fit the content, and deciding on theme-based activities to address the objectives. Alternatively, they can simply arrange instruction around a particular book, rather than threading it through a thematic unit. For example, the book *Mouse Mess* (Riley, 1997) may be extended through an alliteration activity with the children using laminated paper "mischievous mice" to "make a mighty mouse mess."

Multiple Classroom Contexts

In SEEL instruction, all of the classroom strategies and procedures can be used to provide children with varied exposure to and practice with literacy skills in functional contexts (Richgels, 2001) and are addressed regularly in three contexts: large-group, small-group, and daily routines.

Large-Group Activities

All children participate in large-group sessions during which the SLP or the teacher introduces themes, provides motivational experiences, and introduces and teaches skills. Typically, the teacher introduces books tied to the curricular theme and comments on the story, demonstrates story elements, manipulates materials, and provides children with occasional turns.

The routines and predictable actions typical with large-group sessions facilitate easy management of behavior and materials. Participation within large-group contexts allows children to practice skills with fast turns, multiple responses, and playful interaction.

Small-Group Activities

For activities that are freer and more flexible than large-group experiences, small-group contexts are ideal, taking place in centers or stations, free play times (with enticing, adult-mediated activities), or other times during which children rotate through a series of activities. Small-group activities can extend or revisit earlier phonological awareness skills or provide opportunities to practice multiple examples of target skills (Adams, 2001), particularly as needed to support children who are struggling (Foorman & Torgesen, 2001; Kaderavek & Rabidoux, 2004; Kaderavek & Justice, 2004).

Classroom Routines

The SLP or teacher can playfully highlight and reinforce literacy skills during classroom routines that typically are considered "noninstructional": snack time, transitions, welcome, circle time, putting away and getting out materials, cleaning up, and getting ready to leave. Thus, the targeted skill is transferred to less supported or more authentic contexts, where interactions and language tend to be more complex or varied than in typical "teaching" contexts. Children learn more quickly when the activities designed to support literacy skill development engage their minds, emotions, and bodies. SEEL's methodologies are designed to provide for these needs through multiple, meaningful literacy experiences.

Sample SEEL Unit

The activities unit presented in Figure 6-2 illustrates how SLPs and teachers can plan theme-based instruction to take place in multiple contexts. The unit is planned for a "bears" theme, utilizing large-group, small-group, and classroom routines. The sample unit represents one week of instruction, although instructional periods for such units can be as long as one month, depending on the theme and the SLP's or teacher's preference.

Planning Instructional Activities

Within each unit, instructional activities are planned using several general engagement strategies, along with explicit teaching methods. Relevant, meaningful, and interactive activities provide the appropriate support and practice for effective skill learning.

Engagement Strategies

Regardless of the specific activity, strategies are employed to make instruction engaging, to feature: (1) variety, (2) sensitivity to children's input, and (3) playfulness and enthusiasm (Richgels, 2001; Ukrainetz, Cooney, Kyer, Kysar, & Harris, 2000).

Varying the Presentation

Variety, ranging from attractive hands-on materials to unexpected or interesting events, engages children and holds their attention (Adams, 2001; Pellegrini, 2001; Verhoeven & Snow, 2001). Opportunities for talk about the literacy target (e.g., rhyming word, initial sound) occur in a range of presentation contexts, allowing repetition and multiple turns to participate without seeming overly redundant.

Sensitivity to Children's Input

During SEEL activities, the SLP or teacher continually responds to and values the children's contributions and incorporates their ideas.

ACTIVITIES

Monday	Tuesday	Wednesday	Thursday	Friday
		Large-Group Context		
Introduce bear theme; tell *Lost* (McPhail, 1993), a story about a bear who crawls in a snack truck and falls asleep in the truck; highlight the problem (got lost in the city), attempts (a boy takes him to a park, goes to the library to get a map, takes a bus back to the forest), consequence (gets back home on the bus), and response (bear decides to take the boy back to his home in the city).	Rhyme with bear in a "care for a bear" activity: comb the bear's hair, share the bear, put the bear in a chair, give the bear something to wear, fix a tear, etc.; blend onsets with key "air" rime words (e.g., b-ear = bear; ch-air = chair).	Engage in shared reading of a language experience text based on the "stuck in a truck" activity: "The bear got in a truck. He got stuck in the truck. Then a duck got in the truck. The duck got stuck in the truck. Then the truck got stuck. The truck got stuck in muck. The bear and the duck were in the truck and the truck got stuck in muck. Yuck! What bad luck!"	Tell *My Friend Bear* (Alborough, 2001), a story about a real bear who looks for his big stuffed bear and is frightened by a boy looking for his small stuffed bear; highlight key ideas (real versus not real; big versus small); emphasize rhyme words from the story (snug; hug; Eddie, Teddie, Freddy; jiggled, giggled, wiggled; hairy, beary; wave, cave; scare, bear).	Engage in a shared reading about pretending to go back to see the bear: "We wanted to see the bear. We went back to see the bear. We got our back packs. We got a snack. We put the snack in our pack. We followed the tracks back. We found the bear. We gave the bear a snack. Then the bear followed us back on the tracks. The bear came back with us to the city."
		Small-Group Context		
Enact *Lost* and highlight story grammar elements; use props to stand for characters, locations, and objects (map, bus, park, library).	Engage in a rhyme extension activity based on getting stuck in a truck; pretend to get a toy or cutout bear and duck stuck in a truck;	Follow a map to get the bear back to the forest or the boy back to visit the bear; use letters symbolically to stand for places (*B* = bus stop;	Enact *My Friend Bear*; put *B*s and *S*s on the children to be big and small bears, or *R*s and *S*s to be real or stuffed; highlight story grammar elements	Make a big, beautiful, birthday /b/ banner for the bear (put on balloons, *B*s, bows, bits of bread, buttons, etc.).

Figure 6–2. Sample preschool theme-based instruction: "bears" unit.

use "muck" (water and flour) to get the bear, truck, and duck stuck in yucky muck.	P = park; T = tree; S = snack store; H = home; F = forest).	and main ideas (the bear and boy are afraid of each other but then become good friends).	Take a pretend bus to visit the bear and point out letters along the way (tape targeted letters on the path from the sink to the snack table).

Transitions

Generate a rhyme with *bear* to take a turn to move from large group to small group.	Pretend to take the bear back to his home; decide how to go, and pick a *B* for bus; *P* for plane, *T* for truck, or *S* for sled or skates.	Highlight words that begin with /b/ as children get to be big burly brown bears that bump and bound as they go from small group to snack; or have the children identify a *B* to be the bear that bumps and bounds and bounces.	

Snack Time

Make a place for a bear to sit and label it with *B*; feed the bear paper bits of bread, butter, bacon, etc., and label the paper items with *B*s.	Use *S* and *B* to sort small and big pieces of paper food for the bear.	Make a menu with bear's food choices: fish, honey, berries, crackers (pretend and real choices); signal the foods with letters (*F* for fish, *P* for pretzels; *B* for berries); use letter cards to request snacks.	Pack a /b/ basket for the bear's picnic; include things to eat, do, and play with that begin with /b/ (bread, bananas, balloons, bubbles, etc.).

Get ready to take the bear back: "You will need your cap and a map. Snap the cap's strap. Put the cap and map on your lap. Take a nap. Done with your nap? When I give you a tap, wake from your nap and go with your map and cap."

Talk about what bears like to eat; taste honey and syrup (bear's favorite snack); take a poll to see if children like honey or syrup better; have children mark *H* for honey or *S* for syrup.

For example, in one SEEL session enacting Nancy Shaw's (1989) rhyming story *Sheep in a Jeep*, the teacher commented on the actions of the "sheep" (the children) as they climbed into a cardboard jeep: "The sheep get in the jeep. Sheep in jeep." A child then added, "And he beeped." The teacher expanded the script: "And he beeped in his jeep. The sheep beeped in his jeep."

Being Playful and Enthusiastic

The SLP or teacher demonstrates engagement via gestures, facial expressions, pitch, rhythm, and volume—interacting playfully with exaggerated actions. Entertaining examples facilitate active processing for the children.

Explicit Instructional Steps

Three instructional steps are needed to ensure explicit instruction for any SEEL activity (Adams, 1990; 2001; Torgesen et al, 2005). First, the behavior or skill requested of children is identified and modeled, and explicit labels expose children to metalinguistic talk about the features of the phonological system. For example, the SLP may say: "We will play with words that rhyme with *cat*. This fat cat has a hat and a mat, and you will get to pat the fat cat; *fat*, *cat*, *hat*, and *mat* rhyme." The literacy target is modeled by exposing children to many salient examples.

Second, the children playfully practice the literacy target, interacting and responding verbally or nonverbally. The SLP or teacher supports the children by providing choices, giving cues, and stating correct responses in playful, sensitive ways. For example, if the children are to think of a word that rhymes with *cat*, the SLP or teacher may use a few available objects to point to (hat, mat) or give a gesture (pat). The SLP or teacher also may begin to produce a rhyme word for the children to complete. Support is gradually reduced as children can give correct responses independently.

Third, the SLP or teacher reviews the skill and extends it to other contexts. For example, as the children prepare to leave, the SLP may hold up a hat and say, "I have a hat. Is it for a cat? Is this hat for this cat? [pretending each child is a cat]—*hat*, *cat*. *Hat* and *cat* rhyme." Thus, he or she calls attention to examples in authentic but playful contexts.

These three steps may vary slightly depending on skill and context; however, following the sequence will ensure that all activities are explicitly taught and practiced. Appendix 6–A provides an example of the three instructional steps.

SEEL Instruction along the Phonological Awareness Continuum

Meaning-based instruction is used to teach skills within each phonological awareness component—rhyming, alliteration, sound blending and segmenting, letter-sound associations—and to support children's transition from phonological awareness to phonics skills. This section illustrates how SEEL instruction operates within each skill area and across different classroom contexts. The instructional steps are embedded within the contexts and activities to make instruction explicit, with specific examples illustrating how meaning-based instruction within each component looks and feels in an early childhood setting.

Rhyming

In rhyme instruction, interactions center on targeted key words expressed in rhymed phrases. In addition to expressing content in rhyme, the SLP or teacher uses rhymed phrases for communication (questions, commands, comments, requests for actions, expressions), altering intonation, gestures, and facial expressions. Rhyme is made salient by using rhythmic intonation, stressing the rime endings, using buildups and breakdowns in which phrases are elaborated and then reduced (e.g., "I see the tree, see tree, see bee, a bee sees me"), and pulling out of rhyme on occasions to label the sound play as *rhyme*.

Large-Group Activities

Rhyme activities that are effective in the predictable context of large groups include dramatic story telling, interactive routines, and creative movement/dance.

Dramatic storytelling. Dramatic storytelling holds children's attention by its emotional appeal, props, character roles, and opportunities for audience participation, including active quick turns. Any good rhyming trade book can be told dramatically and adapted to highlight rhyme patterns. In SEEL, rhymed stories are first read interactively, with SLP or teacher questions and comments framed in simple natural language, because rhyming books tend to include complex vocabulary and sentence structures. Rhymed phrases may be repeated or highlighted. Children then participate in dramatizing the story. For example, for an activity based on Nancy Shaw's *Sheep in a Jeep* (1989), the children may sit in a "jeep" made from a box or from rows of chairs with wheels and a door represented. They act out the SLP's or teacher's rhymed commentary:

> Sheep's jeep. Sheep creep to the jeep [creep in place]. Creep sheep, creep. The sheep drive the jeep [make steering actions]. The jeep creeps . . . Oh, it's steep. The sheep creep up the steep, steep hill. Creep. Creep. Creep, jeep. Oh no, the sheep go to sleep. Sheep sleep. Sheep sleep in the jeep. Beep! Beep! Beep to wake the sheep [pretend to beep the horn]. **Sheep!** Oh no, the sheep crash the jeep. The sheep leap. Leap out of the jeep, sheep. The sheep weep. Weep, sheep, weep. Sweep the jeep. Now, the jeep is in a heap. Sweep the jeep. A heap of jeep [pile wheels and doors on top of the jeep]. Keep the jeep? The sheep keep the jeep [carry off the jeep parts].

In addition to published children's literature, the SEEL curriculum includes many simple teacher-created rhyme stories that can be dramatized.

Interactive routines. Interactive rhyme routines are fairly tightly structured activities with predictable or repetitive actions and clearly signaled roles and turns. An interactive routine used to teach rhyming with *ock* has a sock puppet demonstrate *ock* actions: The sock talks; knocks blocks, rocks, and locks; puts blocks, chalk, clocks, and rocks in socks; and walks away.

Creative movement and dance. In large-group dance and music activities, all can participate in unison, and rhyme phrases are attached to repeated movements or sounds. For example, the class can take a pretend trip on a ship and act out the movements in rhyme.

The ship takes a trip. A ship trip? Trip on a ship? Skip to the ship. Don't trip getting on the ship [take a big, careful step]. Don't trip. A ship trip. Don't trip. Don't slip. Now be the ship. The ship will zip. Go fast and zip around, ship. Zip. Now tip. The ship tips. Now flip. The ship tips, flips, and dips. And drips. Drip. Drip. Drip. The ship drips [sprinkle or shake off water].

Music with gestures can be made with caps (shampoo caps with flaps and water bottle caps) as instruments. As the children flap and snap the flaps on the caps—tap, clap, and slap the caps— they can sing a tune with lyrics made up of *ap* words, including tap, tap, tap; flap, flap, flap; snap, snap, snap; slap, tap and clap; snap and clap, and so on. When the music is over, the children can put their caps in their laps and pretend to nap.

Small-Group Activities

Small-group activities can be freer and more relaxed, including story enactments, scripted play, manipulation of sensory materials, and special projects. The teacher or SLP comments and responds to children's actions in rhyme.

Story enactments. Story enactments can extend dramatic story-telling. In a corner of the classroom, with props provided and an adult available to mediate, the children assume character roles and act out the parts. The adult comments on their actions with embellished and exaggerated rhyme. The story *Sheep Take a Hike* (Shaw, 1996) can be easily elaborated in an enactment, because the story itself focuses on many rhymed endings embedded in complicated sentences. The enactment can focus on *ack* rhyme pairs as the children pack a black backpack for the hike. They pack sacks, pack snacks, and find train or bear tracks. They smack and snack snacks from their backpack as they go and make their own tracks on the (paper) bear or train tracks. The snack pack can have a crack and the snacks fall out, so the pack can lack snacks. Children find things on the tracks: paper tacks, animals that go quack, things to stack, things that crack (Styrofoam food pack trays), toy jacks, things that are black, sacks, snacks that crack. After getting to a paper shack, they decide to go back. They follow tracks back and unpack the backpack, commenting on the *ack* objects as they do.

Scripted or thematic play. Scripted or theme-based rhyme play consists of related actions on objects that fit a particular topic, described with rhyming words. For example, bugs might tug and lug things that rhyme: jugs, mugs, rugs, slugs (small balloons filled with flour). The adult comments in rhyme:

> Bug tug, tug a jug. Oh, tug a mug. Ug, tug, bug! Want to tug the bug or the slug? The bug tugs the rug. Tug, bug! Tug the rug. When the bugs get tired, they snug on a rug. ("Is the bug snug? Want to be a snug bug?")

Or children may try to get pets (paper fish) and/or jets caught in nets. Once the pet is in the net, the children can get the pet wet by sprinkling it with water.

> Get set? Let's get the pet wet. Let the pet in the net. Let the pet get wet. Wet the pet. Get a pet wet in a net. Get this pet wet in a net. Ready set. Let [child's name] get the pet wet.

Manipulation of sensory materials.   SLPs or teachers can interact in rhyme as the children act on sensory materials. Children enjoy manipulating a gooey substance made out of borax, water, and glue. As they play with the *goo* or *gook*, the adult comments: "Ooey, gooey, goo, put ooey goo on you? Ew! Goo on you? Goo on a shoe? Gooey ooey goo on something blue—a blue shoe? Ooey, gooey blue goo on two blue shoes." Children also enjoy playing with sticky dough, called *muck* for the activity. Ducks and trucks get stuck in the muck, and the muck gets stuck on the children's hands. As the children mess in the muck, the adult says, "Yuck, stuck, muck is stuck. The duck is stuck. The truck is stuck. Oh yuck!"

Special projects. Rhymed words and phrases can be used to interact during art, construction, and cooking projects. These interactions can bring out many reasons to communicate: questions, commands, instructions, requests, comments, answers, expressions. For art, children can trace faces, cases, lace, or vases; leave spaces (on the paper); place lace on vases and cases; or place lace or vases on places or in spaces. With modeling clay or "play dough," children can make objects that rhyme with *ake*: "Make a snake, lake, flakes, or cake with play dough; make the fake snake sleep—

shake the snake so he'll wake; break the snake, cake or lake, and rake up the mess.

To cook, the children may make a real or fake cake in rhyme. The SLP or teacher highlights *ake* words as the children take ingredients and shake portions in a bowl. ("Shake. Take and shake. Shake in the cake.") They stir the ingredients ("Make. Make cake. Make the cake"), break or pretend to break eggs ("break"), put the cake in a pretend or microwave oven ("bake, bake the cake"), remove the cake ("take cake"), decorate the cake ("make flake, shake flake, make fake snake for the cake. Put snake or flake on the cake"), serve the cake ("break the cake, break cake, take cake"), and clean up crumbs with a fake rake ("rake the cake").

Games. A space case race can be played in rhyme. The game is set up in a place for a space race, marked with places and space bases and places or spaces for the space cases and space bases to go. Children place their cases on a space to start and make the cases race through space. The children can place faces on the space cases and the space base. The cases "race through space" (an obstacle course on the ground marked with places and spaces) to get to the space base.

Classroom Routines

Interactions within classroom routines (snack time, transitions, free play, departure, clean-up, welcome) can reinforce rhyming skills by transferring them to more authentic and less supported contexts. In authentic classroom routines, the adult periodically pulls out of the game and labels the word play as *rhyming*. Rhyming can be embedded into all classroom routines, but only snack time and transitions are described here.

Snack time. During snack time, events can be expressed in rhyme, and rhymed word games can be played. The adult and the children sitting at a table can think of rhyming words for objects (e.g., "Let's make up a rhyme name for this fork. How about 'bork'?") Real, pretend, or paper food items can be used. Little circles of green paper can be peas and squares of yellow paper can be cheese (e.g., "pegs please, cheese please, pegs and cheeze please, peas on cheese? cheese on peas? cheese on knees? peas on knees? No!").

Cut-out characters may participate in the snack activity—for example, a "friend named Fred who comes to eat bread and puts red spread [jelly] on his bread," or a "queen named Jean who is keen on green beans and gets mean when her green beans aren't clean." Interesting things may happen that can be talked about in rhyme. Paper bugs can be slipped in jugs and mugs, which evoke comments and exclamations such as "Ug, a bug. A bug in my mug. Bug in the jug? Ug!"

Transitions. Transitions may include a number of rhyme interactions as children wait their turn. The rhyme response serves as the child's "ticket" for moving to a new place (e.g., "What rhymes with new?" "How about blue?" "You can go through.") Or, children can earn their chance to move on by performing a movement in rhyme context: a goat with a note that floats on a boat, or a big pig with a wig doing a jig. The SLP or teacher can also pass out pictures or word cards with the challenge to find a classmate who has a matching rhyme.

Alliteration

Children learn alliteration as they are exposed to word lists or phrases that include words with shared first sounds. These learning opportunities are embedded across the day using a variety of classroom formats and routines.

Large-Group Activities

The controlled and predictable context of large-group instruction is appropriate for playful extensions to story themes, and creative movement.

Story extensions. Although few children's books are written in alliteration, some—*No Mail for Mitchell* (Siracusa, 1990), for example—incorporate a few alliterative phrases. An activity based on this book might highlight additional /m/ phrases: "Mr. Mitchell mails many magazines. Mr. Mitchell's mail has *M* marked on the mail. Mail and magazines with *M*'s go to Mr. Mitchell's messy mailbox. This mailbox has Mr. Mitchell's many, marvelous, magnificent magazines and much, much mail." Books without alliteration phrases can be extended with alliteration activities. *Lilly's Purple Plastic Purse* (Henkes, 1996) can generate a *P* activity when children place things that start with /p/ sound in Pam's pretty purple (or pink) plastic purse (a plastic file folder cut into the shape of a purse). A theme from a story can be easily extended or adapted to play with alliteration in a follow-up activity. For an activity based on the book *Dear Bear* (Harrison, 1994), the children may bring things that begin with /b/ to place on the bear's picnic blanket. Any story can be extended by choosing alliterating key words or phrases and putting them in a theme or play context.

Alphabet books based on categories such as animals or foods generally illustrate letter sounds with a few words that begin with that sound; the words and illustrations can be extended to teach alliteration. For example, *I Stink* (McMullan & McMullan, 2002) is about a garbage truck taking things to the dump that begin with the letters in the alphabet. After reading the book, the class could make a pile of trash items that begin with /t/ to put in the trash or the truck (e.g., tracks, tacks, tape, etc.).

Creative movement. In dance or movement, children can depict alliteration phrases with their bodies. They can be "big bumbling, bumpy buses that bounce and break as they bump and bumble along" or "tyrannosauruses that tramp and trek on tracks and tromp on tall trees." SEEL has a core of alliteration phrases with characters (people, animals, vehicles) performing movements or actions that can be expressed with words that alliterate (e.g., "Bear bends backwards before beginning to burrow").

Small-Group Activities

Alliteration activities for the less formal, more personal setting of small groups include hands-on manipulation of materials, art projects, and sorting games and routines.

Hands-on materials. Children can act on interesting objects with motions that begin with the object's first sound. The SLP or teacher can construct alliteration strings to correspond with what the children are doing. Children can create a mixture of maple marshmallow muffins, or they can mix, mash, mush and make much mush. The SLP or teacher comments as the children mix the mess: "Mix the mush, make messy muffins? Mash the mucky mush. Make and mix much, much mushy mash." Action words can be applied to things that start with the same sound. Thus, paper plates, potatoes, pots, pencils, paper, or "play dough" can be pounded, pushed poked, punched, and passed. Foam, fur, furry fabric, felt, flour, flakes, foil, fluff, or fuzzy fleece can be felt and folded. Spools and spouts (cut from tops of water bottles) can spill, spin, splat, or splatter; children can sprinkle spools and spouts on spaces and spots.

Art projects. Art projects adapt well for practicing alliteration. Children can make monster masks by marking *M*s and putting things that start with /m/ on the mask (e.g., macaroni, mud, mustard). They can paint pink paper with pretty pink and purple paint, or paint and paste paper plates with pictures of people and peas and pretzels.

Sorting games and routines. Children can sort objects that start with a particular sound by placing them in containers or locations that start with the same sound. They can fill a sock, sack or suitcase with things that begin with /s/; put things that begin with /b/ in a basket, bottle, box, or bucket; or place things that start with /p/ in a pouch, pocket, or pot. Sorting also can consist of placing things that start with a target sound in a context that begins with the sound: going to the store to buy /s/ items, preparing for a trip to /t/ places, getting dressed with /d/ clothing, or taking /p/ things to a party.

Class Routines

Snack time. Taste tests and opinion polls can create opportunities to play with alliteration during snack time. Taste test choices can be expressed in alliteration phrases: "Please pick plenty of pleasing prickly pretzels." The choices can be real or pretend: "Better buy Barbara's best banana bread" or "Buy big beautiful baked breakfast buns from better bakers." "Silly" phrases can be concocted about real or pretend food items during snack time: "Let's feed Fred's fish fine frosted fish-food flakes." Children can put real and pretend /p/ items on the "pink paper plate": potatoes, peas, pasta, pudding, popcorn, pizza, pop, popsicles, pretzels, and pickles.

Transitions. During transitions, children perform as animals, humans, or even objects in alliteration phrases as they move from place to place: a "pretty pony that prances past posts, pets, and people"or a "zany, zingy zebra that zigs, zags, and zips." Everyone can become one character each day, or each child can choose from a variety of given characters.

While waiting in line, the SLP or teacher and children can pretend to act on objects with alliteration phrases (blow and bump, break or burst, bright blue, beautiful, brilliant bubbles). When the class is preparing to go home, the SLP or teacher can pretend to put things in children's pockets that begin with /p/, cover their coats with things that begin with /k/, or pack a backpack with things that start with /b/.

Sound Blending and Segmenting

Instruction in sound blending and segmenting should occur frequently in brief time periods across a range of classroom contexts. Blending and segmenting activities are similar regardless of the size of the phonological unit (e.g., sentence, compound word, syllable, onset/rime, phoneme). Strategies use familiar words and include representing word parts with tokens, providing a reason to say words in funny ways, chanting or calling out responses while emphasizing parts, and providing contextual supports.

Large-Group Activities

Short blending and segmenting tasks can be attached to large-group activities or conducted to follow up on some other instruction. The content words from other activities or lessons can be used as the stimuli for segmenting and blending.

Routines and games. Pictures of objects can be presented as puzzle pieces that are taken apart in a left-to-right sequence (e.g., "Here is a house. I can take it apart. Here's one part, /h/, and here is a second part, *ouse*") and then blended.

Talking like a robot is another simple routine for teaching blending and segmenting. Robots talk by pausing between the syllables, onset-rime, or phonemes; they may say words slowly or stretch vowels, emphasizing each sound so they can hear the sounds separately. Such talk lends itself to guessing games ("What am I talking about? I see a *s-ock*."). For a large group, the SLP or teacher may bring in a bag of objects for the children to label or talk about, possibly incorporating a theme ("I am a storeowner, and you pay paper pennies for each sound I say. Here is some soup. How many pennies? Drop a penny in the 'cash register' for each sound: /s/ /u/ /p/").

"Push and say" activity. "Push and say" is a blending and segmenting activity where children represent word parts by manipulating tokens (blocks, bottle caps, plastic chips) for each sound part targeted (Blachman, 1991, 2000). The children move the tokens together as they say the sounds, with modeling at first. For example, in blending *sip*, they produce the /s/ while sliding the token designated /s/ toward a token representing the *ip* rime. When the tokens come together, so does the word. Smaller sound units can be represented by smaller tokens or blocks.

Movement, dance, and music. The children can illustrate sentence or word parts by breaking up words with choppy body movements. Children can clap, march, count, or tap out parts of a word, blending sounds to the rhythm of movement or music. They can tap an object (bottle cap, pencil) once for each rhythmic unit spoken in a sentence or word. The children should first model the adult's tapping or clapping and gradually do some on their own.

Small-Group Activities

Word games. A number of small-group word games focus on blending and segmenting—for example, guessing objects from a box or bag from segmented word clues. The SLP or teacher segments the word and has the children blend the segments back together to guess the object. Alternatively, the SLP or teacher may reverse the process: give semantic clues, show an object, and ask the children to segment its name.

For another game, the SLP or teacher shows pictures of items cut into parts, segments the word (into syllables, onset-rime, or phonemes), and asks the children to re-blend the segments. For example, after showing a picture of a table cut into two parts for syllables or four parts for phonemes, the SLP or teacher says the group will break *table* into parts. He or she provides many models of the process of segmenting a word while taking the puzzle apart, and then supplies the first part of game words and has the children finish the process.

If children are given cards with onsets and rimes or letters for phonemes, they can create simple CVC words. For blending, children may pull word parts out of apron pockets: a two-pocket apron for onsets and rhymes or a three-pocket apron for CVC phonemes. The SLP or teacher reads the word parts. All words can be real, or some words can be real and others imaginary. The SLP or teacher comments on the meaning of the real words and laughs at the "silly" words or says, "I don't know what that is!" If some words are imaginary, children can place the cards that make these silly words into a box labeled "silly" and the cards that make real words into a box labeled "real." Children repeat the words and make a tally by placing a tick mark by column "silly" or column "real." If the activity entails working at the onset-rime level, the rime can be kept the same, with the students choosing just the onset consonant(s).

Story and script extension activities. Children can be exposed to segmenting and blending to follow up scripted alliteration or rhyme activities. At the end of an alliteration activity, the SLP or teacher talks about the words the group has played with, doing so in a "silly," segmented way. He or she breaks apart the initial consonant from the rest of the word, holds up the items discussed in instruction, produces the initial consonant in isolation, and then produces the word ending and blends the word parts together: "We went on a p-p-p-p-p-p-icnic and took p-eas, p-eaches, p-udding, p-otatoes, p-ickles, and p-retzels." Then the children have an opportunity to segment one of the target words (e.g., plums, peanuts). Rhyme activities can be used to focus on onset plus rime blending. At the end of a rhyme activity in which children have played with the words *head*, *bed*, *Fred*, *bread*, *red*, *sled*, and *shed*, the SLP or teacher may ask, "What word am I saying? *b* + *ed*." One child can say the initial consonant of a word, and another child can say the rime ending and then put the parts together and say the whole word.

Breaking rhymed words apart at the end of a rhyme play can be used to raise awareness of the initial consonant. For example, after having a dog, hog, and frog jog to a log in the fog, the SLP or teacher can build in choices: "Here is our log. Now let's see who gets to jog to the log." He or she says one of the animals' names segmented (*fr-og, d-og,* or *h-og*); after the children re-blend the word, the animal gets to jog to the log. The children themselves can pretend to be the animals and jog in place.

Class Routines

As natural interactions during classroom routines, SLPs or teachers can communicate in segmented words or engage in blending and segmenting as word play.

Snack time. During snack time, children can be asked to blend words to figure out what the SLP or teacher is saying. The segmented word can be presented with a bit of intrigue: "Guess what we will have for our snack. I'm going to say a word, and you figure out what I am saying. We will have *cra-ckers*." Segmented words can be presented as a guessing game, with the SLP or teacher giving semantic and phonological clues: "I'm thinking of something you wear. It is a *sh-oe*." To segment at the sentence level, sentences dealing with the snack can be broken apart and put together: "We-will-have-cheese-for-snack." Children clap or tap out syllables in multisyllable words or onset plus rime or phonemes, using whatever is available (bottle caps or cups or spoons). SLPs or teachers can segment and blend any individual word and/or sentence that comes up during conversation.

Transition. During transitions, SLPs or teachers can have children clap, march, or count out parts of sentences or words as they are waiting in line. Children can blend or segment a word (with imitative support) or say a word in its segmented parts as a "password" to move to the next station or activity. Blending or segmenting a word may be their "ticket" to make the transfer. Familiar words (e.g. words that have been used frequently that day, their own names, or common clothing items) can be used for children who need more support. As children are waiting, the SLP or teacher can talk in a "funny way": breaking words apart like a robot or stretching sounds out like a snail. The adult can give information or directions in words segmented into syllables or onset-rime: "These people can go to a center—Jo-dy and Ben-ja-min."

Letter-Sound Associations

In SEEL, children make or identify the sounds corresponding to letters to earn a turn to manipulate the letter in interesting ways. When they communicate by letting the sound of the initial letter stand for a word, letter-sound associations become meaningful. It is important to highlight the sound by exaggerating, repeating, extending, or segmenting it. This process of using letter-sounds to represent meaning can be embedded within large-group, small-group, and classroom routine contexts.

Large-Group Activities

In large-group settings, the SLP or teacher arranges predictable and repetitive situations in which a letter and its sound can be used to communicate. When children must produce a letter's sound to experience a desirable object or action that is symbolized by the letter, letters and sounds take on a functional relationship.

Interactive routines and games. There are a number of large-group interactive routines for teaching letter-sound associations. For example, children produce the /f/ sound when shown the letter *F* in order to fill a fish (fish-shaped envelope) full of *F*s, fins, and fish food flakes (with *F*s written on them) to make the fish fat. The SLP or teacher may say, "See the *F*? It says /f/ like the /f/ in 'fish food flakes.' Make the /f/ sound to get *flakes* (or food, or fins, or F's) to fit in the fish." Children also may write the letter for a given sound to receive an object, turn, or experience. In setting up an "*S* store," for example, children write the letter for the /s/ sound to place soup, sauce, and other /s/ objects (and/or pictures of objects) that begin with /s/ in the store. The SLP or teacher also can engage in amusing actions to reward the children for writing the appropriate letters.

Want to see me slide? Make an *S* for /s/ and I'll slide and slip for you. Want me to tiptoe? Make *T* for the /t/ sound in tiptoe. Oh, your *T* says /t/. What sound does your *T* make?

Children can put letters on objects that begin with the letter's sound. They label with *S* all of the things that begin with /s/, for example, and produce the sound /s/ to get letters to use as labels. The SLP or teacher can say, "We need to mark *S* for /s/ on the things that start with /s/." The SLP or teacher repeats and exaggerates the sound as the children write the letter.

Sorting activities can be based on letter-sound associations: Letters are taped to containers; children identify these letters and their sounds, then place letters or objects in each container when the SLP or teacher says its sound. They also paste letters on objects (e.g., *B*s on ball, bottle, bucket; *P*s on pencil, plate, paper; *sh* on shirt or shoe, and so on) after they say the sound the letter makes or as the SLP or teacher comments on the letter and sound: "A *B* says /b/, /b/, /b/; 'ball' begins with *B*, so we can put these /b/ things on the ball or in the bag."

Children can play letter beanbag by throwing a beanbag to the letter that goes with the sound the SLP or teacher produces. In a similar activity, they play a letter-sound lotto or bingo game, marking the letters on cards when the SLP or teacher produces the letter's sound.

Shared interactive reading. In story contexts, children use letter-sound information to represent words. They read the sound a letter makes to identify a recurring key word in repetitive and predictable stories. For example, for an activity based on *Sam's Cookie* (Lindgren & Eriksson, 1982), the children read the word *Sam* each time it occurs by attaching the /s/ to the initial letter in *Sam*. Teacher-created stories or predictable routines also can incorporate reasons to read a recurring key word. The children "read" letter-sound associations as part of shared reading experiences or simple playful story scripts. Children also can differentiate among written words as they "read" using the initial letter. Rhyme stories can be told and then written or dramatized, with the children choosing key words from among several options

Rhyme stories can be converted into letter sound activities in which children use the initial consonant to contrast meanings (Adams, 1990). For example, the SLP or teacher can quickly tell or dramatize the "make a cake" story in which the storyteller wakes, decides to make a cake, takes a cake mix or recipe, takes and shakes ingredients, and bakes the cake. He or she gives the children some choices by displaying the words *wake, bake, make, take, shake,* and *rake* or letters *W, B, M, T, SH,* and *R* and asking, "What part should I pretend to do: make, wake, bake, take, shake, or rake? If you want me to wake, find the *W* for /w/ in w-w-w-wake." Alternatively, the children can tell the story by reading initial letters to indicate words.

Small-Group Activities

Scripted role-play experiences. Within scripted role play, the SLP or teacher sets up letter-sound associations to represent words that are used to communicate. As children participate in goal-directed activities, they have reasons to convey ideas and make requests in print. While the children act on letters as props, the SLP or teacher explains that the sound of the letter is the reason the letter is representing a particular word. In post office play, the children act on *M*s as signs, nametags, or labels for things that start with the /m/ sound (mail, mailboxes, magazines, money, mail carrier, and a person's name such as Mike or Mary). They also can place *P*s on the post office, the place to put packages, a character named Peter, and the corner of envelopes to represent postage. A theme can be selected to target a specific letter-sound association (i.e., items to slip into an s-s-uitcase). Thus, almost any role play situation can be adapted to fit targeted letter-sounds.

Art and cooking projects. Children can practice letter-sound association as they make projects. They can decorate art objects with a letter while they make the letter sound (e.g., *S*s on signs, *M*s on masks, *P*s on pretty plates and placemats, *F*s on flags, *H*s on hats, etc.), as well as pictures of objects that start with the letter sound. They can apply the same process to make props needed for other activities (e.g., put *M*s for /m/ in money on pieces of paper, *M*s for /m/ in mug on paper cups, *T*s for /t/ on paper for tickets). The SLP or teacher talks about the relationship between the letter and its sound as the children make the item: "We'll know this is money because money starts with /m/ and *M* makes /m/. We write *M* for /m/ in *money*."

In art or cooking projects, children can request materials or actions by using letters that go with certain sounds. For example, the SLP or teacher and children can ask each other to make different things with "play dough":

> Want me to make a lake, cake, rake, or snake? Find the *C* that makes the /k/ /k/ /k/ sound if you want me to make a cake. I found an *R* for the /r/ to ask you to make a r-r-rake.

Cooking projects also may use letter-sound associations to convey directions. Children make play or real soup, batters, or salads by "reading" recipes that give the ingredients or amounts in letters. Big and small spoonfuls and cupfuls are signaled by *B* for b-b-b-ig and *S* for s-s-s-mall: "This *B* says /b/ for big, so you pick a big cup to use."

Taste tests, surveys, and menus. Taste tests and surveys provide opportunities to make requests and signal choices by selecting a letter to stand for a sound. In a taste test, children may get small pieces of a food item by marking the letter that makes that item's first sound: an *F* for /f/ to get free fun fish food (fish crackers); a *T* for /t/ to "try tasty toast (or taco or tortilla) treat"; an *S* for /s/ in "sample several salty snacks." Letter-sound association also can represent preferences and opinions: what children like to eat (e.g., *P* for /p/ in pizza or *M* for /m/ in meat) or what type of pet they would like to have (*F* for /f/ in fish, *D* for /d/ in dog, *C* for /k/ in cat, *H* for /h/ in horse).

Hands-on manipulation of letters. Children can manipulate a letter in humorous or interesting ways while saying its sound or listening as the SLP or teacher says its sound. They can fold *F*s, stretch (fabric) *S*s, tape *T*s to a trunk, or poke *P*s or punch them. They must make the letter-sound associations in order to get a turn. Children generally enjoy performing a movement that begins with a letter as the SLP or teacher holds the letter up and says the sound: When the SLP or teacher holds up a *D* and makes the /d/ sound, for example, children dance as long as the sound continues; when the letter and sound change to *H*, the children hop.

Class Routines

Snack time. During snack time, children can act on (move, stack, hold) letters when the SLP or teacher says a letter's sound, or mark a letter in order to get a treat, a turn, or an object. Children may mark the letter that makes the /s/ sound to get a snack, /n/ to get nuts, /d/ to get a drink. This also can be done as the reverse process: "Put the treat by the letter that *treat* begins with"; "Put the pitcher by the letter that *pitcher* begins with."

To review letters during snack time, the SLP or teacher can incorporate reasons to "read" letters previously taught. For example, the SLP or teacher holding up the letter *P* may ask:

> Do you think we are going to have popcorn or crackers for snack? Here is a clue. Look at the *P*. What sound does it make? The sound for this *P* will give you a clue about what we are having for snack.

The items can be imaginary, paper, or real, but children will need to be warned that the snack may be different, and the presentation must be done in a playful manner.

Snack time is a good opportunity to hide letters and let the children search for the letter that goes with the sound the SLP or teacher makes. Alternatively, the SLP or teacher can pass out letters as little "gifts" at snack time. The children have to say the sound before they get the letter.

Transition. During transition times, children can pick letter cards or get letter stickers, which tell them what to do, where to go, or how to move. Children who select a *B* and say the letter's name get to pretend to be a big burly brown bear. The SLP or teacher can put letters on children and have a short exchange about the letter's sound. The letter can serve as a direction: "If your letter says /t/, you can turn around and tip-toe. If your letter says /m/, you can march."

Phonics

Phonics instruction is addressed in this chapter because of the reciprocal relationship between phonological awareness and reading. Learning to read heightens children's awareness that words are composed of phonemes, and an awareness of phonemes in words supports learning to read (Blachman, 1994; Byrne & Fielding-Barnsley, 1995; Cunningham, 1990; Ehri et al., 2001). In SEEL, phonics instruction extends logically from phonological awareness. Phonological awareness activities focus on rhyme, alliteration, and blending of initial and final sound patterns, and these skills are mapped onto print during letter-sound association activities. When letters are associated with alliteration and rime endings, they can lead to reading short-vowel, regularly spelled CVC words (e.g., *get, wet, pet, net, set, let, jet, bet*), which constitute the foundation for reading early decodable texts (Adams, 2001; Culatta, Culatta, Frost, & Buzzell, 2004; Goswami & Bryant, 1992; Hiebert & Martin, 2001).

Large-Group Activities

The large-group context provides opportunities to introduce phonic patterns, strengthen letter-sound associations and word recognition, and teach the decoding process.

Interactive routines. Predictable interactive routines can be created around a theme using key content words so that children have reasons to read and recognize target phonic patterns. The SLP or teacher arranges for an experience that exemplifies the patterns, then supports children in making letter-sound associations and reading key words before, during, and after the activity. For example, making paper pizzas can be used to practice *ip* words: "We're going to make a pizza with words that end in *ip*. Let's read the words we'll use—*flip, dip, tip, lip,* and *rip.*" As the children make the pizza, they read "flip" or "we flip the pizza" to flip the dough; "snip" or "we snip off the tip" to open a sauce packet (folded wax paper with red paint); "tip and drip" or "we tip and drip the sauce" to put the sauce on the dough; and "rip" or "we rip strips" to rip yellow and green paper into pretend cheese and pepper strips. The children then put the strips of cheese and pepper on the pizza and place it to their lips. After the activity, the children read words to choose which parts of the activity they want to act out in gestures (e.g., dip, tip, clip, snip, drip, flip) and engage in a simple word analysis activity where onsets are combined with the *ip* rime ending to make different words.

Shared reading. After children experience an interactive routine such as the pizza-making activity, they read, with support, controlled texts based on the experience during whole-group shared reading (R. Culatta et al., 2004). In SEEL, a written version of the pizza-making activity is displayed on chart paper or via an overhead or computer projector and read with the children. The pizza-making text may read as follows:

> We made pizza out of paper. We got to flip the pizza dough. We got to clip open the sauce package. We got to tip the sauce and let it drip on the pizza. We got to rip strips of cheese. We got to rip strips of pepper. We put the strips of cheese and pepper on the pizza. Yum! We put the pizza to our lips. But we did not eat the pizza. It was not a real pizza. It was made out of paper!

With short routines, the shared reading of a text can occur immediately after the event. For example, the SLP or teacher may present a quick-paced "draw-talk" story about a bed that turns into a sled, drawing skis or runners on the bed at the appropriate time. The SLP or teacher first tells and draws the story and then displays the written text:

> Ms. Brown made a bed into a sled. First, she made a bed. Then she made the bed red. Then she made the bed into a sled. Then she put Ed in the bed. Ed drove the bed sled. Then he sped away in the bed sled.

In shared reading, the SLP or teacher reads the text along with the children and implements strategies to support decoding (Fountas & Pinnell, 1996; Richgels, 2001). The instructor can point to the target letter or letters and wait for children to respond, begin to form the letter's sound, comment on the feature ("here is an *S* that makes /s/"), segment and blend word parts into words, and adjust the pace of the reading to fit the children's abilities. The SLP or teacher also comments on the meaning and engages children in re-reading the text.

Interactive writing. In interactive writing activities, the SLP or teacher and children write together and then read their co-constructed stories (McCarrier, Pinnell, & Fountas, 2000). The SLP or teacher guides the children in creating decodable texts about experiences that highlight target patterns. The dictated versions are supported by the SLP's or teacher's narrations during the experience, which incorporate many examples of a target pattern as well as predictable elements that keep the text meaningful. In scaffolding the children's dictation of a story about making rag bags with tags that are used to clean as they wag and drag the rags, the SLP or teacher can review the experience:

> Remember you each got a bag. And you got to rip rags and put the rags in the bag. You made a tag for the rag bag. Then you got to clean with a rag. You got to wag and drag the rag to clean the room.

He or she then guides children's dictation with questions ("What did you get to do?" "What did you do to make a rag bag?"); suggestions ("Could you say you put a rag in the bag?"); alternative wordings ("Want to say you made a tag or a flag for the bag?"); and cloze or sentence completion frames ("Then you took the bag and put on a . . . "). The children's dictated oral telling of the experience becomes a sequentially organized written version containing the key words (Tierney & Readence, 2000).

Songs, chants, fingerplays. Songs, chants, fingerplays, and movement routines can be used to teach target phonic patterns, orally with gestures and actions and in writing for the children to read. The children read the verses from cue cards on chart paper, and they produce or illustrate the chant or song with actions and gestures line by line. After each element is read and acted, the entire song or chant can be read as a poem. For example, the children can work up a fingerplay or action-gesture song with *ap* music or rhythmic chant. Using shampoo caps as instruments, they can tap, clap, snap, flap, clap on their laps, and clap-and-tap, with order and rhythm signaled by how close or far apart the words are written on the page.

Small-Group Activities

The small-group context, being more intense and individualized than large-group situations, permits SLPs or teachers to differentiate instruction and provide supplemental opportunities for children with language delays, differences, or deficits to acquire literacy skills (Foorman & Torgesen, 2001; Justice & Kaderavek, 2004; Kaderavek & Justice, 2004).

Routines and scripts. Routines and scripts are effective for teaching phonic skills in small-group as well as large-group contexts. SLPs or teachers pre-teach targeted words, arrange for children to read words to make choices or give commands during the activity, and afterwards review the words the children have encountered. Before or after the activity, children can represent target word-family words with word wheels or flip books in which the initial onset changes while the rime ending stays the same to automatize letter-sound associations and support decoding and word recognition. As with the large-group context, small-group routines and scripts also are turned into controlled texts with the opportunity for shared reading instruction (Fountas & Pinnell, 1996).

Although the SEEL program has hundreds of routine or script-based decodable texts, only a few examples are presented here to illustrate the process. In activities that focus on *ap* words, children can wrap things like water bottle caps; caps to wear with flaps, straps and snaps; maps, snaps, and shampoo bottle caps that flap and snap or plain water bottle caps:

> What can you wrap that ends in *ap*? You can wrap a cap. You can wrap a cap that has a flap and a strap. You can wrap a snap. You can wrap a cap. You can wrap a bottle cap that makes a snap and has a flap.

The SLP or teacher also can show off a cap with flaps and straps and things tucked inside, like the one made in a rhyme activity, and then read:

> There was [or I had] a cap in my [or my teacher's] lap. There was a map in the cap. There was a strap on the cap. There was a flap on the cap. There was a snap on the cap. There was a [bottle] cap in the cap that went snap and had a flap. We took the things out of the cap. Then we put back the flap, the [bottle] cap, the map, the snap, and the strap. Then we were tired so we put the cap on our laps and took a nap.

The children also could read about making a cap out of scraps of paper or cloth, in an activity similar to the one they experienced when they were learning to rhyme:

We made a cap with scraps of paper [or cloth]. We cut a scrap to make a flap to flap over lap. We put on a flap with a "snap" [sound]. We put on another flap with a "snap." We put on a strap. We put on another strap. We put on a snap. Then we put the cap on our lap and took a nap.

Art and movement activities. In a dip art activity, the children rip strips (of paper or cloth), clip the tip of a strip, clip the strip (with paper or binder clip), grip the clip or strip, dip the strip (in paint), let the strip drip, and zip the strip across the paper. The SLP or teacher supports the children in reading words and phrases as they create the artwork and then, with shared reading support, create a decodable text about the experience. For example, after creating some dip art, the students could engage in a shared reading of the following text that describes their art activity:

How to Make a Dip Drip Painting

First you get a strip.

Then you grip the strip and rip, rip, rip.

Then you put a clip on the strip.

Then you grip the clip.

And you dip the strip.

And you let the strip drip, drip, drip.

1, 2, 3 and zip the strip!

Now you have a dip drip painting.

Construction of language experience stories. Children's own telling of any of the structured phonics experiences can be turned into a language experience decodable text. Like the large-group experiences, small-group activities can be presented with models or story frames on which children can co-construct a language experience story. Although children create some interesting variations, controlled or decodable texts usually emerge.

An easy activity can be developed as children watch the SLP or teacher blow up a balloon with a picture of a cat (or bat or rat) drawn on it. With each breath the SLP or teacher uses to blow up the balloon, the children say: "Make the cat fat!" When the cat is fat, the children pat the cat, put hats on the cat, and make the cat a mat to sit on. The language experience text (written on chart paper) would look something like this:

> We got to see [Mr. Smith] make a cat fat. The cat got fat and we got to pat the cat. Then we made hats for the cat. The fat cat tried on all the hats. Then we made a mat and the cat sat on the mat.

Classroom Routines

Snack time. Conversations and activities during snack time can help children recognize meaning in print and thus support the teaching of reading. Notes and messages can be distributed and read that fit the snack context and use as many target words as possible. Invitations, menus, social notes, and announcements fit particularly well. The SLP or teacher also may model aspects of the writing process: "think-alouds," writing ideas, or observations. Children sometimes enjoy reading and writing words on things other than paper: napkins, paper plates, Styrofoam packing materials, snack wrappers, paper cups. Target words written on sticky notes, small pieces of paper, or labels can be put on or under cups and plates. Sight words such as *is*, *there*, or *a* can be reinforced by writing predictable messages: "There is a bug under your cup." "There is a cat on your chair." Reading instruction also can be incorporated into the snack activity by playing simple phonic games. Word-family words can be written on cards that the children or an adult can pull out of a box on the table and read.

Transitions. Transition time can be used to practice reading target word patterns. Words or phrases written on pieces of paper can be the "ticket" to leave. The SLP or teacher can remind the children about an experience that highlighted a target word pattern and let the children read a few of these word-family words before leaving to go to the next activity: "Remember when you made a ragbag and put a tag on the rag bag and we got to wag the rags as we cleaned the room? Well, now we get to read those words." The words can be presented as a list with the rime endings lined up in a column or on a flipbook or word wheel. Each child can quickly read, with support, three or four targeted words.

Summary

To improve the reading and academic outcomes of children with communication difficulties, young children must be provided with intense and systematic literacy instruction that also provides them with hands-on and interactive experiences (Bowman, Donovan, & Burns, 2001; Neuman et al., 2000; Snow et al., 1998). Furthermore, all children appear to benefit from access to interesting, interactive and playful activities to increase motivation and provide frequent opportunities to learn and practice literacy skills (Lyon, 1999; Verhoeven, 2001; Yopp, 1992).

The SEEL program embodies these principles to provide explicit and interactive literacy instruction for young children. SEEL focuses on teaching children the critical phonological awareness and early phonics skills that will lead them to later reading success. SEEL uses multiple instructional contexts and activities that provide frequent and varied exposure to literacy skills. These varied instructional experiences promote engagement during repeated practice of specific literacy targets. The SLP and the teacher can serve as collaborators in implementing this curricular program, with the teacher conducting some activities and the SLP (or other support personnel) supporting and amplifying beyond what the teacher can do. With this type of developmental curriculum, appropriate instructional strategies, and opportunities for differentiated instruction, SLPs and teachers will be able to provide all children with the instruction they need to be successful in school and beyond.

References

Adams, M. (2001). Alphabetic anxiety and explicit, systematic phonics instruction: A cognitive science perspective. In S. B. Neuman & D. K. Dickinson (Eds.), *Handbook of early literacy research* (pp. 66–80). New York: Guilford Press.

Adams, M. J. (1990). *Beginning to read: Thinking and learning about print*. Cambridge, MA: MIT Press.

Baker, L., Dreher, M. J., & Guthrie, J. T. (Eds.). (2000). *Engaging young readers: Promoting achievement and motivation*. New York: Guilford Press.

Ball, E. W., & Blachman, B. A. (1991). Does phoneme awareness training in kindergarten make a difference in early word recognition and developmental spelling? *Reading Research Quarterly, 26,* 49-66.

Bird, J., Bishop, D., & Freeman, N. (1995). Phonological awareness and literacy development in children with expressive phonological impairments. *Journal of Speech and Hearing Research, 36,* 446-462.

Bishop, D., & Adams, C. (1990). A prospective study of the relationship between specific language impairment, phonological disorders and reading retardation. *Journal of Child Psychology and Psychiatry, 31,* 1027-1050.

Blachman, B. (1991). Getting ready to read: Learning how print maps to speech. In J. F. Kavanagh (Ed.), *The language continuum: From infancy to literacy* (pp. 41-59). Parkton, MD: York Press.

Blachman, B. (Ed.). (2000). *Phonological awareness* (Vol. III). Mahway, NJ: Lawrence Erlbaum Associates.

Blachman, B. A. (1994). Early literacy acquisition: The role of phonological awareness. In G. P. Wallach & K. G. Butler (Eds.), *Language learning disabilities in schoolage children and adolescents* (pp. 253-274). Boston: Allyn & Bacon.

Blank, M., & White, S. (1992). A model for effective classroom discourse: Predicated topics with reduced verbal memory demands. *Australian Journal of Special Education, 16,* 23-39.

Bowman, B., Donovan, M. S., & Burns, M. S. (2001). *Eager to learn: Educating our preschoolers.* Washington, DC: National Academy Press.

Brady, S. A., & Fowler, A. E. (1988). Phonological precursors to reading acquisition. In R. L. Masland & M. W. Masland (Eds.), *Preschool prevention of reading failure* (pp. 204-215). Parkton, MD: York Press.

Byrne, B., & Fielding-Barnsley, R. (1995). Evaluation of a program to teach phonemic awareness to young children: A 2- and 3-year follow-up and a new preschool trial. *Journal of Educational Psychology, 85,* 488-503.

Catts, H. W., Fey, M. E., Zhang, X., & Tomblin, J. B. (2001). Predicting reading disabilities: Research to practice. *Language Speech and Hearing Services in Schools, 32,* 38-50.

Catts, H. W., & Kamhi, A. G. (2005). *Language and reading disabilities* (2nd ed.). Boston: Allyn & Bacon.

Center for Research on Education, Diversity and Excellence. *The five standards for effective pedagogy.* Retrieved May 6, 2005, from: www.crede.org

Culatta, B., Aslett, R., Fife, M., & Setzer, L. A. (2004). Project SEEL: Part I. Systematic and engaging early literacy instruction. *Communication Disorders Quarterly, 25*(2), 79-88.

Culatta, B., Kovarsky, D., Theadore, G., Franklin, A., & Timler, G. (2003). Quantitative and qualitative documentation of early literacy instruction. *American Journal of Speech Language Pathology*, *12*, 172–188.

Culatta, B., Setzer, L. A., Wilson, C., & Aslett, R. (2004). Project SEEL: Part III. Children's engagement and progress attainments. *Communication Disorders Quarterly*, *25*(3), 127–144.

Culatta, R., Culatta, B., Frost, M., & Buzzell, K. (2004). Project SEEL: Part II. Using technology to enhance early literacy instruction in Spanish. *Communication Disorders Quarterly*, *25*(2), 89–96.

Culturally and Linguistically Appropriate Services. (2001). *Review guidelines for material selection*. Early Childhood Research Institute. Retrieved on July 26, 2003, from: clas.uiuc.edu

Cunningham, A. E. (1990). Explicit versus implicit instruction in phonemic awareness. *Journal of Experimental Child Psychology*, *50*, 429–444.

Cunningham, A. E., & Stanovich, K. E. (1998). What reading does for the mind. *American Educator*, *22*(Spring/Summer), 8–15.

Dickinson, D. K., McCabe, A., Anastasopoulos, L., Peisner-Feinberg, E. S., & Poe, M. D. (2003). The comprehensive language approach to early literacy: The interrelationships among vocabulary, phonological sensitivity and print knowledge among preschool-aged children. *Journal of Educational Psychology*, *95*(3), 465–481.

Dickinson, D. K., McCabe, A., & Clark-Chiarelli, N. (2004). Preschool-based prevention of reading disability. In C. A. Stone, E. R. Silliman, B. J. Ehren, & K. Apel (Eds.), *Handbook of language and literacy: Development and disorders* (pp. 209–227). New York: Guilford Press.

Dickinson, D. K., & Sprague, K. E. (2001). The nature and impact of early childhood care environments on the language and early literacy development of children from low-income families. In S. B. Neuman & D. K. Dickinson (Eds.), *Handbook of Early Literacy Research* (pp. 263–280). New York: Guilford Press.

Ehri, L., Nunes, S., Willows, D., Schuster, B., Yaghoub-Zadeh, & Shanahan, T. (2001). Phonemic awareness instruction helps children learn to read: Evidence from the National Reading Panel's meta-analysis. *Reading Research Quarterly*, *36*(3), 250–287.

Foorman, B. R., & Torgesen, J. K. (2001). Critical elements of classroom and small-group instruction promote reading success in all children. *Learning Disabilities Research & Practice*, *16*(4), 203–212.

Fountas, I. C., & Pinnell, G. S. (1996). *Guided reading*. Portsmouth, NH: Heinemann.

Gillon, G. T. (2004). *Phonological awareness: From research to practice*. New York: Guilford Press.

Goswami, U. (2001). Early phonological development and the acquisition of literacy. In S. B. Neuman & D. K. Dickinson (Eds.), *Handbook of early literacy research*. New York: Guilford Press.

Goswami, U., & Bryant, P. (1992). Rhyme, analogy, and children's reading. In P. Gough, L. Ehri, & R. Treiman (Eds.), *Reading acquisition* (pp. 49–63). Hillsdale, NJ: Lawrence Erlbaum Associates.

Goswami, U., & Bryant, P. E. (1990). *Phonological skills and learning to read*. Hillsdale, NJ: Lawrence Erlbaum Associates.

Guthrie, J. T., Wigfield, A., & VonSecker, C. (2000). Effects of integrated instruction on motivation and strategy use in reading. *Journal of Educational Psychology, 92*(2), 331–341.

Gutierrez-Clellen, V. (1999). Mediating literacy skills in Spanish-speaking children with special needs. *Language, Speech, and Hearing Services in Schools, 30*, 285–292.

Harrison, J. (1994). *Dear bear*. New York: Learner Publishing Group.

Henkes, K. (1996). *Lily's purple plastic purse*. New York: Greenwillow Books.

Hiebert, E. H., & Martin, L. A. (2001). The texts of beginning reading instruction. In S. B. Neuman & D. K. Dickinson (Eds.), *Handbook of early literacy research* (pp. 361–376). New York: Guilford Press.

Justice, L. M., & Kaderavek, J. N. (2004). Embedded-explicit emergent literacy intervention I: Background and description of approach. *Language, Speech, and Hearing Services in Schools, 35*, 201–211.

Kaderavek, J., & Rabidoux, P. (2004). Interactive to independent literacy: A model for designing literacy goals for children with atypical communication. *Reading and Writing Quarterly, 20*(3), 237–260.

Kaderavek, J. N., & Justice, L. M. (2004). Embedded-explicit emergent literacy Intervention II: Goal selection and implementation in the early childhood classroom. *Language, Speech, and Hearing Services in Schools, 35*, 212–228.

Lindgren, B., & Eriksson, E. (1982). *Sam's cookie*. New York: Harper-Collins.

Lyon, R. (1999). Reading development, reading disorders, and reading instruction: Research-based findings. *Language Learning and Education, ASHA Division 1 Newsletter, May*, 8–16.

McCardle, P., Scarborough, H. S., & Catts, H. W. (2001). Predicting, explaining, and preventing children's reading difficulties. *Learning Disabilities Research and Practice, 16*(4), 230–239.

McCarrier, A., Pinnell, G., & Fountas, I. (2000). *Interactive writing*. Portsmouth, NH: Heinemann.

McGee, L. M., & Richgels, D. J. (2000). *Literacy's beginnings: Supporting young readers and writers* (3rd ed.). Needham Heights, MA: Allyn & Bacon.

McKenna, M. (2001). Development of reading attitudes. In L. Verhoeven & C. Snow (Eds.), *Literacy and motivation: Reading engagement in individuals and groups* (pp. 135–158). Mahwah, NJ: Lawrence Erlbaum Associates.

McMullan, K., & McMullan, J. (2002). *I Stink*. New York: Joanna Cotler.

National Reading Panel. (2000). *Teaching children to read: An evidence-based assessment of the scientific research literature on reading and its implications for reading instruction* (NIH Publ. No. 00-4754). Washington, DC: National Institute of Child Health and Human Development.

Neuman, S., Copple, C., & Bredekamp, S. (2000). *Learning to read and write*. Washington, DC: National Association for Education of Young Children.

Pellegrini, A. D. (2001). Some theoretical and methodological considerations in studying literacy in social context. In S. B. Neuman & D. K. Dickinson (Eds.), *Handbook of early literacy research* (pp. 54–65). New York: Guilford Press.

Perfetti, C. (1985). *Reading ability*. New York: Oxford University Press.

Rand, M. (1993). Using thematic instruction to organize an integrated language arts classroom. In L. M. Morrow & J. K. Smith & L. C. Wilkinson (Eds.), *Integrated language arts: Controversy to consensus* (pp. 177–192). Boston: Allyn & Bacon.

Richgels, D. J. (2001). Invented spelling, phonemic awareness, and reading and writing instruction. In S. B. Neuman & D. K. Dickinson (Eds.), *Handbook of early literacy research* (pp. 142–158). New York: Guilford Press.

Riley, L. (1997). *Mouse mess*. New York: Scholastic.

Scarborough, H. (1990). Very early language deficits in dyslexic children. *Child Development, 61*, 1728–1743.

Scarborough, H. (2001). Connecting early literacy and literacy to later reading (dis)abilities: evidence, theory, and practice. In S. B. Neuman & D. K. Dickinson (Eds.), *Handbook of early literacy research* (pp. 97–110). New York: Guilford Press.

Shaw, N. (1989). *Sheep in a jeep*. Boston: Houghton Mifflin.

Shaw, N. (1996). *Sheep take a hike*. Boston: Houghton Mifflin.

Siracusa, C. (1990). *No mail for Mitchell*. New York: Random House.

Snow, C., Burns, S., & Griffin, P. (1998). *Preventing reading difficulties in young children*. Washington, DC: National Academy Press.

Storch, S. A., & Whitehurst, G. J. (2002). Oral language and code-related precursors to reading: Evidence from a longitudinal structural model. *Developmental Psychology, 38*(6), 934–947.

Tierney, R., & Readence, J. E. (2000). Teaching reading as a language experience. In *Reading Strategies and Practices: A Compendium* (5th ed., pp. 198–228). Boston: Allyn & Bacon.

Torgesen, J. K., Al Otaiba, S. A., & Grek, M. L. (2005). Assessment and instruction for phonemic awareness and word recognition skills. In H. W. Catts & A. G. Kamhi (Eds.), *Language and reading disabilities* (pp. 127–156). Boston: Pearson Education.

Torgesen, J. K., & Mathes, P. (1999). What every teacher should know about phonological awareness. In B. Honig, L. Diamond, & R. Nathan (Eds.), *CORE reading research anthology: The why of reading instruction* (pp. 54–61). Navato, CA: Arena Press.

Treiman, R. (1992). The role of intrasyllabic units in learning to read and spell. In P. B. Gough, L. C. Ehri, & R. Treiman (Eds.), *Reading acquisition* (pp. 65–106). Mahwah, NJ: Lawrence Erlbaum Associates.

Troia, G. A. (2004). Phonological processing and its influence on literacy. In C. A. Stone, E. R. Silliaman, B. J. Ehren, & K. Apel (Eds.), *Handbook of language and literacy* (pp. 271–301). New York: Guilford Press.

Ukrainetz, T., Cooney, M., Kyer, S., Kysar, A., & Harris, T. (2000). An investigation into teaching phonemic awareness through shared reading and writing. *Early Childhood Research Quarterly, 15*(3), 331–352.

Verhoeven, L. (2001). Prevention of reading difficulties. In L. Verhoeven & C. Snow (Eds.), *Literacy and motivation: Reading engagement in individuals and groups* (pp. 123–134). Mahwah, NJ: Lawrence Erlbaum Associates.

Verhoeven, L., & Snow, C. (2001). Literacy and motivation: Bridging cognitive and sociocultural viewpoints. In L. Verhoeven & C. Snow (Eds.), *Literacy and motivation: Reading engagement in individuals and groups* (pp. 1–20). Mahwah, NJ: Lawrence Erlbaum Associates.

Wagner, R., & Torgesen, J. K. (1987). The nature of phonological processing and its causal role in the acquisition of reading skills. *Psychological Bulletin, 101*, 199–212.

Wagner, R., Torgesen, J. K., & Rashotte, C. A. (1994). Development of reading related phonological abilities: New evidence of bidirectional causality from a latent variable longitudinal study. *Developmental Psychology, 30*, 73–87.

Whitehurst, G. J., & Lonigan, C. J. (1998). Child development and emergent literacy. *Child Development, 69*, 335–357.

Whitehurst, G. J., & Lonigan, C. J. (2001). Emergent literacy: Development from prereaders to readers. In S. B. Neuman & D. K. Dickinson (Eds.), *Handbook of early literacy research* (pp. 11–29). New York: Guilford Press.

Yopp, H. K. (1992). Developing phonemic awareness in young children. *The Reading Teacher, 45*(9), 696–706.

APPENDIX 6–A

Lesson Plan for Teaching Children to Rhyme with "ack"

1. State the literacy target and model it for the children:
   Put the backpack on your back with the "ack" things inside.
   Say: "See this black backpack on my back? *Black backpack* and *back* rhyme. We will rhyme with *pack*. Maybe we'll find things that rhyme with *pack* in my black back pack—like *snack*, *sack*, *tack*, *track*, and *jack*."

2. Provide playful practice:
   a. Take the "ack" things out: Pull out one item at a time and let the children act on it or see it. Give the children quick turns with some of the items, or provide enough of some items for each child to hold. Interact in rhyme as the children see and act on the items.
   b. "Sack back": Pull out small sacks and give one to each child. Pull out a large sack, and ask the children to give back the small sacks so they can be put away in the large sack. The children can hand the sacks to the teacher or place them in the large sack, but the teacher says "sack back" and "pack sack" each time a sack is put in place. "Sack back, pack the sack, *pack* and *sack* rhyme!"
   c. "Snack": Show or pass out paper snacks or small pretzels. Ask, "Snack?" and say "snack, snack, snack" while passing out the snacks or taking out many examples of snacks from the pack.
   d. "Snack sack": Pack snacks in snack sacks. Carry out an *ack* conversation: "Snack sack? Pack snack in sack. Snack in snack sack. Pack snack, snack in the sack. *Snack* and *sack* rhyme! Pack your snack, pack-snack. *Pack* and *snack* rhyme! (Other "ack" items can be packed as well.)
   e. "Track, back, Jack": Show or pass out tracks. Lay out tracks in a line, saying "track" each time you set one down. Walk on the tracks to take the tracks back to the children, or let a toy train or Jack (puppet) take the tracks. Ask, "Want Jack

back?" Have the children tell Jack to come back. Say, "Back, Jack. Take track back." Gesture for Jack to come back on the track.

   f. "Black": Prepare small pieces of black paper. Ask the children, "Want something black?" Say "black" as you hand each child a small piece of black paper.

   g. "Cracker Jack": Copy pictures of the Cracker Jack box. Pass out paper copies, or use a real box and give each child a real or pretend Cracker Jack.

   h. "Stack toy jack": Show jacks (one at a time). Ask, "Stack jack?" Try to stack the jacks. Comment when they fall, "Jacks don't stack."

   i. "Pack, crack": Bring out packing material that cracks (Styrofoam and bubble pack). Say, "This will crack. Crack! [as it is snapped]" Give each child a quick turn to crack the bubble pack. Now break the Styrofoam packing material into small pieces. Say: "I can whack the pack to make it crack—whack and crack the pack."

3. Review literacy target:

   a. "Put things back": Say, "Now we will pack the black backpack. We'll put things back in the black backpack."

   b. Ask if items rhyme. Go through item by item: "Does *snack* rhyme with *pack*?" Try to put something back that doesn't rhyme with pack. "Shall I pack the shoe in the black backpack? Does *shoe* rhyme with *pack*?" (Shake head "no" if children need support.)

Chapter Seven

Using Emergent Writing to Develop Phonemic Awareness

Teresa A. Ukrainetz

Overview

Phonemic awareness is an important part of literacy. Children must learn to segment and manipulate the sounds of speech, so that they can map these sounds with letters in reading and writing. For many children, the ability to attend to phonemes begins in preschool, thus representing an important emergent literacy skill. At the same time, preschoolers are making strides in the many other dimensions of literacy, such as print concepts, letter knowledge, word reading, spelling, and language skills. This chapter describes how children's writing emerges over the preschool and kindergarten years, how phonemic awareness develops during this same period, and how these two literacy skills build on each other. Also described is how writing, from nonsense letters to conventional spelling, can be used as a tool to develop phonemic awareness.

Learning to Write

The Many Tasks of Learning to Write

Even as early as the preschool years, children learn what they can do with writing, what it looks like, and how it is produced to represent ideas. As they become older, they learn how to step away from their writing and consciously reflect on it as an object of communication and craftsmanship. From preschool into the elementary grades, learning to write involves learning the functions, forms, and processes of print (McGee & Richgels, 2004; McLane & McNamee, 1990).

Children must learn the varied functions or purposes of writing: to aid memory, to organize thoughts, to communicate information, to express emotions, to maintain social connections, and to document events. Less abstractly, they will come to know that writing is used for grocery lists, phone numbers, class attendance, e-mail communication, garage sale ads, and diaries. In school, writing is composed into the formal discourse of stories, posters, essays, and reports.

Children also must learn the forms of print: upper and lower case letters, block and cursive. Modern children must be able both to shape letters by hand and to find letters with appropriate fingering on a keyboard. They must know how letters are grouped to indicate words, sentences, and paragraphs. They must learn a punctuation system that represents stress, intonation, and pauses. They learn how to lay out letters, stories, and reports. In this print-busy world, they also learn to add bullets, color, shape, and graphics to increase the salience and appeal of their messages.

Finally, children must learn the processes of writing. At the word level, they learn that print represents language and ideas; that letters represent sounds (i.e. alphabetic principle); that there are systematic correspondences between sounds and letters; and that, the alphabetic principle notwithstanding, many words have limited correspondence between individual letters and sounds (e.g., *Wednesday* versus /wɛnzdeɪ/). Over time and with experience, children acquire a huge store of visual images of print words for rapid, accurate spelling and reading. At the text level, children learn how to map ideas on paper; and how this mapping varies with purpose (e.g., a storybook versus a birthday card). They learn how to generate ideas, put the ideas into words, put those words on paper, and craft the words into a message. They also must learn how to express their ideas in written monologues, without the benefit of a supportive conversational partner. Eventually, they are expected to achieve the daunting task of writing about abstract ideas in formal academic prose of particular discourse genres, for a hypothetical reader with presumed understandings and purposes.

Acquisition of Spelling Skills

The roots of the many skills of writing are apparent in children's emergent literacy development, during which they gradually accumulate the knowledge and skills that they will bring to formal reading and writing. Given models, opportunities, and tools, well before formal reading and writing instruction, young children will begin to explore and use writing and begin to represent meaning with print. They also will gradually learn to spell and compose primitive narratives and reports. They may even critique and revise their work to share it proudly with an admiring audience. With these early print representations, preschoolers have embarked on the complex act of writing.

The central task for the novice writer is to break into the mystery of spelling. The writings children produce can be organized into levels of sophistication. There are typically considered to be five levels, first documented by Gentry (1978) and summarized in Richgels (2001): precommunicative, semi-phonetic, phonetic, transitional, and conventional. The distinctions among the semi-phonetic, phonetic, and transitional levels are subtle, so in this chapter they are collapsed here into one grouping called phonetic spelling, resulting in a three-level approach: pre-communicative, phonetic, and conventional.

Precommunicative writing consists of marks on paper that do not represent ideas in a consistent way that can be shared with others. The earliest manifestation of pre-communicative writing is scribble with print patterns, such as lists, lines, and word-length chunks of scribble. Slightly further along on the road to writing are "symbol salads," which are combinations of letters, numbers, and shapes (Bear, Invernizzi, Templeton, & Johnston, 2000). Nonsense writing also may be seen, which involves random collections of letters only. Nonsense writing that is placed in horizontal strings, grouped into word-length units, or produced left-to-right, shows awareness of print organization. Even with scribble, children may show understanding of the symbolic function of writing, telling listeners what the messages mean or (more challenging for the adults), asking the "reader" what message is held in the scribble (Clay, 1975). The arrangement of preschoolers' scribble and nonsense letters can sometimes be recognized as discourse genres, such as birthday messages, birthday lists, calendars, and poems. These genre indications may be subtle and require context (e.g., a mother also writing birthday cards), talk (e.g., about birthdays), and actions (e.g., placing the paper in an envelope) to identify them (McGee & Richgels, 2004).

As children emerge from this precommunicative level, they typically will show a holistic understanding of some printed words. In reading, this is apparent through children's recognition of environmental print, such as on stop signs and cereal boxes. In writing, children may show advanced writing of some frequently occurring words, such as *the* and *mom*. They write these words as logographs, holistic units that represent ideas, without awareness of the correspondence between individual letters and phonemes. Children often learn to write their own names through this strategy (Hildreth, 1936; McGee & Richgels, 2004). They understand early on that print can represent their names. Their earliest name representation may be be only a single shape, such as a particular squiggle. With print experience, children move to letter-like symbols. These become recognizable letters that are constantly used but may be scrambled or scattered on the page. Conventional signature representations follow. These memorized units may occur alongside much more rudimentary spelling understandings for other words.

For most words, spelling progresses in a developmental sequence in which phonetic features are increasingly represented. This type of spelling, called *phonetic spelling*, shows children's growing understanding of the alphabetic principle and phoneme-grapheme correspondences. Phonetic spelling sometimes is called "invented spelling" because children are using their own hypotheses regarding how to represent the sounds of spoken words with letters. When children first begin to use phonetic spelling, they often make a number of errors in their spelling renditions, similar to the developmental "errors" seen among children as they master expressive phonology. For example, children often represent only the most salient parts of words, such as beginning and ending consonants (e.g., BG for *big*). They also may use but confuse letters that correctly represent some feature of the phoneme, such as place of articulation (e.g., D for /t/). Sometimes children write words using letters based on the name of the letters (e.g., C for *see*). Also, vowels may be overlooked initially, so that a child may write CT for *cat*. If they are noticed, vowels may be marked, but the markings are not specific. For example, the child may distinguish lax and tense vowels (e.g., /i/, /u/ versus /ɛ/, /ʊ/) with letters (e.g., E versus I) but may spell all of the lax vowels with one vowel. Particular trouble with vowels is not surprising in view of the fact that vowel spelling is very complicated: Spoken vowels are not perceived categorically (e.g., "Was that an /i/ or an /u/ or something in between?"); their pronunciation varies across dialects and idiolects; and, even if agreement can be obtained on what vowel is said, the relationship between letters and vowels is complex and inconsistent. Fortunately for the emergent writer, words often are readable in context despite missing or incorrect vowels. Figure 7–1, showing a 5-year-old's protest message, demonstrates how multiple levels of spelling can be present within a single message: with memorized words, phonetic spelling, letter names, salient phonemes, missing vowels, and vowel markers.

When children begin to use phonetic spelling, writing becomes more meaningful and useful. Discourse genres become more recognizable. For example, a 5-year-old boy (my nephew Lukas) composed a grocery list that was organized as a vertical listing of individual letters representing the beginning sound of each grocery item, such as P for *peas*. He distinguished *peas* and *pumpkins* by a small and a large P, respectively. He was able to use the list to guide the subsequent shopping trip, although the individual letters were not sufficient to cue recall (for either of us) the next day.

Toward the end of the phonetic phase of spelling, children continue to use invented spelling for some words (particularly those that are morphologically complicated or unfamiliar), but children also have learned many of the conventions of spelling, such as writing TION for /ʃʌn/ (e.g., in *nation*) and knowing that GH can represent /g/ or /f/ or silence (e.g., *ghost*, *cough*, or *through*). At this level, children combine memorized chunks and patterns with

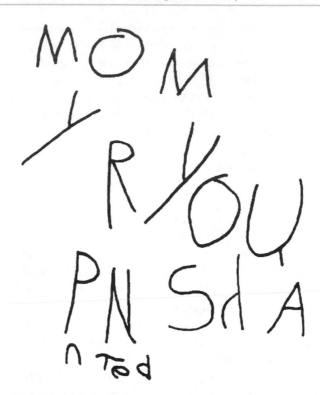

Figure 7–1. A 5-year-old's written message uses multiple levels of spelling to say "Mom, why are you punishing me? Ted." (Reprinted with permission from *Literary's Beginnings* [4th ed., p. 90] by L. M. McGee and D. J. Richards, 2004. Boston: Pearson.)

phonetically based spellings. On occasion, these phonetically based spellings may reveal pronunciations for which adults have lost awareness. For example, CHRIE for try (Read, 1971, p. 13) involves, in addition to the memorized IE pattern and the phonetically based R, a nonconventional spelling that reflects the affrication with which *try* is sometimes pronounced (/tʃrai/). As we become more accustomed to spelling, our perceptions can become distorted to match spelling (Ehri & Wilce, 1986), so for the word *butter*, the spelling makes us think we say /bʌtɚ/ when we really say /bʌdɚ/.

The final level children achieve as writers is *conventional spelling*. Children primarily use correct spelling at this level, although errors will still occur. Each new word a child aims to write is initially analyzed for its phonological features, as the child seeks the corresponding letters or letter chunks to represent the sounds in the word. Children may have difficulty holding long, multisyllabic words in memory while they seek conventional letter representations. With repeated decoding and encoding, the words become permanent detailed print images that can be read or spelled fluently without going through the sound-letter route. This mental store of visual orthographic images is critical for fluent writing and reading (see Apel & Masterson, 2001; Apel & Swank, 1999). Reading and writing experiences will continue to expand and refine this mental store of images. Unfortunately, even as children are encountering many exemplars of conventional spelling, they also are encountering variable spellings of some words, such as popular reductions of *night* to *nite* and *through* to *thru*. English spelling, with its many borrowings and inventions, is already difficult, and these variations only complicate the situation. It is not surprising that conventional spellers, even some who are fluent composers of extended writing, will continue to make spelling errors into adulthood.

This description of writing development suggests an orderly unfolding like that of oral language. As with learning to talk, children observe models, take guidance, and invent their own rule-based solutions. Precommunicative writing is carried out by some toddlers and preschoolers. Their writing products show their emerging understanding that print represents ideas in a constant manner, the purposes to which writing is put, and the way in which letters represent individual sounds. By kindergarten, children have some memorized words and are using phonetic spelling for many words. Conventional spelling appears alongside invented spelling in kindergarten. Over the course of first and second grades, conventional spelling increasingly takes over from invented spelling. Thus, there is a developmental aspect with a set of expectancies for children's writing. However, unlike for spoken language, these levels are *not* a set of invariant developmental milestones that all children will travel to attain.

Development of literacy is notably subject to learning experiences, and the learning experiences for writing tend to be particularly limited and highly variable among children. The companion act of reading can occur anywhere at any time, from the morning cereal box to street signs to classroom posters to bedtime story-books. Children are constantly exposed to potential acts of reading. By contrast, writing experiences are more constrained: under supervision, sitting at a table, with designated pen and paper. Writing experiences also are more diverse, with some families and preschools encouraging learning of the functions, forms, and processes of writing across many daily activities and other care-givers limiting writing experiences to letter formation during a structured lesson.

As a result of this diversity in learning experiences, the development of writing is not an orderly event in which all children move at the same time through the same developmental levels. Children who are provided emergent literacy instruction may enter into purposeful use of phonetic spelling and sight words before kindergarten. Some preschoolers may even move into invented spelling largely on their own. By contrast, children whose preschool experiences have consisted of only copying or isolated letter practice may not explore precommunicative writing. If in kindergarten and first grade children are allowed to use only the small set of words they have learned to spell correctly, there is little need for phonetic spelling.

Accordingly, the question arises: Are early writing experiences and preconventional explorations necessary or even helpful to young children, especially because kindergarten and first grade will provide them with more formal instruction in conventional spelling and writing? The accumulated literature suggests that they are. Preschoolers and kindergartners who have had wider and deeper literacy experiences, including writing explorations, are far more likely to meet with success in reading and writing than children who have been limited to alphabet learning exercises (Adams, 1990; Richgels, 2001). Children who are encouraged to explore learn that writing is enjoyable and functional—that they can express ideas and communicate with others via the written word. They learn the forms of text: how to write a job list versus a birthday greeting. Of greatest importance, exploration of phonetic spelling improves children's ability to notice the sounds in words and find reasonable spellings. Teachers cannot teach every word that must be spelled or every rule of spelling, so children who are equipped to sound out and spell words will manage better in their writing compositions.

There is evidence that invented spelling is beneficial for reading and writing. Richgels (1995) documented that children who enter kindergarten as users of invented spelling show better reading and writing outcomes than those who do not. Although these children may have entered kindergarten with other advantages that accounted for their better performance, other studies have shown a cause-and-effect relationship. For example, Ehri and Wilce (1987) showed that combined phonetic spelling and phonemic awareness instruction provides additional advantages to children's literacy development compared with phonemic awareness instruction alone. Kindergartners who were taught to phonemically segment words with phonetic letter tiles were better able to read nonsense and unfamiliar words than those who were taught to segment with colored blocks. Ehri and Wilce directly taught phonetic spelling. By contrast, Clarke (1988) investigated the effects of children's own invented spelling. Clarke compared two first grade classrooms in which invented spelling was encouraged and two first grade classrooms employing more traditional instruction in which word lists, dictionaries, dictating stories, and copying teacher models were promoted. In their writing samples, the traditional instruction group showed fewer spelling errors than the invented spelling group but produced much shorter stories. At year's end, the two groups spelled high-frequency irregular words comparably, but the invented spelling group did better on lower-frequency, regularly spelled words and on several word reading measures. Additional analyses showed that this effect was primarily due to the advantage afforded children entering first grade with lower literacy achievement. These children, who had less incoming spelling knowledge, benefited most from the explicit guidance and encouragement to reflect on the sounds in words and to invent reasonable spellings for them.

As children learn to write, they come to know the many forms, purposes, and processes of graphic representation. Word spelling and text writing come together to allow the elaborated and sophisticated acts of language and literacy occurring in school. The foregoing shows how the process and product of children's graphic representations reveals their emerging understandings of writing and spelling. Clarke's (1988) study and others have shown the benefits of encouraging young children to work out their best guesses for spelling. How writing can be applied as a tool to support the literacy skill of phonemic awareness is explored next.

Phonemic Awareness Through Writing

Phonemes and Graphemes: A Reciprocal Relationship

Phonemic awareness is the understanding that spoken words can be split into component phonemes which can be isolated and manipulated. For instance, children with phonemic awareness realize that *name* consists of three phonemes and that the beginning sound is /n/.

Phonemic awareness is one of five critical components of reading, along with word decoding, vocabulary, comprehension, and fluency (National Reading Panel [NRP], 2000). Phonemic awareness allows children to understand the alphabetic principle, notice the regular ways in which letters represent sounds in words, and generate possibilities for words in context that are only partially sounded out (Torgesen, Al Otaiba, & Grek, 2005). Phonemic awareness is one of the strongest kindergarten indicators for identifying the likelihood of a later reading disability (Catts, Fey, Zhang, & Tomblin, 2001; Catts & Kamhi, 2005). Fortunately, phonemic awareness is a very teachable skill, and many studies have demonstrated that instruction in phonemic awareness improves children's reading and spelling (Ehri et al., 2001; NRP, 2000). Providing explicit instruction in phonemic awareness is now recommended from the early grades for all children, with particular attention to young children at risk for reading difficulties.

There are many tasks that tap phonemic awareness. Beginning phoneme *isolation* is the easiest (e.g., /b/ is the beginning phoneme in *bat*) and can be accomplished by many 3-year-olds (Chaney, 1992; Maclean, Bryant, & Bradley, 1987). Phoneme *matching* is harder (Lonigan, Burgess, Anthony, & Barker, 1998), requiring the child to remember and compare several words (e.g., does *man* begin with the same sound as *dog, cow*, or *mouse?*). Phoneme *blending* (e.g., /b/-/a/-/t/ makes the word *bat*) is needed for reading written words. Phoneme *segmenting* (e.g., *bat* is made up of /b/-/a/-/t/), the inverse of blending, is needed to isolate all the sounds in a word so it can be spelled. Phoneme segmenting is more difficult than isolating, matching, or blending (Wagner, Torgesen, & Rashotte, 1994).

Phonemic awareness is a curious phenomenon. It is an oral language skill, but one that is not required for oral communication. It is an important literacy skill specifically required for encoding and decoding printed words in an alphabetic writing system, but it does not involve letters. Improving phonemic awareness improves word spelling, but word spelling also helps to improve phonemic awareness. Phonemic awareness helps conventional spellers deal with occasional unfamiliar words and helps emergent spellers deal with all of their spelling challenges. Of importance, there is a reciprocally beneficial relationship between phonemic awareness and spelling.

The positive influence of spelling on phonemic awareness often is not recognized. This direction of the relationship is readily seen in the following illustration.. Look away from this text and segment the word *supercilious* into phonemes. Do you "see" the printed word while you listen to yourself say it? As you segment the phonemes, your *working memory* will be operating on the sound representation within your *phonological loop* but also will place the spelling of this word in your visual *sketchpad*, to use Baddeley's (1986) description of memory processes. Referring to that sketchpad aids you in this task. Good spellers can even invent a graphemic visualization of nonsense words or foreign words to assist their phonological processing resources.

Now examine the process of spelling for a preschooler or kindergartner. For example, a child has drawn a picture of a cat and would like to label it. She is at the invented level of spelling in which she knows sounds are represented by letters. She mutters /k/-/k/-/k/ to herself as she casts about for an appropriate letter. She settles on a K. She skips over the vowel to the next salient sound. She says /t/-/t/-/t/ and selects D. Her end product is the invented and incorrect but decipherable "KD" written above her whiskered animal. Through this spelling exploration, the child has independently segmented beginning and ending phonemes in a word. She is becoming aware of phonemic segmentation through her spelling.

Phonemic awareness is not a precursor that must be achieved before children learn to spell. Children gradually acquire knowledge of spelling at the same time as they gradually become aware of the sounds of speech. In fact, spelling and phonemic awareness are quite synchronous. When formal reading and spelling instruction started in first grade, older studies found that phoneme segmentation was also just emerging in 7-year-olds (Fox & Routh, 1975; Liberman, Shankweiler, Fischer, & Carter, 1974). In the modern approach, formal literacy instruction occurs in kindergarten, and both phoneme segmentation and invented spelling are expected at this younger age. For the child to be ready for kindergarten, beginning sound awareness and some alphabet knowledge are now expected by the end of preschool (McGee, 2004).

Although a range of programs are available that promote preschoolers' phonological awareness, whether in tandem with alphabet instruction or in absence, preschoolers typically are not considered developmentally ready for the critical level of phonemes. Instead, phonological awareness instruction often begins with larger units of sound, such as syllable and rhyme, and even nonspeech sounds such as those of doorbells (e.g., Adams, Foorman, Lundberg, & Beeler, 1998). Although larger units are easier to teach, it is not clear that most of such instruction is necessary or even helpful. Listening skills can be acquired directly through speech tasks, without spending time on identifying doorbells and bird tweets. Syllable clapping instruction can lead to confusion when children must move from syllables to phonemes (Nuspl & Ukrainetz, 2006). Rhyming is the only one of these skills that combines well with phonemes: Rhyming books draw attention to the sounds of language, and rhyming pairs contrast in their beginning phonemes.

Early studies showed that competence in tasks such as segmenting sentences into words, clapping syllables, and rhyming occurred developmentally earlier than that for phoneme tasks (e.g., Fox & Routh, 1975; Maclean et al., 1987). When the memory demands of the tasks are controlled, however, and with use of simple instructions, the developmental ordering of syllable, rhyme, and phonemes actually is slight and overlapping (Anthony, Lonigan, Driscoll, Phillips, & Burgess, 2003). Simple varieties of syllable, rhyme, and phoneme tasks all can be achieved by the age of 4 years (Bryant, Bradley, Maclean, & Crossland, 1989; Chaney, 1992; Fox & Routh, 1975; Liberman et al., 1974; Maclean et al., 1987).

Awareness of syllable, rhyme, and phonemes thus all begin about 4 years of age. Of these three units, only phonemes are directly and strongly related to reading performance (Gillon, 2004). In addition, preschoolers can learn phonemic awareness without previous instruction in rhyme and syllable (Byrne & Fielding-Barnsley, 1991; Gillon, 2000; Ukrainetz, Cooney, Dyer, Kysar, & Harris, 2000), and some evidence suggests that rhyme and syllable instruction may not even provide additional benefit (Nuspl & Ukrainetz, 2006). Thus, phonological awareness instruction can be initiated at the phoneme level and taught within the context of shared writing activities, even for preschoolers. Young children can learn to talk about sounds in words as they explore how to map the sounds on paper.

Message Writing as the Context for the Skill of Phonemic Awareness

Best practices in language and literacy intervention reflect the understanding that "language serves communication ends and is learned in the course of communicative events" (Johnston, 1985, p. 126). Rather than using an approach that breaks down a task to permit training on simple components within structured hierarchies of contrived tasks, developmentally appropriate intervention occurs within whole, real, complicated activities. At the same time, language and literacy patterns are amplified and learning is systematically supported to aid and accelerate learning. This approach to intervention has been variously labeled as activity-based, hybrid, and naturalistic. I prefer the term *contextualized skill intervention*, which captures the duality of both meaningful contexts and explicit skill targets (Ukrainetz, 2006a).

Contextualized skill intervention can be applied to phonemic awareness, particularly through the avenue of writing. Writing messages intended for readers provides a purposeful context for skill development. Children know why it matters to break spoken words into sounds and to represent ideas and sounds with print. The attention to words and awareness of individual phonemes that occurs during the process of spelling words, particularly in inventing phonetic spellings, leads to improvements in phonemic awareness, spelling, and reading (Clarke, 1988; Ehri & Wilce, 1987). The act of inventing spelling can be especially useful as "a holistic way for teachers and others who are interested in emergent literacy to assess and facilitate children's phonemic awareness" (Richgels, 2001, p. 143).

Phonological awareness instruction, which typically is composed of structured, hierarchical, decontextualized procedures, has been criticized for its lack of developmentally appropriate, emergent literacy features (International Reading Association [IRA] and

National Association for the Education of Young Children [NAEYC] [IRA/NAEYC], 1998; McFadden, 1998; McGee & Purcell-Gates, 1997; Teale & Yokota, 2000). Such instruction stands in stark contrast with the rest of the preschool literacy curriculum, which occurs through exploration within purposeful daily life activities with a minimum of direct instruction. Even language intervention, which must be more explicit, systematic, and frequent than regular instruction, involves active learning within meaningful activities (Johnston, 1985; Pretti-Frontczak & Bricker, 2004; Rice, 1995). IRA/ NAEYC recommends not teaching phonological awareness until children are ready for formal instruction. However, as described in the previous section, it makes sense to explore ways of teaching phonemic awareness using meaningful, contextualized approaches that build on children's other emergent literacy achievements, including knowledge of the alphabet. "Sound talk" embedded in the composition of purposeful messages provides such an approach. Sound talk, also called phonemic referencing, is discussed later in this chapter as a means for providing scaffolded interactive experiences with children to promote phonemic awareness via writing. This approach can be used for all young children, including those with language impairment who require more systematic attention for facilitating emergent literacy skills.

Children with language impairment need more structured instruction than that occurring during the course of writing instruction in the regular classroom. Intervention involves providing individualized, explicit, and systematic guidance (McFadden, 1998; Ukrainetz, 2006b). Even for preschoolers, phonemic awareness can be explicitly targeted as a treatment objective within shared reading and writing activities. In this approach, advanced phonemic skills are addressed in tandem with earlier skills in a horizontal skill sequence. By contrast, a *traditional skill sequence* is vertical, wherein skills are ordered in difficulty and one skill is taught at a time until mastery. In a horizontal approach, however, multiple phoneme-level subskills are taught concurrently within a single, meaningful activity with a routine sequence of events and differential scaffolding.

As discussed previously, spelling draws on a range of phonemic awareness abilities, including isolating, segmenting, and blending the beginning, middle, and ending sounds in words. Even though some of these tasks are easier than others, they are beneficially taught together to form the purposeful whole of spelling words. For example, in a single instructional interaction, a clinician can combine both segmenting and blending tasks in a horizontal manner, rather than targeting one skill until mastery and then moving on to the other skill. To introduce segmenting, for example, an instructor may ask a child to engage in beginning sound isolation: "Tell me the sounds in *baby* so I can write them—what is the beginning sound?" To focus on blending, the instructor may engage a child in beginning sound matching: "What have I written, /b/ /i/? No, not *bow*, but those both start with /b/." With use of a horizontal approach to intervention, segmenting and blending can go back and forth within an activity: "What am I saying, /b/-/i/? Yes, bee— you write the word. Say the sounds as you write. What is the beginning sound?"

Teaching several subskills focused principally at the phoneme level within a single activity provides many benefits over a vertical, hierarchical approach to instruction (Ukrainetz, 2006b):

- Shortening the time required to get to phoneme-level awareness
- Recognizing the overlapping emergence of phonemic awareness subskills
- Providing additional practice on easy subskills
- Providing increased exposure to difficult subskills
- Employing easier subskills to scaffold more difficult subskills
- Showing how component subskills are orchestrated into the greater whole of segmenting words
- Increasing flexibility in applying different subskills as needed
- Providing a variety of difficulty levels for mixed abilities within a group

Research supports use of this instructional approach of teaching multiple phonemic awareness subskills concurrently, without previous instruction in larger units of sound (Ukrainetz et al., 2000). In one study of 36 children, consisting of 5- and 6-year-olds matched by ability level, the children were randomly assigned to treatment and control conditions. Children in the treatment group received phonemic awareness instruction in small groups for

20 minutes three times per week for 7 weeks. Instruction employed word stimuli that arose naturally during shared book reading and emergent message writing completed by the child working with an instructor. Specifically, the instructor and the children read rhyming books and identified the rhyming words in the verses (e.g., "Silly Sally goes to town, dancing backwards, upside down" from *Silly Sally* [Wood, 1992]). They then isolated the beginning and ending sounds in the rhyming words and counted the sounds in each word. For the message writing, the instructor and the children drew pictures and wrote accompanying captions. In the writing activity, the instructor modeled conventional spelling, while the children wrote at their own emergent levels of spelling. During the message composition, the instructor talked aloud about her own and the children's writing. She elicited from the children beginning and ending sounds and had the children match the number of letters to the number of sounds in words. Results of this study showed significantly greater progress for the treatment group children on beginning isolation, ending isolation, and segmentation. Additionally, parents of the treatment group children reported greater incidence of interest in literacy activities after the intervention. Children with lower literacy abilities showed patterns of achievement similar to those in the full sample. Although their gains were less than those of the higher-achieving children, they tripled their mean pretest performance.

Scaffolding Phonemic Awareness

Achieving phonemic awareness is a challenge for many young children, especially for those who are not yet at phonetic levels of spelling. It is critical to provide developmentally sensitive learning support for preschoolers and kindergartners to progress in phonemic awareness during reading, writing, and other literacy activities. Phonemic awareness can be taught within authentic print experiences in a developmentally sensitive manner that is consistent with other aspects of emergent literacy instruction. But such instruction is challenging, because, unlike rhythmic syllables and rhyme, phonemes are difficult to segment, and some, such as stops, cannot truly be isolated from the surrounding vowels. To make this instruction successful for young children, a key intervention element is *scaffolding*.

Systematic support via scaffolding enables a child to participate in and learn from developmentally advanced activities (Vygotsky, 1978). Some phonemic awareness skills are within the independent developmental level of preschoolers, such as identifying the beginning sound in words (e.g., /b/ in *ball*). However, with scaffolding, preschoolers also can show assisted performance in more difficult tasks such as phoneme segmentation (Nuspl & Ukrainetz, 2006). Early supportive exposure and practice lead to greater understanding and increases in independent performance, moving development forward. Children equipped with early understandings of phoneme isolation, segmentation, and blending are then ready to take advantage of formal kindergarten and first grade instruction in word reading and spelling.

Scaffolding is the temporary provision of support aimed at assisting a learner to internalize the behavior and talk modeled by the instructor. It involves working on an emerging skill within complex contexts, with both strategic support from the instructor and active involvement from the child (Greenfield, 1984; Wood, Bruner, & Ross, 1976). With scaffolding, an activity occurs many times, with the child moving from almost total dependence on the instructor to independence. The support provided is like the guided participation or apprenticing characteristic of daily life activities, such as learning to tie one's shoe or change the oil in a car (Rogoff, 1990).

Like that employed for other language domains, scaffolding of phonemic awareness includes several important techniques (Ukrainetz, 2006a, 2006b). *Structural scaffolds* are modifications of the environment that simplify and focus learning (Hart & Risley, 1975; Kaiser, Yoder, & Keetz, 1992). *Linguistic scaffolds* are adult behaviors that provide the learner new information. These include modeling, prompting, and expanding (e.g., Camarata, Nelson, & Camarata, 1994; Girolametto, Pearce, & Weitzman, 1996). *Response scaffolds* are hierarchies of response prompts that help the learner answer questions (e.g., Hart & Risley, 1975; Kaiser et al., 1992). *Regulatory scaffolds* are used to help the child self-reflect, organize, and intentionally learn (e.g., Feuerstein, 1980; Lidz & Pena, 1996). Table 7–1 provides examples of these four types of scaffolding.

Scaffolding is an important feature of both language and literacy intervention. In addition to using scaffolding to provide *systematic support* to children to improve their learning, intervention

Table 7–1. Critical RISE Elements of Treatment Applied to Phonemic Awareness within the Meaningful Context of Emergent Message Writing

Critical Element	Description
Repeated opportunities	Two comments per word for a 10-word message equals 20 trials across isolation, blending, and segmenting phonemes.
Intensity	Writing is used as one of multiple phonemic awareness activities, delivered to groups of 1 to 3 children for 60 minutes per week for 8 to 10 weeks.
Systematic support	• Structural scaffolds; e.g., use fingers to count the number of sounds in words before writing, or use letters to represent the number of sounds in words during writing. • Linguistic scaffolds, e.g, stress the target sound in the word, or expand a partial phoneme segmentation into a full segmentation. • Response scaffolds; e.g., wait for a response, or provide a Cloze question. • Regulatory scaffolds; e.g., call a child by name to focus attention before asking a question, or ask the child to identify what he or she is listening for.
Explicit skill objective	Maintain a clear focus on phonemic awareness over letter formation, letter choices or message content.

Source: Based on Ukrainetz, T. A. (2006b). Scaffolding young children into phonemic awareness. In T. A. Ukrainetz (Ed.), *Contextualized language intervention: Scaffolding preK–12 literacy achievement* (pp. 429–468). Eau Claire, WI: Thinking Publications.

should have three other features as listed in Table 7–1. Specifically, high-quality intervention should *explicitly* target a small number of literacy skills with *repeated* opportunities for learning and practice in an *intense* service delivery structure (Gillam, Loeb, & Friel-Patti,

2001; Torgesen et al., 2001). These key elements are represented by the acronym RISE: repeated practice opportunities, intense service delivery, systematic learning support, and explicit attention to target skills (Ukrainetz, 2006a).

The interactive scaffolding possibilities that occur within RISE are preplanned by the SLP, but enactment is dynamic and responsive to child needs. To achieve learning gains greater than those in daily life, scaffolding should be systematically provided in a way that keeps the child challenged but not frustrated. Matching the degree and nature of support to child need is critical for successful instruction. This matching can occur by varying the number of scaffolds provided or the directiveness of the scaffolds. High-directiveness scaffolds involve step-by-step support from the clinician with very little child responsibility (Schneider & Watkins, 1996). Low-directiveness scaffolds simply highlight elements. Table 7–2 presents a systematic way of quantifying the amount of support in phonemic awareness instruction. This rating table provides a way to plan systematic support and keep data on a child's progress toward mastery and independence. Segmentation scaffolding is the most difficult of these to quantify because of the many ways the child can be helped, the judgment of whether the child is in advance or in unison with the support, and the possibility of getting part of the word correct but still needing help with the rest.

From relevant studies (Ukrainetz et al., 2000; Nuspl & Ukrainetz, 2006), a few generalizations are possible concerning children's performance outcomes. First, typically developing preschoolers can be expected to achieve independent isolation of beginning sounds (e.g., identifying the initial sound in *dog*) after a fairly short instructional period. Second, blending phonemes seems to be an all-or-none phenomenon: Children will repeatedly not be able to do this task; then suddenly, it will make sense and they will be able to consistently produce words by blending phonemes (e.g., /d/ /a/ /g/ = *dog*). Third, for phoneme segmentation (e.g., identifying each of the phonemes in *dog*), preschoolers gradually will improve from total dependence to partial performance, but they often will continue to need moderate support. Nevertheless, they make gains in understanding the concept of segmenting phonemes. For example, at the end of intervention in the study by Nuspl and Ukrainetz (2006), preschoolers segmented *fat*, *brag*, *liver*, and *seashell* into the following: /fæ/ /æ/ /t/, /br/ /æ/ /g/, /l/ /ɪ/ /ver/, and /si/ /ʃ/ /ɛl/.

Table 7–2. Levels of Scaffolding for Isolating and Segmenting Phonemes in Writing

		Example Clinician-Child Interaction		
Level	Scaffolding	Beginning Phoneme Isolation	Phoneme Blending	Phoneme Segmentation
0 None	Question asked with no support provided	"We want to write the word *ball*. What is the first sound in *ball?*" [correct answer]	"So what I have I written? You tell me word, /b/-/r/-/ε/-/d/." [correct answer]	"You count the sounds in *man*. I am listening." [correct answer]
1 Low	Question asked with target sound stressed or word repeated	"What is the first sound in *ball?*" [first sound stressed] [correct answer] or [correct letter answer] "B is the letter. What is the sound?" [correct sound]	"So what I have I written? You tell me word, /b/-/r/-/ε/-/d/." [no answer] "Listen to the sounds: /b/-/r/-/ε/-/d/." [correct answer]	"You count the sounds in *man*. Get ready. Count the sounds in *man*." [slowly but not separated] [at least two sounds correct].
2 Moderate	Target sound stressed or word repeated plus another prompt	"What is the first sound in *ball?*" [wrong answer—/k/] "No, listen again, and watch my lips [points to mouth and repeats sound]: b-b-b-all?" [correct sound]	"/b/-/r/-/ε/-/d/" [no answer] "What have I written? /b/-/r/-/ε/-/d/." [wrong answer—beans] "Close, that starts with /b/. Listen again [onset-rime]: /br/-/ed/." [correct answer]	"You count the sounds in *man*. Get your fingers up and say it with me: /m/-/æ/-/n/." Instructor uses fingers and/or silent mouthing while child says each aloud. [at least two sounds correct]

Example Clinician-Child Interaction

Level	Scaffolding	Beginning Phoneme Isolation	Phoneme Blending	Phoneme Segmentation
3 High	Answer provided after prompting	"What is the first sound in b-b-ball?" [wrong answer—ball] "No, just the sound. Listen again, and watch my lips." [points and repeats sound] "b-b-ball?" [no answer] "It is /b/. You say /b/." [imitated answer]	"/b/-/r/-/ɛ/-/d/." [no answer] "What have I written? /b/-/r/-/ɛ/-/d/." [wrong answer—beans] "Close, that starts with /b/. Listen again [onset-rime]: /br/-/ed/." [no answer] "Bread, it is bread." [imitated answer]	After an effort at partial support with finger counting, sound prompting, and/or mouthing, instructor has child chant sounds in unison with instructor. [imitated answer]
4 Full	Question asked and answer provided with no prompting	"What is the first sound in ball?, say it with me: /b/." [imitated answer]	"What am I saying? /b/-/r/-/ɛ/-/d/" /b/-/r/-/ɛ/-/d/ is bread." [imitated answer]	"Let's count the sounds in man. Fingers up and say it with me: /m/-/æ/-/n/." [imitated answer]

Although none of these were fully correct, these were impressive performances that showed an emerging concept of segmenting phonemes. Children with language impairments can be expected to need more support for a longer period of time, but they too will learn these complex phonemic skills when provided ongoing scaffolding

With scaffolding deployed within a RISE format, developmentally challenging tasks such as phoneme isolation, phoneme blending, and phoneme segmentation can be taught to preschoolers and kindergartners. Repeated opportunities for intensely scheduled, systematically supported, explicit skill instruction within meaningful print activities, such as message writing, can lead to sizable gains in phonemic awareness. These gains in understanding may be demonstrated through increases in fully correct or partially correct performance in independent situations, or by decreases in the instructor scaffolding needed by the child to achieve correct performance.

Phonemic Referencing During Writing Activities

As has been discussed, SLPs can exploit the relationship between the development of spelling and phonemic awareness by using writing as a structural scaffold to develop preschoolers' and kindergartners' phonemic awareness. Children learn that spoken words are composed of a certain number of particular phonemes that can be isolated and manipulated. Letters are a visual representation that both assist in this task and reveal the purpose of isolating sounds from the speech stream. This section presents writing activities and procedures that teach phonemic awareness within this context.

Across a number of studies, Justice and colleagues (e.g., Justice, Skibbe, & Ezell, 2006) use the term *print referencing* to describe adults' intentional, explicit, repeated attention to print within a shared storybook reading. *Phonemic referencing*, also called sound talk, describes a similar approach but with speech sounds rather than with letters. Phonemic referencing can easily be applied within shared book reading and emergent writing activities (McFadden, 1998; Ukrainetz, 2006b); the latter context is focused on in this chapter. This approach to teaching phonemic awareness has four central features:

■ Phonemic awareness is taught *through* print, not before or separate from print instruction. Naturally occurring spelling is used as a context for talking about the sound structure of words. The SLP models conventional spelling, and children apply their level of emergent spelling.

■ Phoneme-level instruction occurs in a *horizontal* rather than a vertical skill arrangement. Young children experience guided interactions in isolating and matching beginning and ending phonemes, and segmenting and blending phonemes concurrently within a session.

■ Instruction provides an *explicit* skill focus with repeated opportunities for learning and practice of phonemic awareness. Phonemic awareness is the skill taught. Children's ideas, language, letter formation, spelling, and writing layout are accepted with little comment.

■ Systematic *scaffolding* occurs. Young children are scaffolded into competence across a range of task difficulties, with differential support matching developmental difficulty and child need. Scaffolding is provided at levels that ensure every child is challenged but not frustrated.

Teaching sounds through writing requires no commercial kits and no special materials. All that is needed is a message to write, paper, and pencil. Phonemic referencing in writing involves generating discourse to write, then writing it, with a lot of talk about speech sounds occurring during the writing. Writing can occur as SLP writing to child dictation or the child writing with SLP guidance. In both, the key element is a "think-aloud" process focused on phonemes that occurs before composing (e.g., "You want to write *Hello Mom*—let's count the sounds in *hello* first"), during composing (e.g., "You write *hello*. What is the first sound? What letter shall you write?"), and after composing (e.g., "You wrote *Hello Mom*. I hear the same sound at the beginning and the end of *Mom*. What is it?"). In the think-aloud process, repeated opportunities for learning and practice are required, but every word need not be discussed exhaustively. Fifteen opportunities can be provided by asking two pre-writing questions, then during composition, engaging in four beginning sounds, one middle sound, one ending sound, a blending item, and three sound segmentation items. After the writing process is concluded, the SLP can engage in three additional sound talk questions while re-reading the work.

There are many messages that can be written: a verse from a story just heard, a grocery list, a note to Dad, a story, or a picture caption. The message can be a self-contained writing activity or can be embedded in a larger event such as playing house. The actual product of writing, which may be simply a string of nonsense letters, is much less important than the process of referencing the sounds in words as they are represented on paper.

In these activities, children are encouraged to spell as best they can. This includes the use of invented spelling. Clarke's (1988) study of invented spelling in the classroom showed that this led to better word spelling and reading, in part by developing children's phonemic awareness. Children began to notice the sound composition of words as they searched for letter representations; teachers encouraged inventiveness but also modeled and guided conventional spelling. It should be noted that direct instruction in phonetic spelling is not recommended (Adams, 1990), despite Ehri and Wilce's (1987) beneficial experimental results. An analogy can be made to over-regularizing past tense (e.g., "runned"). Over-regularizing verbs is a positive temporary development that shows young children are attempting to talk about the past and thinking about the regularities of language. However, they must eventually deal with irregular verbs. While children are problem-solving through the inconsistencies of language, adults provide good models and support development. Spelling is the same. Emergent writing allows preschoolers and kindergartners to express themselves, to puzzle out the mysteries of spelling, and to have a visual tool for talking about sounds in words. Children actively struggle with the mysteries of spelling amidst good models and adult guidance that assist them toward conventional spelling.

Phonemic referencing can occur through three procedures: child dictation to the instructor, child emergent writing, and "kid writing" lessons. For *dictation*, the child tells his or her message to the instructor, who writes it down. In the example presented in Figure 7–2, the instructor is an SLP. To promote phonemic awareness through dictation, the SLP talks to the child about her thinking as she writes. She demonstrates how to be aware of sounds in words, isolating and segmenting phonemes for the purpose of writing. She elicits the child's assistance in this venture. In the example given, the SLP says /t/ /u/ as she writes *to*. The SLP elicits the child's isolation and segmentation of the phonemes in each word, such as asking what is the beginning sound in *zoo*. The SLP helps the child count the sounds of the words, using fingers to represent each

SLP:	Tell me what you want to say and I'll write it down.
John:	"I went to the zoo today."
SLP:	I /w̲-ɛ-n-t/ —what's the beginning sound I need?
John:	/w/.
SLP:	Yes, /w/. /w-ɛ-n-t̲/. What's the ending sound?
John:	/t/.
SLP:	Yes, /t/. Whew, four sounds in that word. That's lots to write. "To," /t/-/u/. That's easy, /t-t-t/ and /uuu/, just two sounds [writes them as says them]. "The zoo," /z/-/u/ [stretched out]. What's the beginning sound I need?
John:	/u/.
SLP:	Listen again, /zzz-u/.
John:	/z/.
SLP:	Yes, /z/. I like /z/ words—zoo, zebra, zoom. Then the ending sound?
John:	/u/.
SLP:	You got it—/u/. Last word, "today": /t/-/u/-/d/-/ai/. You count those sounds, fingers out.
John:	/t/-/u/-dai/. Three.
SLP:	Hmm . . . let me check. /t/-/u/-/d/-/ai/. I count four. /d/ /ai/ are two sounds. Four sounds, four letters. Hmm . . . it's written with five letters—oh well, sometimes spelling is strange. We wrote: "I went to the zoo today."

Figure 7–2. The clinician can take dictation from the child for phonemic referencing. (Adapted from Ukrainetz, T. A. [2006]. Scaffolding young children into phonemic awareness. In T. A. Ukrainetz [Ed.], *Contextualized language intervention* [pp. 454–455], Eau Claire, WI: Thinking Publications.)

phoneme. The SLP and the child then talk about the number of letters required.

With *emergent writing*, children write their own meaningful messages in a way that makes sense to them. Figure 7–3 shows a child's rendition of a football cheer that allowed talk about phonemes.

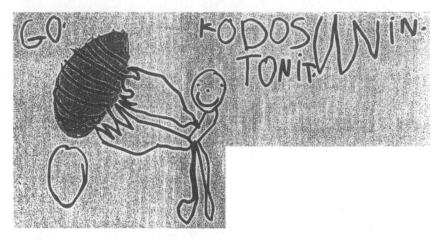

Figure 7–3. A 5-year-old's emergent writing of "Go Cowboys, win tonight!" as an example of source for phonemic referencing. (© Copyright 2006 by T. A. Ukrainetz.)

Figure 7–4 shows the SLP's comments as a child emergently writes. Unlike when the SLP writes to dictation, the spelling may not be correct. In a phonemic awareness lesson, the developmental spelling level of the child is acceptable, whether it is nonsense letters, phonetic, or conventional spelling. The emphasis in the lesson is not on correct sound-letter correspondence but on facilitating the child's awareness that words are composed of phonemes.

The amount and nature of sound talk from the clinician will vary with children's competence. Some children will need a lot of help and others little. Writing takes time, so an SLP can attend to two or three children for some sound talk time before they all complete their message. When a child finishes his message, the SLP can ask the child about his writing for a particular word, asking him to isolate or segment sounds, and compare his count with his number of letters. If the letters and sounds don't match (e.g., *bee* and /bi/), the SLP can comment that spelling doesn't always make sense.

A more structured way of teaching phonemic awareness through invented spelling is a *"kid writing" lesson* (L. M. McGee,

SLP:	What are you going to write?
John:	"I went to the zoo today."
SLP:	Okay, write that. How many sounds in the first word, "I"? [said short and quickly]
John:	One?
SLP:	Yes—I only hear one sound in "I."
John:	[Writes a P, then looks at SLP.]
SLP:	Good—one sound, one letter. What's next?
John:	"Went to the zoo." [Writes a nonsense string of letters.]
SLP:	Lots of letters for lots of sounds: "went to the zoo." How about "today"? What's the beginning sound?
John:	/t/. [Writes D.]
SLP:	Yes, "today" starts with /t/ sound. Better add some letters for the rest of the sounds in "today."

Figure 7–4. Phonemic referencing around a child's emergent message writing. (Modified slightly from McFadden, T. U. [1998]. Sounds and stories: Teaching phonemic awareness in print contexts. *American Journal of Speech-Language Pathology, 7,* 11. © 1998 by American Speech-Language-Hearing Association. Reprinted with permission.)

personal communication, February 12, 2004). This lesson bridges a group of children between self-directed invented spelling exploration and conventional writing. A group of children are directed to listen to the beginning and ending sounds in words while helping the teacher write (Figure 7-5). If correct and incorrect best spelling guesses are offered, the SLP validates the contributions but takes the correct answer (e.g., "Those are all good guesses, but T is the best guess").

In all cases, the SLP's writing expectations should fit the child's developmental level. While the SLP models correct spelling in his or her own writing, children should be encouraged to write

SLP:	What is the message we want to write for Valentine's Day?
Children:	"I love you."
SLP:	[Draws three lines on a strip of paper.] "I – love – you." [Pointing to each line.] Here are three spaces for those words. How should we write the first word, "I"? What sound do we hear?
Amari:	/ai/.
SLP:	Yes, /ai/. That's all. That's a very short word, just one sound. What letter should we use, Amari?
Amari:	A.
SLP:	A—one sound, one letter. "I love . . . ." Next is "love." John, what is the beginning sound in "love"?
John	/l/.
SLP:	/l/, yes. What letter should we use?
John:	L.
SLP	L—I will write that. Now listen for the ending sound. What is the ending sound in "love"?
Deepa:	/l/.
SLP:	/l/ is the beginning sound. Let's listen again: "lovvve." [drawn-out /v/]
John:	/v/.
Deepa:	/v/.
SLP:	/v/. What letter, Deepa?
Deepa:	I don't know.
SLP:	Use your best guess. This is kid writing. Kids can use their best guess to write sounds if they don't know.
Deepa:	B.
SLP:	I'll write that. Last word for "I love you": "you." What is the beginning sound?
Amari:	/j/—write a U.
SLP:	"You": /j/-/u/. There are two sounds. But we can write U for kid writing. One letter, two sounds. Now it is your turn to write "I love you" on your cards. Use your best guesses for each word—beginning and ending sounds.

Figure 7–5. The children can direct the writing for a "kid writing" lesson to promote phonemic referencing. (Adapted with permission from Ukrainetz, T. A. [2006]. Scaffolding young children into phonemic awareness. In T. A. Ukrainetz [Ed.], *Contextualized language intervention: Scaffolding preK–12 literacy achievement* [pp. 454–455]. Eau Claire, WI: Thinking Publications.)

as best they can. For children who are only at the level of nonsense letters, lining up the number of letters with the number of sounds is sufficient (e.g., TNX for *sun*). For children at the phonetic level of writing, alignment of a phoneme with a reasonable letter may be expected (e.g., /m/ can be written as N, but not A).

Children often are concerned about spelling and letter formation issues, particularly if the classroom environment has allowed only copying and correct spelling. An alphabet strip can be available to provide a model of how to form letters. Children who spell conventionally may ask for spellings or may criticize others who do not use such orthographic rules as LL, TH, or silent E. Correct spellings can be offered or accepted, but the SLP should emphasize that "kid writing" is readable and appropriate in this lesson. Spelling instruction will happen too, but not during this lesson. The objective is to keep an explicit skill focus on sound analysis, with spelling expectations matched to each child's individual level.

Intervention sessions can be brief single activities 4 or 5 times per week or longer sessions comprising three or four activities 2 or 3 times per week. In either format, teaching should occur across a variety of activities. Within a session or across sessions, the instructor or SLP can alternate phonemic referencing in message writing with other phonemic awareness activities, such as name talk, contrived games, and shared verse book reading (Ukrainetz, 2006b). Talking about the sounds in children's names provides brief transition activities (e.g., "Before we start reading this book, let's count the sounds in each of our names"). Contrived games with picture cards or objects, such as finding two picture cards that begin with the same sound, provide many opportunities to practice a single subskill such as matching beginning sounds. Shared book reading involves more dispersed practice opportunities, but with the benefit of a meaningful activity that shows the purpose for phonemic awareness. Engaging in periods of rhyme-alone instruction is not necessary or recommended, but rhyme can be embedded into phoneme instruction. The onset portion of a rhyme usually (but not always) is a single phoneme (e.g., *bad-sad-glad*), so beginning phoneme isolation is occurring when rhymes are identified. In addition, in verse books such as *Silly Sally* (Wood, 1992) or *Sheep in a Jeep* (Shaw, 1986), the rhyme and rhythm of the lines draw attention to the sounds of words. Like shared book reading, message writing provides a purposeful context for thinking about the sounds in words. As with the contrived games, many response opportunities can occur in a short period of time.

Of all of these activities, message writing is most naturally linked to phonemic awareness—the message writer must think about each sound of a word as letters are laboriously selected and formed. The important element in message writing is to talk about the sounds, not write in silence. In combination, name talk, contrived games, shared verse book reading, and message writing provide variety, interest, learning flexibility, and complementary advantages for phonemic awareness intervention.

Conclusion

An important component of early literacy programs is phonemic awareness, particularly for children with language impairment. Preschoolers and kindergartners can embark on phonemic awareness development in addition to gaining print knowledge through adult guidance within purposeful literacy activities. Emergent writing experiences can be used as a tool to promote attention to the sounds of speech, and children's efforts to invent spellings are particularly powerful in improving their awareness of the sounds of spoken words. For children with language impairment, repeated opportunities for scaffolding the explicitly presented skills of isolating, segmenting, and blending phonemes can occur around the formation of meaningful written messages. This contextualized skill approach teaches children not only how to manipulate phonemes but why all this talk about sounds in words is important, moving novice writers further along the road of literacy.

References

Adams, M. J. (1990). *Beginning to read*. Cambridge, MA: MIT Press.

Adams, M. J., Foorman, B. R., Lundberg, I., & Beeler, T. (1998). *Phonemic awareness in young children: A classroom curriculum*. Baltimore: Paul H. Brookes.

Anthony, J. L., Lonigan, C. J., Driscoll, K., Phillips, B. M., & Burgess, S. R. (2003). Phonological sensitivity: A quasi-parallel progression of word structure units and cognitive operations. *Reading Research Quarterly*, *38*, 470-487.

Apel, K., & Masterson, J. J. (2001). Theory-guided spelling assessment and intervention: A case study. *Language, Speech, and Hearing Services in Schools*, *32*, 182-196.

Apel, K., & Swank, L. K. (1999). Second chances: Improving decoding skills in the older student. *Language, Speech, and Hearing Services in Schools*, *30*, 231-242.

Baddeley, A. (1986). *Working memory*. Oxford: Oxford University Press.

Bear, D., Invernizzi, M., Templeton, S., & Johnston, F. (2000). *Words their way*. Upper Saddle River, NJ: Prentice-Hall.

Bryant, P. E., Bradley, L., Maclean, M., & Crossland, J. (1989). Nursery rhymes, phonological skills and reading. *Journal of Child Language*, *16*, 407-428.

Byrne, B., & Fielding-Barnsley, R. (1991). Evaluation of a program to teach phonemic awareness to young children. *Journal of Educational Psychology*, *83*, 451-455.

Camarata, S. M., Nelson, K. E., & Camarata, M. N. (1994). Comparison of conversational-recasting and imitative procedures for training grammatical structures in children with specific language impairment. *Journal of Speech and Hearing Research*, *37*, 1414-1423.

Catts, H. W., Fey, M. E., Zhang, X., & Tomblin, J. B. (2001). Estimating the risk of future reading difficulties in kindergarten children: A research-based model and its clinical implications. *Language, Speech, and Hearing Services in Schools*, *32*, 38-50.

Catts, H. W., & Kamhi, A. G. (2005). *Language and reading disabilities* (2nd ed.). Boston: Allyn & Bacon.

Chaney, C. (1992). Language development, metalinguistic skills, and print awareness in 3-year-old children. *Applied Psycholinguistics*, *13*, 485-514.

Clarke, L. K. (1988). Invented versus traditional spelling in first graders' writings: Effects on learning to spell and read. *Research in the Teaching of English*, *22*, 281-309.

Clay, M. (1975). *What did I write? Beginning writing behavior*. Portsmouth, NH: Heinemann.

Ehri, L. C., & Wilce, L. S. (1986). The influence of spellings on speech. In D. B. Yaden & S. Templeton (Eds.), *Metalinguistic awareness and beginning literacy* (pp. 101-113). Portsmouth, NH: Heinemann.

Ehri, L. C., & Wilce, L. S. (1987). Does learning to spell help beginners learn to read words? *Reading Research Quarterly*, *20*, 163-179.

Ehri, L. C., Nunes, S. R., Willows, D. M., Schuster, B. V., Yaghoub-Zadeh, Z., & Shanahan, T. (2001). Phonemic awareness instruction helps children learn to read: Evidence from the National Reading Panel's meta-analysis. *Reading Research Quarterly, 36,* 250–287.

Feuerstein, R. (1980). *Instrumental enrichment.* Baltimore: University Park Press.

Fox, B., & Routh, D. K. (1975). Analyzing spoken language into words, syllables, and phonemes: A developmental study. *Journal of Psycholinguistic Research, 4,* 331–342.

Gentry, J. R. (1978). Early spelling strategies. *Elementary School Journal, 79,* 88–92.

Gillam, R. B., Loeb, D. F., & Friel-Patti, S. (2001). Looking back: A summary of five exploratory studies of Fast ForWord. *American Journal of Speech-Language Pathology, 10,* 269–273.

Gillon, G. T. (2000). The efficacy of phonological awareness intervention for children with spoken language impairment. *Language, Speech, and Hearing Services in Schools, 31,* 126–141.

Gillon, G. T. (2004). *Phonological awareness: From research to practice.* New York: Guilford Press.

Girolametto, L., Pearce, P. S., & Weitzman, E. (1996). Interactive focused stimulation for toddlers with expressive vocabulary delays. *Journal of Speech and Hearing Research, 39,* 1263–1273.

Greenfield, P. M. (1984). A theory of the teacher in the learning activities of everyday life. In B. Rogoff & J. Lave (Eds.). *Everyday cognition: Its development in social context* (pp. 117–138). Cambridge, MA: Harvard University Press.

Hart, B., & Risley, T. (1975). Incidental teaching of language in the preschool. *Journal of Applied Behavior Analysis, 8,* 411–420.

Hildreth, G. (1936). Developmental sequences in name writing. *Child Development, 7,* 291–302.

International Reading Association (IRA) and National Association for the Education of Young Children (NAEYC). (1998). Learning to read and write: Developmentally appropriate practices for young children. *Young Children, 53*(4), 30–46.

Johnston, J. (1985). Fit, focus, and functionality: An essay on early language intervention. *Child Language Teaching and Therapy, 1,* 125–134.

Justice, L. M., Skibbe, L., & Ezell, H. (2006). Using print referencing to promote written language awareness. In T. A. Ukrainetz (Ed.), *Contextualized language intervention: Scaffolding preK–12 literacy achievement* (pp. 389–428). Eau Claire, WI: Thinking Publications.

Kaiser, A. P., Yoder, P. J., & Keetz, A. (1992). Evaluating milieu teaching. In S. F. Warren & J. Reichel (Eds.), *Communication and language inter-*

vention series: Vol. 1. Causes and effects in communication and language intervention (pp. 9–47). Baltimore: Paul H. Brookes.

Liberman, I. Y., Shankweiler, D., Fischer, F. W., & Carter, B. (1974). Explicit syllable and phoneme segmentation in the young child. *Journal of Experimental Child Psychology, 18,* 201–212.

Lidz, C. S., & Pena, E. D. (1996). Dynamic assessment: The model, its relevance as a nonbiased approach, and its application to Latino American preschool children. *Language, Speech, and Hearing Services in Schools, 27,* 367–372.

Lonigan, C. J., Burgess, S. R., Anthony, J. L., & Barker, T. A. (1998). Development of phonological sensitivity in two- to five-year-old children. *Journal of Educational Psychology, 90,* 294–311.

Maclean, M., Bryant, B., & Bradley, L., (1987). Rhymes, nursery rhymes, and reading in early childhood. *Merrill-Palmer Quarterly, 33,* 255–281.

McFadden, T. U. (1998). Sounds and stories: Teaching phonemic awareness in print contexts. *American Journal of Speech-Language Pathology, 7,* 5–13.

McGee, L. M. (2004, December). *The role of wisdom in evidence-based preschool literacy curriculum.* Paper presented at the Presidential address to the National Reading Conference, San Antonio, TX.

McGee, L. M., & Purcell-Gates, V. (1997). "So what's going on in research on emergent literacy?" *Reading Research Quarterly, 32,* 310–318.

McGee, L. M., & Richgels, D. J. (2004). *Literacy's beginnings: Supporting young readers and writers* (4th ed.). Boston: Pearson.

McLane, J. B., & McNamee, G. D. (1990). *Early literacy.* Cambridge, MA: Harvard University Press.

National Reading Panel. (2000). *Teaching children to read: An evidence-based assessment of the scientific research literature on reading and its implications for reading instruction.* Washington, DC: National Institute for Child Health and Human Development. Retrieved November 30, 2003, from: http:www.nichd.nih.gov/publications/nrp/fin dings.htm

Nuspl, J. J., & Ukrainetz, T. A. (2006). *Preschool phonemic awareness instruction with and without prior syllable training.* Presented at the Symposium on Research in Child Language Disorders, Madison, WI, June 2,3.

Pretti-Frontczak, K., & Bricker, D. (2004). *An activity-based approach to early intervention* (3rd ed.). Baltimore: Paul H. Brookes.

Read, C. (1971). Pre-school children's knowledge of English phonology. *Harvard Educational Review, 41,* 1–34.

Rice, M. L. (1995). The rationale and operating principles for a language-focused curriculum for preschool children. In M. L. Rice & K. A. Wilcox (Eds.), *Building a language-focused curriculum for the preschool classroom: Vol. 1, A foundation for lifelong communication* (pp. 27–38) Baltimore: Paul H. Brookes.

Richgels, D. J. (1995). Invented spelling ability and printed word learning in kindergarten. *Reading Research Quarterly, 30*, 96–109.

Richgels, D. J. (2001). Invented spelling, phonemic awareness, and reading and writing instruction. In S. B. Neuman & D. K. Dickinson (Eds.), *Handbook of early literacy research* (pp. 142–155). New York: Guilford Press.

Rogoff, B. (1990). *Apprenticeship in thinking: Cognitive development in social context*. New York: Oxford University Press.

Schneider, P., & Watkins, R. V. (1996). Applying Vygotskian developmental theory to language intervention. *Language, Speech, and Hearing Services in Schools, 27*, 157–170.

Shaw, N. (1986). *Sheep in a jeep*. Boston: Houghton Mifflin.

Teale, W. H., & Yokota, J. (2000). Beginning reading and writing: Perspectives on instruction. In D. S. Strickland & E. M. Morrow (Eds.), *Beginning reading and writing* (pp. 3–21). New York: Teachers College Press.

Torgesen, J. K., Al Otaiba, S., & Grek, M. L. (2005). Assessment and instruction for phonemic awareness and word recognition skills. In H. W. Catts & A. G. Kamhi (Eds.), *Language and reading disabilities* (pp. 127–156). Boston: Allyn & Bacon.

Torgesen, J. K., Alexander, A. W., Wagner, R. K., Rashotte, C. A., Voeller, K. K., & Conway, T. (2001). Intensive remedial instruction for children with severe reading disabilities. *Journal of Learning Disabilities, 34*, 33–58.

Ukrainetz, T. A. (2006a). Assessment and intervention within a contextualized skill framework. In T. A. Ukrainetz (Ed.), *Contextualized language intervention: Scaffolding preK–12 literacy achievement* (pp. 7–58). Eau Claire, WI: Thinking Publications.

Ukrainetz, T. A. (2006b). Scaffolding young children into phonemic awareness. In T. A. Ukrainetz (Ed.), *Contextualized language intervention: Scaffolding preK–12 literacy achievement* (pp. 429–468). Eau Claire, WI: Thinking Publications.

Ukrainetz, T. A., Cooney, M. H., Dyer, S. K., Kysar, A. J., & Harris, T. J. (2000). An investigation into teaching phonemic awareness through shared reading and writing. *Early Childhood Research Quarterly, 15*, 331–355.

Vygotsky, L. (1978). *Mind in society: The development of higher psychological processes*. Cambridge, MA: Harvard University Press.

Wagner, R. K., Torgesen, J. K., & Rashotte, C. A. (1994). Development of reading-related phonological processing abilities: New evidence of bidirectional causality from a latent variable longitudinal study. *Developmental Psychology, 30,* 73–87.

Wood, A. (1992). *Silly Sally.* San Diego, CA: Harcourt-Brace.

Wood, D., Bruner, J. S., & Ross, G. (1976). The role of tutoring in problem solving. *Journal of Child Psychology and Psychiatry, 17,* 89–100.

Chapter Eight

Integrating Phonological Sensitivity and Oral Language Instruction into Enhanced Dialogic Reading

A. Lynn Williams

Overview

Learning to read involves two related but interdependent skills: decoding and reading comprehension. Children must develop competency in both skills to be fluent and accurate readers, and early literacy interventions can systematically promote children's precursory decoding and reading comprehension skills, including phonological sensitivity and oral language. This chapter presents a modification of a shared book reading method that addresses both sets of precursors, termed the *Enhanced Dialogic Reading* (EDR) approach. This is an alternative format to train phonological sensitivity and oral language interactively within the dialogic reading approach.

To provide the basis for an understanding of both skills and their role in learning to read, the first part of the chapter describes domains of emergent literacy and presents a model of emergent literacy for guiding use of enhanced dialogic reading. The second part of the chapter describes shared storybook reading as an intervention context, with particular attention given to dialogic reading as a method to facilitate oral language skills. The third part describes intervention activities that focus on facilitating phonological sensitivity skills using play-based activities that are based on children's literature, and the fourth part addresses the rationale for training both decoding (phonological sensitivity) and comprehension skills (oral language) interactively. The final section discusses implementation of a program for training both phonological sensitivity and oral language in the EDR approach.

What Is Emergent Literacy?

Emergent literacy is a term used to indicate that literacy acquisition represents a continuum of skills, knowledge, and characteristics that ultimately lead to later reading and writing. This concept assumes that reading, writing, and oral language develop in tandem and are mutually supportive from an early age. It further assumes that these skills develop from children's interactions with adults in meaningful activities that involve talking and print but do not involve formal reading instruction.

Emergent literacy comprises three primary domains that are related to later reading and writing skills: oral language, print knowledge, and phonological processing. According to Lonigan (2003), these three skills form the foundation for the ease, rate, and proficiency with which children will learn to read and write once they begin kindergarten and first grade. In addition, preschool children's skills in these three domains can predict how well they will read in first grade. The focus of this chapter is on two of these domains—oral language and phonological processing—and readers are referred to Chapter 10 for strategies to support print knowledge.

Oral language is a crucial component of a child's reading success. It encompasses the vocabulary and language structures (syntactic and narrative) that are important in understanding the meaning of words, the structure of stories, and the concepts that are presented in stories. In essence, oral language helps children understand what is being read. Consequently, oral language is important in reading comprehension, but has no direct impact on decoding skills. However, vocabulary increases may facilitate phonological sensitivity indirectly in that they affect the segmental representation of the lexicon.

Phonological processing skills encompass several different abilities, including phonological memory, phonological access, and phonological sensitivity, and all refer to how the brain processes the phonological structures of language. Most readers are likely to be aware of the term *phonological awareness*, which describes the conscious attention to phonological structures, as expressed through rhyming and blending activities, for example. Some experts (e.g., Stanovich, 2000) prefer the term *phonological sensitivity* as a replacement for phonological awareness, because the former term precludes the need for an "awareness" of manipulations of phonological structures, as well may be the case when children detect rhyme patterns among words. According to Wagner and Torgesen (1987), phonological processing ability encompasses phonological awareness, or phonological sensitivity, and also includes coding of phonological information in working memory and retrieving phonological information from long-term memory. Figure 8–1 illustrates the division of abilities that comprise phonological processing skills.

Although all three components (phonological memory, access, and sensitivity) comprise phonological processing skills, almost all of the research in this area has focused on phonological sensitivity. It is this component of phonological processing skills that is addressed in this chapter.

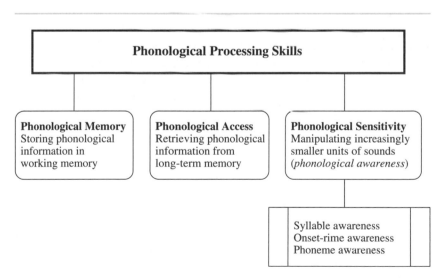

Figure 8–1. Components of phonological processing skills.

Inside-Out and Outside-In Processes

Whitehurst and Lonigan (1998) described the components of emergent literacy as comprising two interdependent sets of processes referred to as *outside-in* and *inside-out* processes—terms that help describe how these components develop, influence each other, and result in learning to read.

The inside-out processes represent the child's understanding of the rules for translating print into the appropriate sounds and for coming to understand the alphabetic principle. It represents the decoding aspect of reading. The inside-out processes include the child's knowledge and understanding of letters (alphabet knowledge), sound structures (phonological sensitivity), the relationship between letters and sounds (alphabetic knowledge), print units and organization (print awareness), and the cognitive strategies incorporated by the child to help him or her actually read. Thus, components of inside-out skills include alphabet knowledge, phonological sensitivity, alphabetic knowledge, and print awareness.

The outside-in processes involve children's understanding of what they read. These processes represent the child's knowledge of the world, semantic knowledge, and narrative knowledge. The outside-in processes allow the child to understand the sentence concepts and the context in which these concepts are occurring. Components of emergent literacy that are considered to be outside-in processes include language skills—specifically, vocabulary knowledge, syntactic knowledge, and narrative understanding.

Both inside-out and outside-in processes are related to reading development, but at different points in the reading acquisition process. Inside-out emergent literacy skills are critically important in the earliest stage of learning to read when the focus is on decoding text. At least for some children, these skills must be explicitly taught so that they emerge in a timely manner. Outside-in emergent literacy skills (language) may play a greater role in the stage at which children begin to read more complex text for meaning and pleasure than in the initial stage of learning to decode. These two domains of emergent literacy are summarized in Table 8–1.

Table 8–1. Two Domains of Emergent Literacy: Inside-Out and Outside-In Processes

	Inside-Out Processes	*Outside-In Processes*
Description	Represents children's knowledge of the rules for translating print into sounds	Represents children's knowledge of the world, semantic knowledge, and narrative knowledge
Emergent literacy components	Phonological sensitivity Alphabet knowledge Print awareness	Oral language
Relation to Reading	Decoding	Comprehension
Facilitating activities	▪ Requires explicit teaching – Phonological awareness – Alphabet knowledge – Print knowledge	▪ Language and print-rich environment ▪ Meaningful adult-child interactions ▪ Shared storybook reading

Source: Adapted from G. J. Whitehurst and C. J. Lonigan [1998]. Child development and emergent literacy. *Child Development, 69*, 848–872.

Shared Storybook Reading as an Intervention Context for Emergent Literacy

Shared storybook reading provides one intervention context for facilitating the outside-in emergent literacy process of oral language. To heighten its focus to improve emergent literacy skills, shared storybook reading expands from simply reading a story to a child to a more interactive reading activity that recruits children's active participation and exposure to important language concepts and structures. Although shared storybook reading has been used largely for facilitating language skills, including vocabulary skills (Anderson-Yockel & Haynes, 1994; Lonigan & Whitehurst, 1998) and increased participation in the book reading activity (McDonnell, Friel-Patti, &

Rollins, 2003), other aspects of emergent literacy have been targeted in numerous studies, including print awareness (Justice & Ezell, 2000; Whitehurst, Crone, Zevenbergen, Schultz, Velting, & Fischel, 1999; Whitehurst, Epstein, Angell, Payne, Crone, & Fischel, 1994) and phonemic awareness (McFadden, 1998). These studies suggest that the interactive strategies adults incorporate into their shared reading interactions with children can significantly improve a range of emergent literacy abilities.

Morgan and Goldstein (2002) listed several benefits of shared storybook reading, including the following:

- Ease of implementation
- Value as a widely accepted form of teaching
- Repetitive modeling for the child
- Targeting of multiple skills
- Ease of monitoring treatment outcomes
- Facilitation of positive interaction patterns for adult and child

There are two primary approaches to using shared storybook reading as an approach for heightening children's oral language abilities: specific commenting and dialogic reading. Although the two approaches are similar, *specific commenting* has a more narrow focus on facilitating decontextualized language through specific comments. This approach has been shown to be effective in engaging children in abstract thinking and promoting language and interaction during adult and child storybook reading (Hockenberger, Goldstein, & Haas, 1999).

Dialogic reading was developed by Whitehurst and his colleagues (Arnold, Lonigan, Whitehurst, & Epstein, 1994; Lonigan & Whitehurst, 1998; Valdez-Menchaca & Whitehurst, 1992; Whitehurst, Falco, Lonigan, Fischel, Valdez-Menchaca, & Caulfield, 1988; Whitehurst & Lonigan, 1998) to focus more broadly on language skills, especially vocabulary. The dialogic reading approach was designed to increase children's language development based on appropriate scaffolded interactions between the adult and child during interactive book-reading. According to Crain-Thoreson and Dale (1999), dialogic reading provides a systematic approach for parents or teachers to use to engage their children in discussions about the text. In this approach, the role of the child as a passive listener is shifted to a more active one by the adult incorporating specific question strategies and interaction strategies.

The specific question strategies consist of five different types of prompts or questions for the adult to incorporate while reading a book: completion, recall, open-ended, "Wh-" questions, and distancing questions, represented by the acronym CROWD. These are detailed in Table 8–2. When using these prompts and questions, the adult follows the child's answers with additional questions and provides a model if the child requires it.

The specific interaction strategies provide a framework for adults to interact with the child while discussing the story. These strategies are used to prompt the child to respond to the book, evaluate the child's response, expand the child's response, and repeat the initial prompt to check the child's learning, represented

Table 8–2. Descriptions and Examples of CROWD Questions (Based on Lonigan and Whitehurst, 1998)

CROWD Questions	Example*
Completion questions request a "fill-in" response that can be used to ask questions about the structure of language used in the book.	"The cow said 'Cock-a-doodle- _____ [moo].'"
Recall questions relate to the story content of the book.	"Do you remember how the rooster taught the cow to crow?"
Open-ended questions are used to increase the amount of talk about a book and to focus on the details of the book.	"What is happening on this page?"
Wh- questions are used to teach new vocabulary.	"What does 'crowing' mean?"
Distancing questions help the child bridge the material in the book to real-life experiences.	"How do you think the cow felt about all the animals laughing at her?"

*Examples are based on shared reading of *Cock-A-Doodle-Moo!* by Bernard Most.

by the acronym PEER (see Table 8–3). Sophisticated responses are encouraged by expanding on the child's utterances and increasing the complexity of the questions asked by the adult. When using CROWD and PEER strategies, the adult uses both praise and encouragement to scaffold children's active engagement and participation.

The CROWD and PEER strategies for the dialogic reading approach have been used in studies with both teachers and parents to facilitate children's vocabulary, language, and literacy (Crain-Thoreson & Dale, 1999; Justice & Ezell, 2000; Lonigan & White-hurst, 1998; Valdez-Menchaca & Whitehurst, 1992; Whitehurst et al., 1994). Collectively, these studies demonstrate that the dialogic reading approach has several benefits. Adults can check for children's understanding of vocabulary through questions and build on vocabulary through the use of the book's illustrations; adults can create links from the children's personal experiences and relate them back to the story; and the repetition and expansion of words and concepts facilitate children's language acquisition. Studies consistently show that participation in dialogic reading sessions for an extended period, either in one-on-one reading sessions or in small groups, improves children's receptive and expressive vocabulary skills and their grammatical complexity as measured by mean length of utterance (MLU).

Table 8–3. Descriptions and Examples of PEER Interaction Strategies (Based on Lonigan and Whitehurst, 1998)

PEER Interaction Strategy	Example
Prompt or initiation by adult for the child to respond to the book	"What is the cow doing?"
Evaluate the child's response	"You're right. She is waking up the pigs."
Expand the child's response	"The pigs woke up and they're laughing at the cow."
Repeat the initial question to check that the child understands the new learning	[Reading the book the next time] "What is the cow doing? Do you remember?"

Training Phonological Sensitivity Skills Using Children's Books

Phonological sensitivity, as noted previously, includes the ability to manipulate increasingly smaller units of sounds; these units include syllables, intrasyllabic structures (onset, rime), and phonemes. Examples of these different levels of phonological sensitivity are provided in Table 8–4, along with different tasks used to assess or train each level.

A number of studies have shown the importance of phonological sensitivity to children's acquisition of reading and spelling, particularly with regard to the decoding skills necessary for conventional literacy (see Lonigan, Burgess, & Anthony, 2000). Specifically, phonological sensitivity, along with letter knowledge, is consistently shown to be the most robust independent predictor of decoding skills from preschool to late kindergarten/early first grade. It is not surprising, then, that educators of young children have looked for guidance in the instruction of phonological sensitivity skills. Concerns such as the following are common:

- What type of instruction is appropriate?
- How much time should be devoted to these activities?
- How are these instructional activities developed and implemented?

Depending on the approach selected, the answers will vary but tend to fall into one of two categories: (1) structured activities and (2) play-based activities. Both current evidence and my own clinical experience support the use of a play-based approach that will, in part, draw upon the structure provided by storybooks—a context that has been shown to provide facilitating effects for both oral language skills (e.g., Whitehurst et al., 1988) and emergent literacy skills (e.g., Justice & Ezell, 2002).

What Type of Instruction Is Appropriate?

Although structured instructional activities have been shown to be effective in individual and small-group settings, they often are not practical for classroom-based instruction involving relatively larger

Table 8–4. Levels of Phonological Sensitivity with Examples of Sound Manipulation Tasks

Level of Phonological Sensitivity	Example/Tasks of Sound Manipulation
Syllable awareness	1. Compound word segmentation (*cowboy* = "cow" + "boy") 2. Syllable segmentation (*doggy* = [da] + [gi]) 3. Syllable deletion (*sandwich* – "sand" = "wich") 4. Syllable counting ("How many beats are in the word 'dinosaur'?")
Onset-rime awareness	1. Rhyme identification ("Do these words rhyme: *fish dish?*") 2. Rhyme generation ("What rhymes with 'cat'?") 3. Onset-rime segmentation (*cat* = /k/ + /æt/)
Phoneme awareness	1. Sound matching ("Which word starts with the same sound as *cat*: 'fish,' 'cow,' 'shoe'?") 2. Sound identification ("What sound is at the beginning of 'dog'?") 3. Sound segmentation (*cat* = /k/ + /æ/ + /t/) 4. Sound deletion (*sand* – /s/ = "and") 5. Sound blending (/d/ + /a/ + /g/ = *dog*) 6. Sound substitution (change the /k/ in "cat" to /b/ = "bat")

numbers of children. Rather, songs, chants, and word-sound games provide an option for a less structured and more play-based approach that can be used in large-group contexts. These enticing activities are ideally suited for developing young children's sensitivity to the sound structure of language (Yopp & Yopp, 2000). Yopp (1992) has suggested that the more playful, gamelike, and amusing the activity, the better. She maintains that phonological awareness instruction should be playful, engaging, interactive, and social in stimulating curiosity and experimentation with language.

How Much Time Should Be Devoted to Instruction?

Actually, in providing phonological sensitivity training, more is not necessarily better. The training studies reviewed by the National Reading Panel (2000) found that studies in which only moderate amounts of time were spent teaching phonological sensitivity (i.e., 5 to 18 hours) resulted in greater effect sizes than were observed in studies involving longer periods of instruction (i.e., 20 to 75 hours). According to Ehri (2004), instruction on phonological sensitivity does not need to be extensive in order to have its greatest impact on reading outcomes. Yopp and Yopp (2000) stated that durations of 10 to 30 minutes per session daily for two to three times per week for a minimum of three weeks up to 2 years have been reported in the research literature; however, these investigators caution that the quality of instruction and the responsiveness of instruction to the children in the classroom should be given greater consideration than the amount of time.

How Do You Develop and Implement Instructional Activities?

A number of factors should be considered in designing and implementing instructional activities to increase children's phonological sensitivity. The following compilation of general guidelines is based on research findings related to the development of instructional activities (Ehri, 2004; Gillon, 2004; Yopp & Yopp, 2000).

- ■ Choose instructional activities that are developmentally appropriate.
- ■ Provide instruction that is explicit and intentional.

■ The level of awareness (i.e., word, syllable, onset-rime, or phoneme) needs to be considered, as well as the type of manipulation (i.e., identification, segmentation, blending, deletion, matching).

  ■ Word and syllable levels require less direct instruction than phoneme analysis.

  ■ Instruction at the syllable level has little effect on manipulation at the phoneme level, although the reverse is evident.

  ■ Teaching phoneme blending and segmentation skills produces greater benefits in reading outcomes.

■ Instructional activities may focus on skill mastery of one phoneme level skill at a time, such as phoneme blending, until the children master it (*skill mastery approach*) or a range of tasks may be addressed at one time to increase sensitivity to a range of phonological units (*multiple-skill approach*).

  ■ Studies show both approaches to be beneficial, but the latter may be more efficient.

■ Phonological sensitivity is facilitated when letters (and letter-sound pairings) are integrated into instructional activities.

■ Phonological sensitivity should be embedded within a broader literacy program.

■ Individual or small-group instruction may be needed for children considered to be at risk or low achievers.

Appendix 8–A includes a collection of activities available to train phonological sensitivity drawn from the education literature, much from the work of Yopp (1992; Yopp & Yopp, 2000). The activities are based on children's books and are organized by the particular skill being trained. Extension activities also are described to expand the story and provide additional phonological sensitivity training. Participation in these activities will encourage children's curiosity about language and their experimentation with it. Yopp (1992) lists several recommendations for implementing the activities, including that the activities should be playful and fun in helping the children develop positive feelings toward learning. Accordingly, drill and rote memorization should be avoided. She also cautions to allow for and be prepared for individual differences in children's abilities to catch on to these phonological sensitivity activities.

Some children will catch on quickly, others will show an emerging understanding of the relationship between the sounds in the activities and their use in speech, and still others will find the activities completely nonsensical but delightful. Finally, these activities do not serve as diagnostic tools, so judgments about individual children's abilities should be avoided. Clinicians should strive to make the tone of the activities fun and informal, rather than evaluative. The activities included in Appendix 8-A can be used within the EDR approach presented in the final section of this chapter.

Why Train Both Oral Language and Phonological Sensitivity?

Lonigan (2003) reported that the results of several multivariate studies examining the prediction of reading skills indicate that emergent literacy skills (i.e., oral language, print knowledge, phonological sensitivity) are modular. That is, oral language intervention will not have a direct effect on decoding or its precursors. Likewise, phonological sensitivity intervention will not result in an increase in oral language skills. Therefore, both aspects need to be addressed simultaneously in order to facilitate the precursors to decoding and reading comprehension required for conventional literacy. Figure 8–2 illustrates the modularity of emergent literacy skills and represents the role of oral language and phonological sensitivity in reading. As shown in the figure, oral language intervention directly affects reading comprehension, whereas phonological sensitivity intervention directly affects decoding skills. The dashed arrow between oral language and phonological sensitivity reflects the possibility that phonological sensitivity may be facilitated indirectly through increased vocabulary development. Reading comprehension and decoding constitute the two skills necessary for conventional literacy, as indicated by their containment within the larger arrow linking these skills to literacy acquisition.

The effect of combining oral language intervention with phonological sensitivity intervention and print knowledge intervention was summarized by Lonigan (2003). In this study, three interventions were implemented separately. Oral language intervention utilized dialogic reading or typical shared reading; phonological

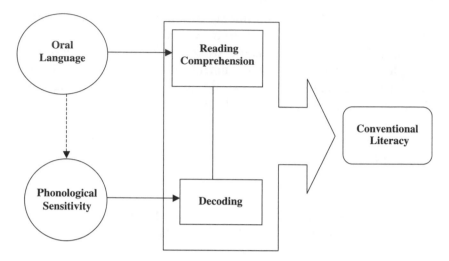

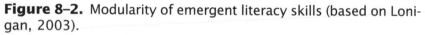

Figure 8–2. Modularity of emergent literacy skills (based on Lonigan, 2003).

sensitivity intervention focused on blending and segmenting skills; and print knowledge intervention focused on teaching letter names and letter sounds to children. Although all interventions were effective for the domain trained, there were no interaction effects, which suggested that combining treatments did not have a synergistic effect across domains. An important point of the combined interventions is that each intervention was implemented independently of the others. The following section describes an EDR approach in which phonological sensitivity intervention is combined with oral language intervention simultaneously.

How to Integrate Phonological Sensitivity Training and Oral Language in an Enhanced Dialogic Reading Approach

This section describes a 5-week parent training program that was implemented in a preschool program for children from low-income families (Davis, 2004). This book reading program emphasized use of strategies to improve both oral language and phonological sensitivity. The EDR approach was based on the dialogic reading approach described by Whitehurst and his colleagues (e.g., Arnold et al., 1994; Whitehurst et al., 1994; Whitehurst et al., 1988; Whitehurst & Lonigan, 1998) but differed with regard to both intensity and focus. Typically, training in dialogic reading involves viewing a 20-minute videotape (Whitehurst, 1992), along with role playing that is provided in two short 30-minute instructional sessions.

For EDR training, parents met for 90-minute sessions for 5 weeks. The weekly training sessions were developed to provide the parents with instruction on the dialogic reading strategies using CROWD and PEER, as well as information on phonological sensitivity. The latter included addressing its importance and role in literacy acquisition, different tasks and activities related to phonological sensitivity, and facilitation of children's phonological sensitivity through dialogic reading activities. Thus, parents were trained to use interactive reading strategies simultaneously with phonological sensitivity training.

The major difference between the EDR approach and dialogic reading was the modification of the CROWD questions to train phonological sensitivity. CROWD questions were modified in the EDR approach to address the different levels of phonological sensitivity (e.g., rhyme identification, rhyme generation, sound awareness, sound substitution) and print knowledge (tracking, print awareness). In Table 8–5, examples of CROWD questions used to train phonological sensitivity and print knowledge with EDR for *The Hungry Thing* are compared with the typical CROWD questions used with the dialogic reading approach. As can be seen in the emphasis on phonological sensitivity of the CROWD questions in EDR, focus on oral language is indirect and largely is encountered through the reading of the books, with some questioning directed at vocabulary and conceptual knowledge.

The focus of each week of the EDR training is summarized in Table 8–6. Notice that the first two weeks focused solely on CROWD and PEER strategies, similar to the dialogic reading approach. Information and training on phonological sensitivity was not introduced until week 3. This gave the parents time to learn the interactive reading strategies before they were presented with a new training strategy for them to incorporate into their weekly book reading activities. Two weeks were devoted to discussions about phonological sensitivity and print knowledge (weeks 3 and 4).

Table 8–5. CROWD Questions to Train Phonological Sensitivity and Print Knowledge: Enhanced Dialogic Reading Versus Dialogic Reading*

CROWD Question Type	Dialogic Reading	Enhanced Dialogic Reading
Completion question	"The Hungry Thing pointed to a sign that said ____ [feed me]."	"'Shmancakes' sounds like 'fancakes' sounds like ____ [pancakes]." "'Foodles' rhymes with ____ [noodles]."
Recall question	"Do you remember who tried to guess what the Hungry Thing wanted to eat?"	"Do you remember what words rhyme with 'gollipops'?"
Open-ended question	"What is happening on this page?"	"How did the little boy always know what the Hungry Thing wanted to eat?"
Wh- question	"What does 'dine' mean?"	"'Thread' rhymes with 'bread'; what is 'thread'?" "Point to a word on this page." "Where would you start reading on this page?"
Distancing question	"When you get hungry, what do you eat?"	"Tell the Hungry Thing what your favorite snack is." "How would you ask the Hungry Thing if he wanted some 'candy'?"

*Examples from *The Hungry Thing* by Jan Slepian and Ann Seidler.

Table 8–6. Weekly Topics in the EDR Parent Training Program

Week	Focus
Week 1	• Introduction and description of dialogic reading approach • CROWD and PEER strategies • Book and activities for the week
Week 2	• Review of shared book reading (CROWD/PEER) • Two additional strategies (slow down and help child as needed) • Book and activities for the week
Week 3	• Phonological sensitivity skills (rhyming, sound matching, isolation, substitution, deletion, and segmentation) • Book and activities for the week
Week 4	• Print knowledge (print tracking; print awareness) • Book and activities for the week
Week 5	• Wrap-up and review (CROWD/PEER strategies; phonological sensitivity; print knowledge) • Book and activities for the week

The final week provided a review of all of the concepts for which training was provided.

A variety of activities were included to present, demonstrate, and review the information each week as an effective way to reinforce the new concepts with the parents, and to facilitate successful application at home with their children. The specificity, focus, and redundancy of the training supported the parents' new learning, which also promoted group cohesion, a sense of understanding and accomplishment, compliance with implementing the home program, and high parental attendance throughout the 5-week training program. The structure of each weekly session was as follows:

■ Review of previous week's book and home activities for parents to report what worked well, as well as what did not work well, with staff response to any questions or concerns [15 minutes]

- Overview of the night's topic [5 minutes]
- Presentation of new information for that week [15 minutes]
- Demonstration videotape of a parent and child reading the selected book for the week using CROWD questions to guide parents in their own readings at home [5 minutes]
- Snack break [15 minutes]
- Distribution of new book with a handout of sample CROWD questions, with corresponding page numbers that were specific to the assigned book for the week [10 minutes]
- Role-play with and between groups of parents to practice reading the assigned book with the sample questions [15 minutes]
- Question-and-answer period (although questions were encouraged throughout the session) [10 minutes]

The books used in the EDR program were selected to address a specific aspect of phonological sensitivity that was targeted each week. Each book had a high density of rhyming words that were used throughout the stories in different ways. For example, *The Hungry Thing* uses rhymes as the way the little boy translated what the Hungry Thing wanted to eat (i.e., "*tickles* sound like *sickles* sound like *pickles*"). When the townspeople try to communicate with the Hungry Thing, they have to say nonsense words that rhyme with the actual word (i.e., "Have some *smello*"). *The Cow That Went Oink* provides frequent opportunities for sound awareness and sound manipulation training, as the cow that oinks practices many times before she finally learns to moo from the pig that moos ("oink—moink—moinkoo—moonk—mook—moo"). The other farm animals' laughter at the cow and pig also offers sound awareness opportunities, as children hear how sounds in words represent the way the different animals laugh (e.g., "quack-ha," "meow-ha," "baa-ha," "cheep-ha"). *The Disappearing Alphabet* incorporates rhymes as well as sound deletions as part of talking about each of the alphabet letters (e.g., "What if there were no letter A? Cows would eat HY instead of HAY"). *Cock-A-Doodle-Moo!* uses sound substitutions and rhyming as the cow who learns to crow in order to wake the farm animals from the rooster who has laryngitis (e.g., "mock-a-moodle-moo," "sock-a-noodle-moo," "rock-a-poodle-moo," "clock-a-doodle-moo," and finally "cock-a-doodle-moo").

In addition to the books, toys were used to supplement and extend the play from each book. Toys were included to provide another context for the story. Kaderavek and Sulzby (1998) suggest that different book reading strategies, such as playing with toys, are important to foster a family's individual style of reading and enjoying the story. Parents were encouraged to extend the activities with the toys by using some of the activities described in Appendix 8–A for phonological sensitivity intervention related to the specific books used in this parent training. For example, the plastic food and paper bags may be used to extend the story of *The Hungry Thing*. The parent and the child can take turns looking into the bag and naming a food item, such as "Ah, mogurt! I love mogurt!" and the child (or parent) can guess what "mogurt" is. Parents reported that the toys extended the children's play related to the stories or provided an alternative to reading if the child was not interested. Table 8–7 lists the books, corresponding toys, and specific aspect of phonological sensitivity that were targeted.

Table 8–7. Books, Toys, and Specific Aspects of Phonological Sensitivity Targeted

Book	Toys	Phonological Sensitivity Target
Cock-A-Doodle-Moo by Bernard Most	Plastic farm animals	Sound substitution and rhyming
The Hungry Thing by Jan Slepian and Ann Seidler	Plastic food	Rhyming and sound substitution
The Cow that Went Oink by Bernard Most	Plastic farm animals	Sound awareness and sound manipulation (addition, deletion)
The Disappearing Alphabet by Richard Wilbur	Plastic or magnetic alphabet letters	Print awareness, alphabet knowledge, and rhyming
Henny Penny by Paul Galdone	Plastic farm animals	Rhyming

Every week, parents were given sample EDR CROWD questions for each book to support their use and success in implementing this approach during home reading activities. Handouts with sample questions were provided for each CROWD question type, along with the page number that corresponded to the specific question. This type of explicit instruction was important in supporting the parents' learning of two new skills simultaneously (interactive reading strategies plus phonological sensitivity training).

To provide an accessible resource for the CROWD questions and PEER interaction strategies, parents were given a bookmark in the first session that summarized CROWD on one side and PEER on the other side, to remind them to use these strategies during the shared reading activities. At the end of each session, a weekly log was given to the parents to report the frequency and type of questions asked, number of times the book was read during the week, and whether the toys were used to extend the play or theme of the book. Parents were encouraged to ask a minimum of 10 questions but no more than 25 questions in order to avoid the child's "tuning out" from excessive questioning.

The effectiveness of this brief but focused parent training program using EDR was reported by Williams and Coutinho (2003). Videotapes of parents reading to their children made before and after the 5-week training program revealed that the parents significantly increased their initiations (questioning) and responses during shared storybook reading. In fact, dramatic changes were observed from the parents' initial readings, which typically involved reading the book from cover to cover with little or no interaction with their children beyond simple pointing or single-word responses to questions. Corresponding with the parents' increase in questions/responses, it was not surprising that the children demonstrated a significant increase in their number of responses during shared storybook readings. Pre- and post-testing also revealed improvement in the children's preliteracy skills, as measured by Phonological Awareness Literacy Screening: PreK (Invernizzi, Sullivan, & Meier, 2001), as well as an increase in their mean length of utterance (MLU) based on 20-minute language samples. Therefore, EDR was effective in training parents to use dialogic reading strategies to facilitate phonological sensitivity, which, in turn, led to an increase in the children's language and phonological sensitivity in a short time period.

Two follow-up studies revealed that the parents continued to use dialogic reading strategies with their children 6 months after the EDR training (Adams, Davis, Norby, Rothrock, Williams, & Coutinho, 2004) and even 18 months after the training when their children were enrolled in first grade (Chalk, Eggers, King, Rouse, Williams, & Coutinho, 2005).

In summary, the EDR approach provided a robust training program to facilitate oral language and phonological sensitivity skills in young children. Although parents were targeted in this training, effective intervention agents with the EDR approach also may include teachers, teacher aides, speech-language pathologists (SLPs), reading resource specialists, and community volunteers.

Some Caveats and Concluding Considerations

As presented in this chapter, shared storybook reading is an effective context to train a variety of language and emergent literacy skills that also is becoming more commonly used by SLPs for providing language intervention. A number of advantages and benefits of shared book-reading were discussed in this chapter, including the positive effects of EDR on children's literacy and language skills, but it is also important to consider some possible negative factors. Scarborough and Dobrich (1994) and Kaderavek and Justice (2002) discussed the fact that some children have a negative attitude toward books and do not like to participate in book reading activities. Kaderavek and Justice reported that about 10% of typically developing children do not like being read to and that this percentage is likely to be much higher among children with language impairment. Forcing children to participate in activities they do not enjoy can result in a negative response toward book reading that Scarborough and Dobrich called the "broccoli effect," in which people become more negatively disposed toward acts they don't enjoy by virtue of being asked to do them. The use of toys, as described in this EDR approach, may provide a better context for training with less time spent interacting and training with the books. Perhaps through positive and fun play-based interactions related to books that encourage and maintain the child's interest, a greater interest in book reading may be developed.

The parent's style of book reading (or that of any intervention agent) is another factor to be considered in shared storybook reading activities. Kaderavek and Justice (2002) discuss strategies to facilitate adult-child interactions during reading that are important considerations, including being sensitive to the child's responsiveness to different types of interaction. In the EDR training program, it was important to stress with some parents not to flood their child with too many questions during the book-reading sessions. Too many questions not only detracted from the flow of the story but also resulted in the interactions becoming interrogating contexts rather than training contexts.

This chapter has highlighted the importance of the distinction between decoding and comprehension in the integration of phonological sensitivity training and oral language within the EDR approach. Nation and Snowling (2004) point out another important distinction between decoding and word recognition: For children to become efficient readers, they must be able to do more than decode words. Specifically, children need to acquire a word recognition system that is automatized. This automatic retrieval of word pronunciations from letter strings is necessary to develop reading fluency for words that have irregular spelling-sound mappings and to be able to read effortlessly and fluently. Development of word recognition is independent of the decoding skills of phonological sensitivity and is influenced by broader aspects of oral language skills, including vocabulary and comprehension. The available evidence not only supports the importance of a variety of skills required for reading, but also underscores the simplicity of dichotomous models of reading, development into decoding and language skills to adequately represent the complexities that are involved in developing fluent, efficient, and accurate reading.

References

Adams, M., Davis, T., Norby, J., Rothrock, W., Williams, A. L., & Coutinho, M. (2004). *A shared storybook parent reading program for low-income preschoolers.* Poster presentation at the annual convention of the American Speech-Language-Hearing Association, Philadelphia.

Anderson-Yockel, J., & Haynes, W. O. (1994). Joint book-reading strategies in working-class African American and white mother-toddler dyads. *Journal of Speech and Hearing Research, 37,* 583–593.

Arnold, D. H., Lonigan, C. J., Whitehurst, G. J., & Epstein, J. N. (1994). Accelerating language development through picture book reading: Replication and extension to a videotape training format. *Journal of Educational Psychology, 86,* 235–243.

Chalk, K., Eggers, T., King, N., Rouse, J., Williams, A. L., & Coutinho, M. (2005). *Enhanced dialogic reading intervention: A follow-up study.* Poster presentation at the annual convention of the American Speech-Language-Hearing Association, San Diego, CA.

Crain-Thoreson, C., & Dale, P. (1999). Enhancing performance: Parents and teachers as book reading partners for children with language delays. *Topics in Early Childhood Special Education, 19,* 28–39.

Davis, S. E. (2004). *An enhanced dialogic reading approach to facilitate typically developing preschool children's emergent literacy skills.* Unpublished master's thesis, East Tennessee State University, Johnson City, TN.

Ehri, L. C. (2004). Teaching phonemic awareness and phonics. In P. McCardle & V. Chhabra (Eds.), *The voice of evidence in reading research* (pp. 153–186). Baltimore: Paul H. Brookes.

Galdone, P. (1968). *Henny Penny.* New York: Clarion Books.

Gillon, G. T. (2004). *Phonological awareness: From research to practice.* New York: Guilford Press.

Hockenberger, E. H., Goldstein, H., & Haas, L. S. (1999). Effects of commenting during joint book reading by mothers with low SES. *Topics in Early Childhood Special Education, 19,* 15–27.

Invernizzi, M., Sullivan, A., & Meier, J. (2001). *Phonological awareness literacy screening—pre-kindergarten.* Charlottesville, VA: Curry School of Education.

Justice, L. M., & Ezell, H. K. (2000). Enhancing children's print and word awareness through home-based parent intervention. *American Journal of Speech-Language Pathology, 9,* 257–269.

Kaderavek, J., & Justice, L. M. (2002). Shared storybook reading as an intervention context: Practices and potential pitfalls. *American Journal of Speech-Language Pathology, 11,* 395–406.

Kaderavek, J. N., & Sulzby, E. (1998). Parent-child joint book reading: An observational protocol for young children. *American Journal of Speech-Language Pathology, 7,* 33–43.

Lonigan, C. J. (2003). *Development and promotion of emergent literacy: An evidence-based perspective.* Invited session at the annual convention of the American Speech-Language-Hearing Association, Chicago.

Lonigan, C. J., Burgess, S. R., & Anthony, J. L. (2000). Development of emergent literacy and early reading skills in preschool children: Evidence from a latent variable longitudinal study. *Developmental Psychology, 36*, 596–613.

Lonigan, C. J., & Whitehurst, G. J. (1998). Relative efficacy of parent and teacher involvement in a shared-reading intervention for preschool children from low-income backgrounds. *Early Childhood Research Quarterly, 13*, 263–290.

McDonnell, S. A., Friel-Patti, S., & Rollins, P. R. (2003). Patterns of change in maternal-child discourse behaviors across repeated storybook readings. *Applied Psycholinguistics, 24*, 323–341.

McFadden, T. U. (1998). Sounds and stories: Teaching phonemic awareness in interactions around text. *American Journal of Speech-Language Pathology, 7*, 5–13.

Morgan, L., & Goldstein, H. (2002). *Shared storybook reading: A review of intervention approaches.* Invited session presented at the annual convention of the American Speech-Language-Hearing Association, Atlanta, GA.

Most, B. (1996). *Cock-a-doodle-moo.* Orlando, FL: Harcourt Brace.

Most, B. (1990). *The cow that went oink.* Orlando, FL: Harcourt Brace.

Nation, K., & Snowling, M. J. (2004). Beyond phonological skills: Broader language skills contribute to the development of reading. *Journal of research in reading, 27*(4), 342–356.

National Reading Panel. (2000). *Report of the National Reading Panel: Reports of the subgroups.* Washington, DC: National Institute of Child Health and Human Development Clearinghouse.

Scarborough, H. S., & Dobrich, W. (1994). On the efficacy of reading to preschoolers. *Developmental Review, 14*, 245–302.

Slepian, J., & Seidler, A. (1993). *The Hungry Thing goes to a restaurant.* New York: Scholastic.

Slepian, J., & Seidler, A. (1993). *The Hungry Thing returns.* New York: Scholastic.

Slepian, J., & Seidler, A. (1967). *The Hungry Thing.* New York: Scholastic.

Stanovich, K. E. (2000). *Progress in understanding reading: Scientific foundations and new frontiers.* New York: Guilford Press.

Valdez-Menchaca, M. C., & Whitehurst, G. J. (1992). Accelerating language development through picture book reading: A systematic extension to Mexican day-care. *Developmental Psychology, 28*, 1106–1114.

Wagner, R., & Torgesen, J. (1987). The nature of phonological processing and its causal role in the acquisition of reading skills. *Psychological Bulletin, 101*, 192–212.

Whitehurst, G. J. (1992). *Dialogic reading in Head Start, KI, and pre-K.* Stony Brook, NY: Author.

Whitehurst, G. J., Crone, D. A., Zevenbergen, A. A., Schultz, M. D., Velting, O. N., & Fischel, J. E. (1999). Outcomes of an emergent literacy intervention from Head Start through second grade. *Journal of Educational Psychology, 91*, 261–272.

Whitehurst, G. J., Epstein, A. L., Angell, A. C., Payne, A. C., Crone, D. A., & Fischel, J. E. (1994). Outcomes of an emergent literacy intervention in Head Start. *Journal of Educational Psychology, 86*, 542–555.

Whitehurst, G. J., Falco, F., Lonigan, C. J., Fischel, J. E., Valdez-Menchaca, M. C., & Caulfield, M. (1988). Accelerating language development through picture-book reading. *Developmental Psychology, 24*, 552–558.

Whitehurst, G. J., & Lonigan, C. J. (1998). Child development and emergent literacy. *Child Development, 69*, 848–872.

Wilbur, R. (1997). *The disappearing alphabet*. Orlando, FL: Harcourt.

Williams, A. L., & Coutinho, M. (2003). *Contexts for facilitating emergent literacy skills*. Seminar presented at the annual convention of the American Speech-Language-Hearing Association, Chicago.

Yopp, H. K. (1992). Developing phonemic awareness in young children. *The Reading Teacher, 45*(9), 696–703.

Yopp, H. K., & Yopp, R. H. (2000). Supporting phonemic awareness development in the classroom. *The Reading Teacher, 54*(2), 130–143.

APPENDIX 8–A

Phonological Sensitivity Activities Based on Children's Books

Sound Matching/Sound Identification Activities	*Extension Activities*

"Old MacDonald Had a Farm"

Children can sing this familiar tune with different words to encourage them to think about sounds in words. A single sound can be emphasized through the entire song, or each verse can focus on a different sound, as shown below:

This song can be used as an extension activity to follow the farm theme from the book *Cock-A-Doodle-Moo!* or *The Cow That Went Oink*.

What's the sound that starts these words:

Turtle, time, and teeth?

[wait for a response from the children]

/t/ is the sound that starts these words:

Turtle, time, and teeth.

With a /t/, /t/ here, and a /t/, /t/ there,

Here a /t/, there a /t/, everywhere a /t/, /t/.

/t/ is the sound that starts these words:

Turtle, time, and teeth!

What's the sound that starts these words:

Chicken, chin, and cheek?

[wait for a response from the children]

Sound Matching/Sound Identification Activities	Extension Activities

/ch/ is the sound that
starts these words:
Chicken, chin, and cheek.
With a /ch/, /ch/ here, and
a /ch/, /ch/ there,
Here a /ch /, there a /ch/,
everywhere a /ch/, /ch/.
/ch/ is the sound that
starts these words:
Chicken, chin, and cheek!

What's the sound that starts
these words:
Daddy, duck, and deep?
[wait for a response from
the children]
/d/ is the sound that starts
these words:
Daddy, duck, and deep.
With a /d/, /d/ here, and a
/d/, /d/ there,
Here a /d/, there a /d/,
everywhere a /d/, /d/.
/d/ is the sound that starts
these words:
Daddy, duck, and deep!

Examples for focusing on
middle and final sounds are
as follows:

Medial:
What's the sound in the
middle of these words:
Leaf and deep and meat?
[wait for a response from
the children]

continues

APPENDIX 8–A. *continued*

Sound Matching/Sound Identification Activities	*Extension Activities*
/ee/ is the sound in the middle of these words: Leaf and deep and meat. With a /ee/, /ee/ here, and a /ee/, /ee/ there, Here a /ee/, there a /ee/, everywhere a /ee/, /ee/. /e/ is the sound in the middle of these words: Leaf and deep and meat! **Final:** What's the sound at the end of these words: Duck and cake and beak? [wait for a response from the children] /k/ is the sound at the end of these words: Duck and cake and beak. With a /k/, /k/ here, and a /k/, /k/ there, Here a /k/, there a /k/, everywhere a /k/, /k/. /k/ is the sound at the end of these words: Duck and cake and beak!	

Source: Yopp, 1992, p. 700.

Rhyming Activities	*Extension of Activity*

The Hungry Thing by Jan Slepian and Ann Seidler

The Hungry Thing is a creature who comes to town with a sign around his neck that says FEED ME. He asks for food from the townspeople using nonsense words. When the Hungry Thing asks for "schmancakes," the townspeople try to determine what schmancakes are. Only the little boy understands what the Hungry Thing wants by using rhyming words ("*Schmancakes* sounds like *fancakes* sound like *pancakes* to me!").

As you read the book, encourage the children to make predictions about what the Hungry Thing wants to eat. For example: "The Hungry Thing wants 'feetloaf.' What can that be?" Pause before reading that the little boy figures out that "*feetloaf* sounds like *beetloaf* sounds like [pause] *meatloaf* to me!"

Note: This wonderful book is no longer in print, but you may be able to locate used copies. It is definitely worth the effort!

To extend the story, use a lunchbag with different pretend food items. Look into the bag and say "Hmmm . . . shamburger! I have a shamburger!" Encourage the children to guess what "shamburger" is. After they guess that "shamburger" is hamburger, show it to the children and ask them how they knew. This can be repeated with different foods.

Reverse this activity by having the children put food into their lunchbag. Each child takes a turn looking into their bag to describe one food item that everyone else has to guess what it is. Now the child is generating a nonsense rhyming word that others translate what it is. Generating the nonsense rhyming word is a more difficult skill than identifying the nonsense rhyming word.

You can create a play center with plastic foods and lunchbags. Children can play with the food and re-enact the story by creating rhymes as they take turns guessing what they have in their bags.

You also can extend the story by placing a FEED ME sign around your neck. Use plastic food or pictures of food that

continues

APPENDIX 8–A. *continued*

Rhyming Activities	Extension of Activity
	you give to the children and then ask for a food item using nonsense rhymes, such as "Feed me the nandwich." The child who holds the food item or picture of the food that you requested can bring it to you where you pretend to gobble it up. Give the children opportunities to take turns being the Hungry Thing.
There are two additional books by the same authors (*The Hungry Thing Returns* and *The Hungry Thing Goes to a Restaurant*) that follow the same storyline with nonsense rhyming words for food items. These books can be read later to extend the training on rhyming and sound substitution.	To broaden the training activities centered with these books, you can use menus and food trays at a center so children may re-enact the themes of these books.

Twenty Kids Have Hats by
Jean Marzollo

This is a rhyming book for counting ("One bear has a chair, but I have a hat. Two ducks have trucks, but I have a hat."). As you read the book to the children, ask them to make predictions or complete the sentence (e.g., "Five pigs have ...."). The children may answer with any rhyming word, such as "wigs," "twigs," or "figs." Then ask the	To extend the theme of the book, have the children help you create a class counting book and illustration of hats for each child in the class. Assign a number to each child who then would dictate to the teacher a rhyme about their number, and then s/he would illustrate their rhyme. For example, Alison would be given the number "one," Sam

Rhyming Activities	*Extension of Activity*
children how they made their guesses. Encourage the children to continue to listen for rhymes and make predictions.	would be "two," and Nora would be "three." Alison might say, "One duck has a truck, but I have a hat," and then she would draw a duck with a truck. Have each child draw a picture of him/herself wearing a hat. Make a book that has each child's rhyme of counting numbers along with their self portrait wearing a hat.

Source: Yopp & Yopp, 2000, pp. 135–136.

Sound Addition or Substitution Activities	*Extension Activities*
Cock-a-Doodle-Moo! by Bernard Most In this book, a rooster cannot crow above a whisper one morning when he wakes up so he can't wake the farm animals who continue sleeping ("z-z-z-cheep!" snore the chicks and "z-z-z-quack!" snore the ducks). The rooster tries to teach the cow to cock-a-doodle-doo so that she can wake up the farm animals. The cow practices crowing by substituting phonemes ("mock-a-moodle-moo!" and "rock-a-poodle-moo!"). The farm animals wake up with a laugh: "oink-ha!", "quack-ha!", "meow-ha!" etc.	Extend this story by asking the children to think about a different scenario. What if the horse tried to teach the cow to neigh? What would the cow's practice at neighing sound like? Put plastic farm animals at a play center along with the book. The children can re-tell the story and play with sounds as they play with the farm animals.

continues

APPENDIX 8–A. *continued*

Sound Addition or Substitution Activities	Extension Activities
After you read the story, ask the children to think about other farm animals. How would the author have a goat snore, or a sheep snore?	
Reread the different ways in which the cow tried to crow. Ask the children to think of other ways to say "cock-a-doodle-doo." You can write their ideas on paper or on the chalkboard, adding letters to the phonemic awareness activity. Write "cock-a-doodle-doo," erase the initial letters, and replace them with letters suggested by the children.	
Continuing with the farm animal theme, sing the song in "Old MacDonald Had a Farm," but add or substitute sounds in the words. For example, "ee-igh, ee-igh, oh!" can be sung as "Bee-bigh, bee-bigh, boh!" or "See-sigh, see-sigh, soh!," etc.	

Source: Yopp, 1992, p. 701; Yopp & Yopp, 2000, pp. 140–141.

Sound/Syllable Segmentation Activities	Extension Activities

Tikki Tikki Tembo by Arlene Mosel

This story is about two Chinese brothers; one has a very long name ("Tikki Tikki Tembo No Sa Rembo Chari Bari Ruchi Pip Peri Pembo"), and the other one has a very short name ("Chang"). After reading and discussing the story, help the children learn to say the two boys' names. When they learn them, ask them to say them again and clap with each syllable that is said. Tikki Tikki Tembo's name will have 21 claps, while Chang's name will only have one clap.

Have the children try clapping the syllables in their own names. Have the group say each child's name and clap as you separate the syllables. "Erica" would be said "Er" (with a clap)-"i" (clap)- "ca" (clap). "Richard" would be said with two claps.

As another activity to provide further practice, place colored pieces of paper in a pocket chart as you say each syllable in a particular child's name. Point to each piece of paper as you say each syllable. Afterwards the children can glue the appropriate number of colored pieces on a piece of drawing paper to represent the number of syllables in their names. For example, Erica takes three pieces of colored paper from a pile and glues them side by side at the top of a piece of drawing paper. Then the children can move around the room with their papers in hand and group themselves with others who have the same number of colored pieces glued on the drawing paper. Ask each child in a group to say his/her name. Encourage all students to say how many syllables as each name is slowly said. Reinforce their work by commenting that

continues

APPENDIX 8–A. *continued*

Sound/Syllable Segmentation Activities	Extension Activities
	they do, indeed, each have the same number of syllables. ("Yes! Jack, Nick, Sam, and Lee each have one beat! Let's go to our next group. Let's say their names [etc.].") You also can develop a bar graph to represent the number of students who have a given number of syllables in their names.
	As a follow-up activity, you can use clapping when taking attendance so that the children clap the number of syllables of each child's name as it is called. Also at dismissal time, you can clap once for anyone with a one-syllable name to leave; clap twice and students with two-syllable names may leave; etc.
Tingo Tango Mango Tree by Marcia Vaughan	
This story is about different animals with names that have several syllables (an iguana named Sombala Bombala Rombala Roh, a flamingo named Kokio Loki Mokio Koh, a parrot named Dillaby Dallaby Doh, a turtle named Nanaba Panaba Tanaba Goh, and a bat named Bitteo Biteo).	Any of the foregoing activities also can be used in following the reading of this story.

Source: Yopp & Yopp, 2000, p. 138.

Chapter Nine

Supporting Storybook Reading Participation for Children Who Use Augmentative and Alternative Communication Systems

Gloria Soto (in collaboration with Elena Dukhovny and Tove Vestli)

Overview

Storybook reading at home and in school has repeatedly been proposed as an exceptionally rich social context to support children's development of early language and literacy skills (e.g., Dorr, Rabin, & Irlen, 2002; Snow, Burns, & Griffin, 1998). Several reasons have been presented in the literature for why book reading is so important to children's language and literacy development (Snow & Ninio, 1986). First, research suggests that storybook reading is an activity that teaches children new vocabulary and linguistic structures (Ninio, 1983), because the language occurring during reading interactions tends to be more sophisticated and includes a greater representational repertoire than is typical for other interactive contexts, such as play (Dickinson & Tabors, 1991; Snow & Ninio, 1986). In fact, existing research shows a relationship between adults' use of conceptually and semantically complex language during story reading and children's production of syntactically complex utterances (Hockenberger, Goldstein, & Haas, 1999). Similar patterns also are seen for preschoolers with mild to moderate disabilities (Davie & Kemp, 2002).

Second, storybook reading creates a context that facilitates periods of extended joint attention. In early stages of storybook reading, parents and children typically focus on identifying and labeling the people and the actions represented in the book illustrations. As children become more active and able, there is a shift of attention toward more complex language functions such as describing, interpreting, predicting, and inferring (Ninio & Bruner, 1978; Snow & Goldfield, 1983). In addition, storybook reading provides children with opportunities to learn about print conventions (Justice & Ezell, 2004), narrative structure (Snow & Goldfield, 1983), and fantasy worlds (De Temple & Hirschler, 2001).

Third, existing research suggests that storybook reading allows young children to participate in rich verbal interactions that are beyond their independent language abilities. This is possible because of the scaffolds provided by the inherent structure of the story, as well as the structure of the interactions between the child and the adult. As children become more competent with the language and more familiar with the role expected of them, they gradually become more active participants in the activity (Justice & Ezell, 1999). The role of adult scaffolding in promoting children's achievement of both language and literacy skills is discussed more thoroughly in Chapter 8.

Storybook Reading as a Context for Augmentative and Alternative Communication Intervention

For all of the reasons outlined above, storybook reading in school and at home is repeatedly proposed as an important intervention context to support the language and literacy skills of young children, including those with significant communication impairments. This chapter discusses storybook reading as an intervention context for children who have to rely on augmentative and alternative communication (AAC) systems to participate. Over the past 3 decades, educators and clinicians have developed and implemented AAC systems in efforts to support these children's emerging speech and language development (Beukelman & Mirenda, 2005; Koppenhaver & Yoder, 1993; Mirenda & Schuler, 1988; Romski & Sevcik, 1996). *Augmentative* refers to the supplementation of, or addition to, natural speech or handwriting to enhance communication (e.g., speech can be augmented through the use of gestures or pointing to the initial letters of words). *Alternative* refers to the substitution of another form of communication for natural speech or handwriting (e.g., the use of manual signs, graphic symbols mounted on a board or in a notebook, or a computer with speech synthesizer or printed output) (e.g., Beukelman & Mirenda, 2005). AAC is an area of clinical practice that attempts to help persons compensate for the permanent or temporary lack of functional speech.

AAC systems often are multimodal—they involve various aided and unaided forms of representation such as gestures, manual signs, traditional orthography, digitized or synthesized speech, and other types of alternative symbols that can be displayed in a number of static or dynamic devices (Heim & Baker-Mills, 1996). These modes are used in combination to convey meaning, supplementing or replacing spoken communication for persons with severe expressive communication impairments. For children who have little or no functional speech as a result of primary motor impairments, the use of graphic pictorial symbols, either mounted on fixed displays or presented on voice communication output aids, is one of the most widely used alternatives (Beukelman & Mirenda, 2005; Sutton, Soto, & Blockberger, 2002; von Tetzchner & Martinsen, 1996). Pictorial symbols are particularly appropriate for preliterate or nonliterate children (or adults) who are unable to use alphabet-based systems (Sutton et al., 2002).

Storybook reading provides a natural language learning context for meaningful communicative interactions, and as such it is an ideal context to support the language and communication skills of children who use AAC (Bellon & Ogletree, 2000; Norris & Hoffman, 1990; Skotko, Koppenhaver, & Erickson, 2004). Storybook reading intrinsically addresses numerous issues that have been identified as problematic for children with significant communication impairments. Specifically, storybook reading activities can be used to establish, monitor, and maintain joint attention (DeLoache & De Mendoza, 1987) and provide routines that render children's communicative efforts more interpretable and effective (Bornstein & Bruner, 1989). They also can be used to select the vocabulary needed for a set of referents represented in the story and to make language patterns more salient (Bellon, Ogletree, & Harn, 2000), to promote conversational turn-taking (Bruner, 1978), and to provide individualized instructional time with adults who naturally scaffold language learning. Research examining storybook reading as an intervention context to facilitate language and literacy in children with significant communication impairments is rapidly emerging (Bellon & Ogletree, 2000; Bradshaw, Hoffman, & Norris, 1998; Crowe, Norris, & Hoffman, 2004).

Participation Patterns of AAC Users During Storybook Reading

For storybook reading to be truly effective, the active participation of the child during the reading of the story by an adult is required. It is not sufficient for the adult to read the story to the child and the child to simply sit passively and listen; rather, there has to be a high-quality interchange between the two for the vocabulary and the events to be understood and remembered (Nelson, 1996). Children's participation usually takes the form of asking questions about the story, pretending to read, and commenting or answering questions about the story (Light & Kelford-Smith, 1993).

Existing research in the field of AAC indicates that children who use AAC have limited opportunities to engage in storybook reading activities and that they tend to take a more passive role in story reading sessions than that enjoyed by typically developing children. In a study specifically designed to investigate the interaction patterns of five preschoolers who used AAC with their mothers during storybook reading, Light, Binger, and Kelford-Smith (1994) found that the mothers dominated the reading interactions and the children seldom participated. In their analysis of the interaction patterns, Light et al. (1994) found that the mothers mostly read the text and the children simply listened. There were very few questions, and those that did occur were framed to require yes/no answers. Moreover, none of the children had access to their aided AAC systems during any of the 10 reading sessions observed. The lack of access to their systems may explain why the children never asked questions or talked about the story. Their participation involved mainly holding the book, turning pages, and pointing to pictures.

In view of these findings, Light and her colleagues made a number of suggestions for enhancing the participation of children who use AAC during storybook reading:

- Ensure that children have access to their aided systems.
- Provide appropriate story-related vocabulary for children to use to ask questions, comment, predict, and help tell the story.
- Pause to give children opportunities to participate.
- Scaffold children's contributions to assist them in reaching a higher level of linguistic participation.

Adult Scaffolding during Storybook Reading With Children Who Use AAC

Recent research indicates that training adults to scaffold the interactions that transpire during shared reading has a positive effect on children's vocabulary development (Dale, Crain-Thoreson, Notari-Syverson, & Cole, 1996), sentence complexity (Crowe, 2000), and print knowledge (Ezell, Justice, & Parsons, 2000; Justice & Ezell, 2000, 2002). Adult scaffolding strategies that seem most influential in improving children's language and literacy skills are those that provide children more specific information about the content of the book (e.g., certain words, certain letters), through adult labeling, defining, describing, and relating words and their attributes (Jordan, Snow, & Porche, 2000). Studies looking specifically at children with significant language delays show that increased use of adult scaffolding can improve children's language production and comprehension during reading activities (e.g., Justice & Kaderavek, 2003; Skotko et al., 2004), as shown through children's increased use of Picture Communication Symbols (Dexter, 1998), the semantic complexity of their language (Bellon & Ogletree, 2000), and their overall communicative competence (Crowe, Norris, & Hoffman, 2000).

A recent study by Koppenhaver et al. (2001) illustrates how parents can engage their children more fully during storybook reading. Koppenhaver and his colleagues were interested in improving the communication skills of six girls with Rett syndrome using this context. Typically, girls with Rett syndrome communicate at a presymbolic level through gestures, vocalizations, and body positioning. To this end, the girls' mothers were trained to interact more effectively with their daughters while they were reading storybooks together. The intervention strategies included the following: (1) attributing meaning to the child's attempt to communicate even if the meaning was uncertain; (2) prompting the use of communication devices or symbols through natural questions, models, and comments, rather than direct commands; (3) providing sufficient wait time and a hierarchy of support after asking a question; and (4) consistently asking questions and making comments that maximized the use of available symbols and voice output messages (Koppenhaver et al., 2001). All of the girls increased their frequency of symbolic communication and their labeling and commenting. In a follow-up analysis of the same data set, Skotko and associates (2004) found that the girls with Rett syndrome became more active and successful participants in storybook reading when their mothers were trained to ask open-ended questions and to model the use of symbols. As these findings show, helping parents to modify the way they share books with children to promote their active engagement is a promising means for providing language and literacy interventions.

Clinical Examples: Implementation of Scaffolding Strategies by Educators and Clinicians With Children Who Use AAC

Surprisingly little information is available in the AAC field regarding strategies used by professionals during storybook reading to elicit the active participation of children who rely on AAC. Recently, Liboiron and Soto (2006) analyzed the scaffolding strategies used by an experienced clinician during a shared book-reading session with a child who used aided AAC. The scaffolding strategies examined by the researchers included comprehension questions, cueing, pointing and gesturing, references to print, constituent questions, binary choices, expansions, cloze procedures, and modeling the use of the speech generating device. In addition, the study examined the level of semantic complexity targeted by the clinician during the session. Although this study provided an interesting examination of strategies used by the clinician, it did not examine the relationship between the clinician's scaffolding strategies and the quality of the language produced by the child during the session. This relationship—specifically, between the scaffolding strategies used by clinicians during storybook reading and the quality of language produced by children who use AAC to communicate—is the focus of the remainder of this chapter.

This section presents clinical examples illustrating the way in which the quality of adult scaffolding influences the quality of the language produced by children who use AAC systems to communicate. The data for the examples were obtained as part of a larger study involving children who are AAC users (Soto, 2004; Soto & Hartmann, 2006).

Sophie

Sophie is 11 years old. She has cerebral palsy and is a proficient and independent AAC user. She has limited mobility and uses a power wheelchair. She accesses locations on her Dynavox 3100 and Intellikeys keyboard using her left fingers and knuckles with about 80% to 90% accuracy. Additional communication skills include vocalizing and gesturing "yes" and "no" as well as using pointing or eye gaze to locate desired persons or objects and to select choices that are presented orally. Her speech-language pathologist reports that she uses more than 100 customized Spanish and English pages and pop-ups to communicate in all settings. Although her literacy skills have not been formally assessed, it is reported that she is able to combine three to four words to create novel phrases or sentences using a "Sentence Starter" pop-up. In addition, she is able to change verb tenses and use different forms of pronouns and nouns. She is mainstreamed in a fifth grade public school classroom for content subjects and remains in a self-contained special education classroom for reading, math, and augmentative communication and assistive technology skills development.

Anna

Anna is 10 years old. She has a primary diagnosis of arthrogryposis with extremely low muscle tone. She also has a surgically repaired cleft palate, with remaining deficits that cause her severe difficulties in articulation. She has limited mobility and uses an electrically powered wheelchair with joystick at school and a manual wheelchair at home. Her overall speech intelligibility is poor without known context. She uses a Dynamyte voice output device, which she operates with her left index finger. She is able to access over 30 locations with 100% accuracy. Anna is able to greet, make requests, and make social comments to her friends and educators. She is working on formulating complete sentences, changing verb and noun endings, and using communicative repairs. She is mainstreamed in a second grade public school classroom for content subjects and remains in a self-contained special education classroom for reading, math, and augmentative communication and assistive technology skills development.

Heidi

Heidi is 8 years old and has muscular atrophy. As a result, she has very limited mobility and uses a wheelchair. She requires round-the-clock nursing care and is assisted in her breathing and swallowing. She communicates using a combination of vocalizations, word approximations, eye gaze, and a Dynavox 3100 voice output communication device mounted to her chair. She operates her device through a toggle switch activated through slight movements of her right forearm to scan a combination of blocks, rows, and columns. The concepts in Heidi's Dynavox are mainly represented graphically with a written gloss, and she also uses the alphabet page to spell the beginning of words to which she does not have access. According to Heidi's teacher, she has an active vocabulary of 257 adjectives, 605 verbs, 23 prepositions, and thousands of nouns. When writing or engaging in academic activity, Heidi can produce full sentences. In conversations, she produces one- or two-word utterances most of the time, and relies on others to fill in the blanks for her. Heidi attends a special education classroom for children with intense augmentative communication supports but is mainstreamed in a regular second grade classroom for most of her day.

Dave

Dave is 5 years old. He has been diagnosed with choreoathetoid cerebral palsy with hypotonia, a physical impairment that causes him to have uncoordinated, rapid, jerky movements that interfere with his speaking, feeding, reaching, and grasping. He requires a wheelchair for transportation, as well as to support his posture. His physical needs necessitate 100% support with life skills throughout all environments. Dave has learned to use the following devices: Tech Talk, Dynavox, and Step by Step. He also has had success working with an icon board, a printed alphabet board, and a computer with an adapted keyboard and joystick. Dave's speech-language pathologist has stated that although he has severe difficulties with his motor skills and expressive speech, he is an eager communicator. His literacy skills have not been formally assessed. Despite the fact that his level of speech intelligibility is very low, he is a very sociable boy and has made friends in his classrooms. Dave attends a special education classroom for children with intense augmentative communication supports and is mainstreamed into a regular education first grade classroom for a good portion of the day.

Language Sampling During Storybook Reading

To assess quality of language during storybook reading sessions, the children were observed in their special education classrooms, and the clinicians were asked to engage in a shared reading involving a familiar and favorite storybook with their clients. All of the clinicians had extensive experience with AAC users in general and with each of their clients in particular. The children under observation—Sophie, Anna, Heidi, and Dave—were encouraged to participate in the sessions in any way possible (such as vocalizations, eye gaze, eye gaze shifting, gestures, signs, and AAC device). The clinicians were not provided with any particular instructions about how to conduct the storybook reading session; rather, they were asked to read with their clients as they typically would. As the story went along, the children and the clinicians interacted to consider the characters, events, specific details, and the causal relations in the story (Merritt & Liles, 1987). Because the clinicians had received no specific instructions on how they should interact with their clients throughout the book reading session, the characteristics of the exchanges varied from clinician to clinician.

Each of the observed reading sessions was digitally videotaped. In order to capture the richness of the multimodal strategies used by the children, the camera focused on the children and a microphone captured the speech output produced by their AAC systems. After the sessions, the videotapes were transcribed verbatim using video transcription software, and the language produced by the children was transcribed using expanded standardized transcription notation systems; this allowed inclusion of features specific to augmented interactions such as gestures, facial expressions, and vocalizations (Müller & Soto, 2002) (see Appendix 9–A for the key to transcription notation).

Coding Children's Storybook Reading Participation

This study used an expanded version of the coding scheme used in Liboiron and Soto (2006), which originally was influenced by the work of Bellon and Ogletree (2000) and Justice and Ezell (2002). The storybook reading sessions were parsed into conversational turns, and four features of each conversational turn were coded as shown in Appendix 9–B. The coding system was studied for its reliability by having a second transcriber independently code 25% of the samples. For all codes, inter-rater reliability was higher than 95%.

To apply these codes to the reading transcripts, adult scaffolding strategies within the conversational turn were first identified and coded as one of the following: print reference, cloze procedure, expansion, binary choice, pointing/cueing, constituent question, or comprehension question.

Second, the level of semantic complexity targeted within each adult turn was identified and coded as identification, labeling, description, interpretation, inference, or metalanguage.

Third, each child's utterance was coded as identification, labeling, description, interpretation, inference, or metalanguage.

Last, the total number of unique words (i.e., different exemplars), the total number of noun-verb clauses, and the total number of yes/no responses used by the children were calculated.

Analyzing the Language Samples

The data were analyzed using two approaches. First, the language samples were coded according to the categories as outlined. After all utterances were coded, the following frequencies were calculated: (1) the number of conversational turns contributed by the child and the clinician within the session, (2) the number of scaffolding strategies in the clinician's conversational turns, (3) the number of specific scaffolding strategies used by the clinician, (4) the number of specific levels of semantic complexity targeted by the clinician, and (5) the number of specific levels of semantic complexity achieved by the child. The raw frequencies were used to derive proportions for each code.

Second, a finer-grained analysis of adult and child moment-by-moment interaction also was conducted using discourse analysis tools. This yielded a closer look at the clinicians' use of scaffolding strategies for encouraging children's participation and eliciting language learning at varying levels of semantic complexity (Bellon & Ogletree, 2000; Moore, 2004).

Relationship Between Clinicians' Scaffolding Strategies and Children's Levels of Linguistic Complexity

The transcripts of the four dyads were analyzed to study the types of scaffolding strategies produced and the levels of semantic complexity targeted by the clinicians, as well as the semantic complexity produced by the children, during the book reading sessions. The analyses indicated that the greatest proportion of clinicians' conversational turns was yes/no questioning across all four dyads. Yes/no questions generated by the clinicians appeared to serve several purposes: to elicit higher-order information (comprehension questions), to elicit lower-order information (constituent questions), to repair communication, and to make side comments. Of importance, however, the clinicians' use of yes/no questions did not elicit children's use of their AAC devices, because all four children had an effective unaided way to indicate yes/no (i.e., verbally or gesturally). Presented next is a brief summary of how each of the children participated in the book reading sessions and of specific scaffolding strategies used by their clinicians.

Sophie

Sophie participated very actively during the book reading session. She produced a total of 66 distinct vocabulary exemplars and 10 noun-verb clauses in 168 conversational turns. Her clinician used a total of 58 yes/no questions and 112 scaffolding strategies in 193 conversational turns. Of these, 28% were cloze procedures, 23% were constituent questions, 16% were pointing/cueing, 8% were expansions, 7% were comprehension questions, 2% were binary choices, and 0.5% were print references.

The strategies used by the clinician targeted labeling 30% of the time. Metalanguage and description also were prevalent strategies, representing 24% and 17% of the clinician's strategies, respectively; indication, interpretation, and inference occurred infrequently, with each representing only 3% of strategies used.

Anna

Anna was very active during the book reading session, using a myriad of communication modes to express herself, including vocalizations, gestures, manual signs, and speech generating device. She produced a total of 97 distinct vocabulary exemplars and 38 noun-verb clauses in 381 conversational turns.

Her clinician used a total of 82 yes/no questions and 185 scaffolding strategies in 390 conversational turns. Of these, 36% were print references, 29% were constituent questions, 18% were comprehension questions, 5% were expansions, 5% were pointing/cueing, 2% were cloze procedures, and 2% were binary choices. The semantic categories targeted were predominantly interpretation (20% of strategies) and description (17%); labeling (10%), indication (3%), inference (1%), and metalanguage (0.5%) occurred at much lower rates.

Heidi

Heidi did not actively participate during the book reading session, at least in part because of an excessive use of yes/no questioning on the part of the clinician; specifically, Heidi's clinician asked 41 yes/no questions in a total of 39 conversation turns. Heidi produced only 2 distinct vocabulary exemplars and no noun-verb clauses within 31 conversational turns. Her clinician used 14 scaffolding strategies in 39 turns. Of these, 79% were print references; she used only 1 expansion, 1 binary choice, and 1 constituent question.

The levels of semantic complexity most frequently targeted by Heidi's clinician were interpretation (57%) and inference (50%); indication, labeling, and metalinguistic each accounted for 7% of turns.

Dave

Dave did not participate very actively during the book reading session despite selection of his favorite book for reading (*The Grouchy Ladybug* by Eric Carle). In 88 conversational turns, Dave produced only 8 vocabulary exemplars and no noun-verb clauses. His clinician used 21 yes/no questions and 54 scaffolding strategies in 92 turns. Of these, 35% were cloze procedures, 20% were print references, 18% were constituent questions, 16% were binary choices, 14% were comprehension questions, and 9% were pointing/cueing. Dave's clinician used no expansions during the book reading session. The strategies used by the clinician targeted primarily description (31% of the time), with labeling (22%), indication (18%), and inference (18%) also serving as prevalent strategies. Interpretation represented only a small proportion of the clinician's strategies (7%), and metalanguage was not focused on at all.

Individual Differences Among Clinicians

Figures 9-1, 9-2, and 9-3 are visual depictions of individual differences among the dyads, in terms of the percentage of targets children responded to by strategy (see Figure 9-1), clinician use of different scaffolding strategies (see Figure 9-2), and clinician targeting of different semantic complexity levels (see Figure 9-3). Examination of the data for the four dyads revealed considerable differences in all areas.

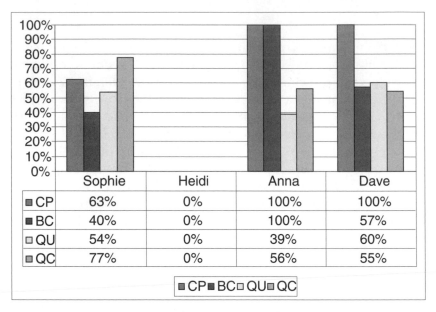

	Sophie	Heidi	Anna	Dave
▪ CP	63%	0%	100%	100%
▪ BC	40%	0%	100%	57%
▫ QU	54%	0%	39%	60%
▨ QC	77%	0%	56%	55%

▪ CP ▪ BC ▫ QU ▨ QC

Key: CP = cloze procedure, BC = binary choice, QU = constituent question, QC = comprehension question.

Figure 9–1. Percentage of semantic complexity targets met per scaffolding strategy, per child

As shown in Figure 9–2, three scaffolding strategies were used most frequently: comprehension questions, constituent questions, and references to the text (print references and pointing/cueing). Of interest, although binary choice was a strategy that clinicians seldom used, it yielded a higher percentage of met targets than that achieved with other strategies the clinicians used more frequently (see Figure 9–1). Some strategies used relatively frequently—specifically, print references, expansions, and pointing/cueing—do not elicit language directly. Rather, they bring the child's attention to important text points and language concepts and frequently are used with other scaffolding that elicit language in more direct ways.

With regard to semantic complexity, adults targeted description and labeling most consistently in the use of their scaffolding strategies, which are relatively contextualized and "lower-level" skills. The level of semantic complexity least frequently targeted was metalanguage, except in Sophie's case.

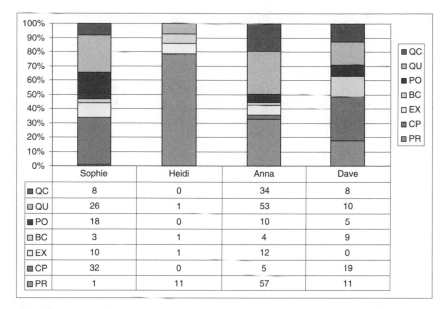

	Sophie	Heidi	Anna	Dave
■ QC	8	0	34	8
▨ QU	26	1	53	10
■ PO	18	0	10	5
▢ BC	3	1	4	9
▢ EX	10	1	12	0
■ CP	32	0	5	19
▨ PR	1	11	57	11

Key: QC = comprehension question, QU = constituent question, PO = pointing/cueing; BC = binary choice, EX = expansion; CP = cloze procedure, PR = print reference.

Figure 9–2. Frequency of scaffolding strategies across dyads.

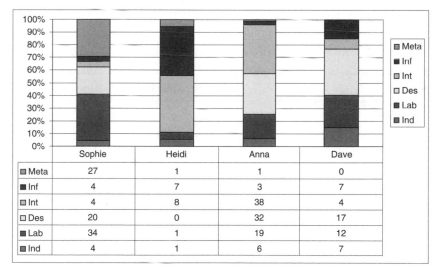

	Sophie	Heidi	Anna	Dave
▨ Meta	27	1	1	0
■ Inf	4	7	3	7
▢ Int	4	8	38	4
▢ Des	20	0	32	17
■ Lab	34	1	19	12
▨ Ind	4	1	6	7

Key: Meta = metalanguage, Inf = inference, Int = interpretation, Des = description, Lab = labeling, Ind = indication.

Figure 9–3. Frequency of adult targets across dyads

The following eight excerpts from video/audiotaped reading sessions (with children's nonverbal responses denoted using the symbols in Appendix 9–A) are provided to illustrate the clinicians' use of different scaffolding strategies to target different levels of semantic complexity:

Excerpt 1: Use of comprehension question targeting interpretation

Anna	Clinician
((points to sentence)) *Goldilocks looked through the window and then she and, and then she peeped through the keyhole . . .*	
	Yeah. I wanted to ask you a question about that. Why do you think she was looking through the window? ((points to picture)) *And peeping through the keyhole?*

Excerpt 2: Use of constituent questions targeting description

Anna	Clinician
	Shall we . . . ((closes book)) *Well, what do you think happened to those three bears?*
((points at bears on the cover)) *Go away.*	
[↑↓↑]	*They go away?* *And then what happens?*
I dunno . . .	

Excerpt 3: Use of pointing/cueing

Anna	Clinician
	Papa bear?
	((points to picture))
	Is that one Papa bear?
↑↓↑	

Excerpt 4: Additional use of pointing/cueing

Dave	Clinician
⇒book	*((point to picture))*
	Look at the picture. That's a . . . what's it called. It's called a boa constrictor. It's going to eat something.

Excerpt 5: Use of cloze procedure targeting description

Anna	Clinician
	((points to picture))
	That's right. So Mama bear's porridge was cold and . . .
And the Papa bear's was hot.	

Excerpt 6: Use of expansion

Anna	Clinician
	What is he doing?
((Opens mouth, brings left hand to neck, and yawns))	
	Yeah, he's yawning . . .

Excerpt 7: Use of binary choice targeting indication

Sophie	Clinician
"The" "bunny"	
	((Nodding)) *That's what I was going to talk about. The bunny*—((Pause. Looking at book. Looks at S.))
((Cont. msg. constr. 4 sec.))	*My turn or your turn?*
((Vocalizes. Points to self.))	
	Your turn? Okay. You go ahead.

Excerpt 8: Use of pointing/cueing used in combination with binary choice

Dave	Clinician
	((points to picture))
	Is the whale on the land or is it in the water?
	Look at the picture—is it in the land or the water?

Improving Communication Opportunities for Children Who Use AAC during Storybook Reading

Previous sections described the scaffolding strategies used by four clinicians during book reading and the quality of language produced by four children who use AAC to communicate. The storybook reading context provided many opportunities for the clinicians to use a range of scaffolding strategies, and substantial numbers of scaffolding strategies were observed across all four participating clinicians. Yet not all of these strategies were used with equal success, and there was a range of individual variation across dyads. Within this range, however, several patterns emerged from the data.

First, the frequency and complexity of the children's language productions during storybook reading seem to have been affected by the communication opportunities provided for them by their clinicians. These communication opportunities came predominantly in the form of scaffolding strategies with direct language elicitation capability—that is, binary choice, cloze procedure, open-ended constituent questions, and open-ended comprehension questions.

Second, different types of scaffolding strategies seem to have affected the quality of the language produced by the children during the book reading session. For this study, the children's language participation was measured by the number of distinct vocabulary exemplars and simple noun-verb clauses that they produced. It seems that the preponderance of yes/no questions by some clinicians may have resulted in a lack of communication opportunities and an impoverished linguistic output. Those adults who used open-ended questions and verbal scaffolds provided more opportunities for children to produce more diverse vocabulary and more complex language.

Third, it appears that children's abilities to meet the targeted level of semantic complexity depended not only on the type of strategy used by the clinician but also on the adult's ability to pause, wait for the answer, and modify the strategy if it was not successful. Pausing to allow children time to formulate their answer has been found to be a very effective strategy to encourage greater storybook reading participation by children who use AAC (Koppenhaver et al., 2001; Skotko et al., 2004). For example, one clinician was able to extend the child's communication opportunity by modifying her original strategy—when the child had obvious difficulty answering a question, the adult cued the child with another question that allowed a more definitive response:

Excerpt 9: Modification of strategy to achieve intended goal

Anna	*Clinician*
	Why?
	Why would she do that?
	((points to picture))
Ahh, I dunno . . .	
	continues

Anna	Clinician
	Well—what do you think?
Ummmm . . . ((points to pictures))	
	What do you think she was _looking_ at?
A teddy bear.	

For the most part, the clinicians who were observed for this study implemented a number of practices that are recommended for use in reading books with children who use AAC, such as providing children with access to their AAC system, modeling key vocabulary, and using scaffolding strategies to foster a higher level of linguistic participation (Light et al., 1994). Yet many of these clinicians utilized a great number of yes/no questions (with a total of 202 observed across the four adults), and most of the clinicians did not provide enough time for their client to respond, with presentation of several questions or scaffolding strategies in quick succession, as seen in Excerpt 10:

Excerpt 10: Stacking questions or scaffolding strategies with inadequate time for response

Heidi	Clinician
	No?
	((turns page))
	Angelina raced as fast as she could to Alice's house. When she got there, Alice had already received a surprise of her own.
	I wonder what it is.
	What do you think it is?
	Do you know?
((head nod, yes))	

An interesting observation from this study is that the participating clinicians often modified their scaffolding strategies to provide various types of support across multiple turns to elicit a particularly difficult response. At times, the combination of two or three strategies eventually enabled the child to meet the intended target:

Excerpt 11: Use of several strategies across different turns

Sophie	Clinician
	Okay . . . well, tell me about it then.
	The—what?
((points again to the picture))	
	Well, you have to tell me about it . . .
((Vocalizes. Blinks. Smiling.))	
	The—what?
((Init. msg. constr. 10 secs)) "*Dress*"	
	Oop, oops. ((guides S.'s hand))
	Clear it. ((pushes key))
	There you go.
((Vocalizing. Init. msg. constr.))	
	Get your finger out. There you go.
"*Roller skate*" "*The*" "*roller skate*"	
	Okay.
	Mm-hm.
((msg. constr.))	
	Oh, you're going to change it, huh?
	Which one should we change it to?

continues

Sophie	Clinician
((reaching for a key))	
	That one? Okay. ((pushes key))
	Roller skates.
	That's right, because there's more than one.
"The" "roller skates"	
	That's right, because there are two of them.
((pointing to book))	
	Well, what about them?
	The roller skates—

Clinical Implications

Storybook reading provides a rich context to support language and literacy growth, and is a particularly important context for providing intervention for children with significant communication impairments. It is important that children who use AAC systems experience storybook reading interactions in sufficient quantity to provide them with frequent opportunities to hear new vocabulary, learn print concepts, and be exposed to a range of syntactic structures. Of equal importance, these reading interactions need to be structured in ways that ensure the active rather than passive participation of these children. Considerable research shows that adult strategies that ensure children's active participation during storybook reading constitute an important mechanism for improving children's language and literacy growth during this activity.

The description of dyadic interactions in this chapter provides a glimpse into what storybook reading interactions involving children with AAC may look like. Until recently, very little literature was available in this area. The descriptions of clinician-child interaction in the study described in this chapter illustrate the diversity of scaffolding strategies available to clinicians for supporting children's participation during storybook reading, as well as some of the difficulties in implementing them in successful ways. Although the observations for the study took place in classrooms, there is every reason to believe that similar results would be seen in clinical settings.

The results of this study, as well as those provided by other researchers conducting studies in this area, point to several criteria for ensuring the quality of storybook reading interactions that involve children with AAC.

Set Appropriate Goals for the Storybook Reading Session

It is important that clinicians set specific and explicit goals for story reading sessions and that these goals be appropriate to the child's developmental needs and abilities. Goals may include, for instance, sustaining joint attention, increasing turn-taking, developing phonological and print awareness, building vocabulary, and generating narratives, as a few examples. By setting specific goals, clinicians can then use strategies that are known to explicitly target those goals; in this regard, storybook reading can be used more systematically as a therapeutic tool. For instance, if the goal of a session is to increase children's turn-taking, the clinician can use strategies that specifically facilitate children's participation in an extended turn-taking interaction. Additionally, the clinician needs to monitor the child's attainment of the goals and adjust the strategies accordingly.

Expect the Child to Participate

It is critical that book reading sessions are organized in ways that enable the child to be an active participant. This can be achieved by using scaffolding strategies that are conducive to the child's production of language, such as using binary choices, using cloze procedures, and asking open-ended questions. If strategies used to elicit active communication by the child are not effective, then the clinician can modify his or her approach. For instance, the clinician may start with a general open-ended question and build cues into the question if the child does not respond, as shown previously in Excerpt 9. If the child is still not responding, the clinician can then use cloze procedure, binary choice, and modeling to prompt a response. Clinicians can use a range of strategies to scaffold children's participation, rather than relying on only one strategy (e.g., the yes/no question).

Give the Child Enough Time to Respond

Pauses are necessary when engaging in interactions with AAC users. Different children need differing periods of time to process questions and produce answers. Clinicians need to be sensitive to the individual needs and abilities of children to provide the most effective wait time (Downing, 2005) and need to know the usual amount of time it takes for a particular child to respond. Such knowledge will help determine how long to wait before giving the child additional information.

Provide Corrective Feedback and Praise

Children who use AAC often mistakenly select the wrong word or symbol. When this happens, the child may need help to correct his or her selection. For instance, if a child points to the wrong picture on the AAC system, the clinician needs to tell the child why the item is incorrect and guide the child toward the correct option. Talking about the correct response and highlighting a certain aspect of the symbol or word may help the child remember the right answer (Downing, 2005). When the child demonstrates the expected response, immediate praise and reinforcement should be provided.

Provide the Child With Story-Relevant Vocabulary

Providing children with access to an AAC system that affords combination of symbols into more complex grammatical forms is an important consideration for helping children develop story-related vocabulary and grammatical structures (see Soto & Hartmann, 2006). As Sutton et al. (2002) noted, the vocabulary available in most AAC devices lacks the morphological and syntactic structures that would make symbol combinations possible. And, Light et al. (1994) have previously indicated, the vocabulary provided cannot be limited to items that allow the children only to label the pictures in the stories or repeat lines in the text of the story. Rather, the vocabulary available must allow children to talk about the story, to ask questions (e.g., "What is that?" "Why?"), to predict outcomes, to re-tell the story in their own words, and to relate the story to their own experiences.

As these suggestions indicate, there is a great deal that clinicians can do to ensure that children who use AAC systems are engaged more fully in storybook reading interactions. Future research on this topic is needed to ensure that clinicians can utilize evidence-based practice when promoting language and literacy for children who use AAC. In view of the importance of this topic, it is likely that, in the relatively near future, clinicians will have increased access to research findings relevant to their work with children who use AAC that specify (1) strategies to foster extended narrative discourse during book reading activities; (2) the reading behaviors of professionals during book reading activities; and (3) the impact of different AAC systems on facilitating active participation during story reading.

In order for the naturally occurring opportunities for language use and literacy development afforded by storybook reading to be fully realized, clinicians may need to carefully study and modify the way they interact with children who use AAC while they are reading. As shown in this chapter, videotaping and discourse analysis are tools professionals can use to become aware of how they interact with children and whether the strategies they are using are effective in meeting their intended goals.

Acknowledgments

We are grateful to the children, parents, and clinicians who generously participated in the study. The research reported in this chapter was made possible in part by a grant from the Spencer Foundation. The data presented, the statements made, and the views expressed are the sole responsibility of the author.

References

Bellon, M. L., & Ogletree, B. T. (2000). Repeated storybook reading as an instructional method. *Intervention in School and Clinic, 36*(2), 75–81.

Bellon, M. L., Ogletree, B. T., & Harn, W. E. (2000). Repeated storybook reading as a language intervention for children with autism. *Focus on Autism and Other Developmental Disorders, 15,* 52–58.

Beukelman, D. R., & Mirenda, P. (2005). *Augmentative and alternative communication: Supporting children and adults with complex communication needs* (3rd ed.). Baltimore: Paul H. Brookes.

Bornstein, M., & Bruner, J. (1989). *Crosscurrents in contemporary psychology.* Hillsdale, NJ: Lawrence Erlbaum Associates.

Bradshaw, M., Hoffman, P., & Norris, J. (1998). The efficacy of expansions and cloze procedures in the development of interpretations by preschool children exhibiting delayed language development. *Language, Speech, and Hearing Services in Schools, 29,* 85–95.

Bruner, J. S. (1978). The role of dialogue in language acquisition. In A. Sinclair, R. J. Jarvelle, & W. J. M. Levelt (Eds.), *The child's conception of language.* New York: Springer-Verlag.

Carle, E. (1996). *The grouchy ladybug.* HarperCollins.

Crowe, L. (2000). Reading behaviors of mothers and their children with language impairment during storybook reading. *Journal of Communication Disorders, 33,* 503–524.

Crowe, L., Norris, J. A., & Hoffman, P. R. (2000). Facilitating storybook interactions between mothers and their preschoolers with language impairments. *Communication Disorders Quarterly, 21*(3), 131–146.

Crowe, L., Norris, J. A., & Hoffman, P. R. (2004). Training caregivers to facilitate communicative participation of preschool children with language impairment during storybook reading. *Journal of Communication Disorders, 37,* 177–196.

Dale, P. S., Crain-Thoreson, C., Notari-Syverson, A., & Cole, K. (1996). Parent-child book reading as an intervention technique for young children with language delays. *Topics in Early Childhood Special Education, 16,* 213–235.

Davie, J., & Kemp, C. (2002). A comparison of the expressive language opportunities provided by shared book reading and facilitated play for young children with mild to moderate intellectual disabilities. *Educational Psychology, 22,* 445–460.

DeLoache, J. S., & De Mendoza, O. A. P. (1987). Joint picturebook interactions of mothers and one-year-old children. *British Journal of Developmental Psychology, 5,* 111–123.

De Temple, J., & Hirschler, J. (1991). *Mother's comments during book reading as a source of narrative structure for preschoolers.* Paper presented at the Boston University Conference on Language Development.

Dexter, M. (1998). *The effects of aided language stimulation upon verbal output and augmentative communication during storybook reading for children with pervasive developmental disabilities.* Unpublished doctoral dissertation, John Hopkins University, Baltimore.

Dickinson, D. K., & Tabors, P. O. (2001). *Beginning literacy with language: Young children learning at home and school.* Baltimore: Paul H. Brookes.

Dorr, A., Rabin, B., & Irlen, S. (2002). Parents, children, and the media. In M. H. Bornstein (Ed.), *Handbook on parenting* (Vol. 5, pp. 349-374). Hillsdale, NJ: Lawrence Erlbaum Associates.

Downing, J. E. (2005). *Teaching literacy to students with significant disabilities.* Thousand Oaks, CA: Corwin Press.

Ezell, H., Justice, L., & Parsons, D. (2000). Enhancing the emergent literacy skills of preschoolers with communication disorders: A pilot investigation. *Child Language Teaching and Therapy, 16,* 121-140.

Heim, M. J. M., & Baker-Mills, A. E. (1996). Early development of symbolic communication and linguistic complexity through augmentative and alternative communication. In S. von Tetzchner & M. H. Jensen (Eds), *Augmentative and alternative communication: European perspectives* (chapter 14, pp. 232-248). London: Whurr.

Hockenberger, E. H., Goldstein, H., & Haas, L. S. (1999). Effects of commenting during joint book reading by mothers with low SES. *Topics in Early Childhood Special Education, 19,* 15-27

Jordan, G. E., Snow, C. E., & Porche, M. V. (2000). Project EASE: The effect of a family literacy project on kindergarten students' early literacy skills. *Reading Research Quarterly, 35,* 526-546.

Justice, L., & Ezell, H. (1999). Vygotskian theory and its application to language assessment: An overview for speech-language pathologists. *Contemporary Issues in Communication Science and Disorders, 26,* 111-118.

Justice, L., & Ezell, H. (2000). Enhancing children's print and word awareness through home-based parent intervention. *American Journal of Speech-Language Pathology, 9,* 257-269.

Justice, L., & Ezell, H. (2002). Use of storybook reading to increase print awareness in at-risk children. *American Journal of Speech-Language Pathology, 11,* 17-29.

Justice, L., & Ezell, H. (2004). Print referencing: An emergent literacy enhancement strategy and its clinical applications. *Language, Speech and Hearing Services in Schools, 35,* 185-193.

Justice, L., & Kaderavek, J. N. (2003). Topic control during shared storybook reading: Mothers and their children with language impairments. *Topics in Early Childhood Special Education, 23,* 137–150.

Koppenhaver, D., & Yoder, D. (1993). Classroom literacy instruction for children with severe speech and physical impairments (SSPI): What is and what ought to be. *Topics in Language Disorders, 13*(2), 1–15.

Koppenhaver, D. A, Erickson, K. A., Harris, B., McLellan J., Skotko, B., & Newton, R. A. (2001). Storybook-based communication intervention for girls with Rett syndrome and their mothers. *International Journal on Disability and Rehabilitation, 23,* 149–159.

Liboiron, N., & Soto, G. (2006). Shared storybook reading with a student who uses AAC: An intervention session. *Child Language Teaching and Therapy, 22,* 69–95.

Light, J., Binger, C., & Kelford Smith, A. (1994). Story reading interactions between preschoolers who use AAC and their mothers. *Augmentative and Alternative Communication, 10*(4), 255–268.

Light, J., & Kelford-Smith, A. (1993). Home literacy experiences of preschoolers who use AAC systems and of their non-disabled peers. *Augmentative and Alternative Communication, 9,* 10–25.

Merritt, D. D., & Liles, B. Z. (1987). Story grammar ability in children with and without language disorder: Story generation, story retelling, and story comprehension. *Journal of Speech and Hearing Research, 30,* 539–552.

Mirenda, P., & Schuler, A. (1988). Teaching individuals with autism and related disorders to use visual-spatial symbols to communicate. In S. Blackstone & D. Bruskin (Eds.), *Augmentative communication: Intervention strategies* (pp. 5.1–17.11, 11–25). Rockville, MD: American Speech-Language-Hearing Association.

Moore, L. (2004). *The role of rote learning.* Unpublished doctoral dissertation, University of California–Los Angeles, Los Angeles.

Müller, E. & Soto, G. (2002). Conversational patterns of three adults using aided speech: Variations across partners. *Augmentative and Alternative Communication, 18,* 77–90.

Nelson, K. (1996). *Language in cognitive development: The emergence of the mediated mind.* Cambridge, UK: Cambridge Press.

Ninio, A. (1983). Joint book reading as a multiple vocabulary acquisition device. *Developmental Psychology, 19,* 445–451.

Ninio, A., & Bruner, J. (1978). The achievements and antecedents of labeling. *Journal of Child Language, 5,* 1–15.

Norris, J., & Hoffman, P. (1990). Language intervention within naturalistic environments. *Language, Speech, and Hearing Services in Schools, 21,* 72–84.

Romski, M., & Sevcik, R. (1996). *Breaking the speech barrier: Language development through augmented means*. Baltimore: Paul H. Brookes.

Skotko, B. G., Koppenhaver, D. A., & Erickson, K. A. (2004). Parent reading behaviors and communication outcomes in girls with Rett syndrome. *Exceptional Children, 70*(2), 145–166.

Snow, C. E., & Goldfield, B. A. (1983). Turn the page please: Situation-specific language acquisition. *Journal of Child Language, 10,* 551–569.

Snow, C. E., & Ninio, A. (1986). The contracts of literacy: What children learn from learning to read books. In W. Teale & E. Sulzby (Eds.), *Emergent literacy: Writing and reading* (pp.116–138). Norwood, NJ: Ablex.

Snow, C., Burns, M. S., & Griffin, P. (1998). *Preventing reading difficulties in young children*. Washington, DC: National Academy Press.

Soto, G. (2004). *Use of narratives at school and home by children who use AAC systems*. Spencer Foundation, Chicago.

Soto, G., & Hartmann, E. (2006). Analysis of narratives produced by four children who use AAC. *Journal of Communication Disorders*. Published online at http://www.sciencedirect.com (print forthcoming).

Sutton, A., Soto, G., & Blockberger, S. (2002). Grammatical issues in graphic symbol communication. *Augmentative and Alternative Communication, 18,* 192–204.

Von Tetzchner, S., & Martinsen, H. (1996). Words and strategies: Conversations with young children who use aided language. In S. von Tetzchner & M. H. Jensen (Eds.), *European perspectives* (pp. 65–68). London: Whurr.

APPENDIX 9–A

Key to Transcription Notation for Aided Conversations

1. Eye Gaze

⇑⇓　　　　Eye gaze upward and downward (equivalent to nodding head)

⇒P　　　　Arrow indicates direction of eye gaze followed by the object or person being looked at; e.g., ⇑P means "looked up at P," and ⇒P means "looked toward P."

2. Head Movement

↑↓↑　　　　Nodding head

←→　　　　Shaking head

↑　　　　　Head orientation upward

↓　　　　　Head orientation downward

3. Other Communication Modes

Word　　　Natural speech

"Word"　　Speech generated by voice output device

"XX"　　　Words or phrases "uttered" via voice output using only one key stroke are contained within quotation marks

((voc.))　　Unintelligible vocalization

((laugh))　Description of other paralinguistic behaviors contained within parentheses

4. Message Construction

((init. msg. constr.))　　Spontaneous message construction initiated during current turn

((msg. constr. cont.))　　Message construction continued across two or more turns

((pre-stored msg.))　　　Activation of pre-stored message

5. Other

(30 sec.)   Time between initiation of one discourse unit and the next

CAPS   Emphatic stress (speech or vocalization only)

[word]   Gloss

Placement of two discourse units on single line (e.g., laugh and establishing eye contact) represents concurrent events.

APPENDIX 9–B

Operationalization of the Coding Scheme

Code	Classification	Definitions
	Scaffolding Strategies	
PR	Print Reference	Adult indexes information at the print, text or book level.
CP	Cloze Procedure	Adult speaks the beginning of an utterance and expects the student to continue the utterance
EX	Expansion	Adult repeats student's utterance and includes an elaboration of syntactically correct language
BC	Binary Choice	Adult usually offers two choices of utterances and/or icons
PO	Pointing/Cueing	Adult points to information at the print, text, book or device level with verbal prompts
QU	Questions Constituent	Adult elicits specific information at lower levels of semantic complexity: In., La., and De
QC	Questions Comprehension	Adult elicits information at a higher level of semantic complexity: Int., Inf., and Me
	Semantic Complexity	
In	Indication	Identifying objects, people or actions by pointing or eyegaze
La	Labeling	Naming of objects, people or actions
De	Description	Description of objects, persons or the relationship between actions or states
Int	Interpretation	Interpretation of goals or states or actions that were not explicitly observable
Inf	Inference	Extended meaning beyond what was present or suggested by the book or context
Me	Metalanguage	Knowledge about language or properties of language

Chapter Ten

Recruiting Children's Attention to Print During Shared Reading

Sharon R. Stewart
Sherri M. Lovelace

Overview

Emergent literacy refers to the skills, knowledge, and attitudes that children acquire before the initiation of formal reading instruction (Whitehurst & Lonigan, 1998). During the emergent literacy period, the child begins to learn about literacy in response to printed language exposure and social-verbal interactions in the child's environment (Hall, 1987), and this learning occurs best in literacy-rich contexts in which the child experiences reading and writing in functional, meaningful settings. Understandings about the functions and forms of literacy developed during this period are critical to success in later literacy learning (e.g., Catts & Kamhi, 1999; Justice & Ezell, 2004; Neuman & Dickinson, 2002; Snow, Burns, & Griffin, 1998; Whitehurst & Lonigan, 1998).

Snow et al. (1998) describe a literacy-rich environment as one in which (1) a high value is placed on literacy; (2) there exists an expectation for achievement; (3) reading materials are available and used for various purposes; (4) children are frequently read to; and (5) there are multiple and varied opportunities for verbal interaction. By observing print-related activities, interacting with skilled learners engaged in literacy-based activities, and practicing reading and writing-related tasks, most children in literacy-rich environments acquire the language skills necessary to understand and interact with print, develop positive attitudes toward print, gain an appreciation for the varied and unique uses of reading and writing, and acquire early knowledge about phonological awareness and print concepts (Adams, 1990; Neuman & Dickinson, 2002; Snow et al., 1998).

In addition to oral language skills, reading outcomes for at-risk children are closely linked to phonological awareness and print concept knowledge (Chaney, 1998; Storch & Whitehurst, 2002; Whitehurst & Lonigan, 1998). Phonological awareness refers to the explicit awareness of and sensitivity to the sound structure of spoken language (Stanovich, 1988). Most children acquire phonological awareness during the preschool period, including skills associated with blending (e.g., c-at = cat) and segmenting (e.g., ball = b-all) sound structures at the word, syllable, onset-rime, and phoneme levels (Justice & Kaderavek, 2004). Typically, phonological awareness follows a developmental progression that proceeds from awareness of larger units, such as words and syllables, to smaller units, including onsets, rimes, and phonemes. Research consistently demonstrates that phonological awareness is important to later reading success and that phonological awareness instruction can be successful for reducing children's risks for reading problems. Therefore, it is not surprising that much of the intervention research for children at risk for reading failure at the emergent literacy stage has addressed phonological awareness (e.g., Catts & Kamhi, 1999; Dickinson & Neuman, 2006; Neuman & Dickinson, 2002; Snow et al., 1998).

Although it has received less attention in intervention research, print concept knowledge is another area important to literacy development and is the focus of this chapter (Lomax & McGee, 1987; Scarborough, 1998). Print concept knowledge includes alphabet knowledge as well as understanding of a range of print concepts, such as how it is organized in various texts. Print concept knowledge provides children with a contextual framework for interpreting printed information (Clay 1993; Snow et al., 1998; van Kleeck, 2003). Although various systems have been used to classify print concepts, the classification system used in this chapter sorts print concepts into three areas: book conventions, print conventions, and print forms.

Book conventions refer to understanding how books are created, how they function, and how they are organized. *Print conventions* refer to knowledge of the organizational scheme of print, which in English involves a left-to-right, top-to-bottom orientation. Knowledge of *print forms* is the understanding that print units, such as words and letters, can be named and differentiated from one another and from other text, such as numbers or scribbles. Table 10–1 lists book convention, print convention, and print form concepts often acquired during the emergent literacy period.

Children at Risk for Reading Problems

Although many children readily acquire the emergent literacy skills necessary for reading success, including competencies in both phonological awareness and print concept knowledge, some do not. This occurs as a result of factors intrinsic to the child, which prevent a child from benefiting from literacy learning opportunities, as well as factors extrinsic to the child, which influence children's exposure to and opportunities for language- and print-related activities. Research indicates that reading problems often stem from influences related to both intrinsic and extrinsic factors (Catts & Kamhi, 1999).

An intrinsic risk factor of considerable interest to the speech-language pathologist (SLP) is the influence of language impairment on children's reading development. It is well established that reading comprehension relates strongly to oral language competencies, and that reading success is correlated with children's abilities in the phonologic, semantic, syntactic, and pragmatic domains of language. Consequently, deficits in any aspect of language can have a negative impact on children's reading, and studies confirm that children with language impairments are at an elevated risk for later reading difficulties (Catts & Kamhi, 1999; Scarborough, 2002; Snow et al., 1998). Scarborough's (2002) recent review of longitudinal studies of reading achievement showed that both a family history of reading problems and a history of language impairment were associated with difficulties in acquiring emergent literacy skills, including phonological awareness, letter knowledge, and print concepts, as well as later reading achievement. Catts and Kamhi (1999) reported that more than half of children with language impairment in preschool or kindergarten demonstrate later reading difficulties, whereas Snow et al. (1998) noted that between 40% and 75% of preschoolers with early language impairment develop reading difficulties, as well as generalized academic problems. Among children

Table 10–1. Examples of Book Convention, Print Convention, and Print Form Concepts

Skill	Concepts for Young Children
Book conventions	How to hold a book (right side up)
	Book handling (turn pages individually from front to back)
	Author (writes the book)
	Illustrator (creates the pictures/illustrations)
	Book title and function
	Beginning/end of book
	Front/back of book
	Page
	Top/bottom of page
	Print and pictures differ in their functions
Print conventions	Read from front to back of book, page by page
	Read left to right across pages and across individual words
	Read top to bottom
	Read by "sweeping" from right end of line to left of next line
	Read from bottom of page to top of next page
	First letter of a word is on the left; last letter is on the right
Print form	Words are separated by spaces
	Words, letters, and numbers are different
	Can point to words individually as they are read
	Words are made up of letters
	Uppercase (capital) and lowercase letter correspondence

with language impairment, those who have more severe and broad-based language deficits constitute the group at highest risk for reading difficulties.

Some studies suggest that even in the context of high-quality literacy-related experiences, print concept knowledge may develop more slowly in children with language impairment than in their typically achieving peers (Gillam & Johnston, 1985; Schuele & van Kleeck, 1987). Although this slower learning is due, at least in part, to intrinsic factors (i.e., presence of language impairment), extrinsic factors also may contribute to children's poor performance. Marvin and Mirenda (1993) found that parents of children with disabilities placed a lower priority on their children's literacy development and provided fewer home literacy experiences than families of nondisabled children in Head Start. In a later study of children with language impairment, Marvin and Wright (1997) found that print-focused interactions with adults were not well supported or encouraged in the home. Marvin and Wright also found that characteristics of adult-child literacy-related interactions differed when children with impairments were compared with typically developing children; parents of children with language impairment were less likely to ask questions during read-aloud activities and to engage in oral story telling, and their children were less likely to ask or answer questions during shared reading. These findings suggest that literacy socialization (i.e., children's interactions during and exposure to early print experiences) and language impairment are related, so that children's inability to interact with adults in a typical fashion may lead to atypical adult interactions around print, which in turn reduce literacy learning opportunities. Such findings may not generalize to all children with language impairment, however; because a study of mother-child interactions during storybook reading revealed significant variability in the type and quality of interactions between parents and their children with developmental disabilities (Rabidoux & MacDonald, 2000).

Role of the Speech-Language Pathologist

Research on the development of language and literacy and their inter-relationships clearly demonstrates that SLPs have an important role in facilitating both language *and* literacy development in young children (American Speech-Language-Hearing Association [ASHA], 2001). Exclusive attention to oral language intervention while leaving written language intervention to others is now recognized as an unnecessary division of professional responsibility that may, in fact, impede children's overall progress. The remainder of this chapter describes how clinical interventions can systematically include attention to both oral language and emergent literacy skills, with a particular focus on print concept knowledge.

Including a focus on emergent literacy skills is increasingly viewed as a fundamental facet of early language intervention because it may reduce children's risk for reading problems in later years. A proactive approach to the prevention of reading problems is preferable to and more efficient than providing intervention after reading disabilities have become apparent (Snow et al., 1998). Research demonstrates that elementary school–age children with reading delays are unlikely to catch up to their age mates for various reasons, including the development of low motivation and poor attitudes toward literacy, difficulties unlearning ineffective compensatory strategies, and problems in acquiring effective reading strategies (Catts & Kamhi, 1999; Dickinson & Neuman, 2006; Snow et al., 1998). By embedding instructional targets that go beyond traditional language skills to include those most directly linked to later reading success, including both phonological awareness and print concept knowledge, SLPs can help ensure that children will be successful in developing the oral and written language skills necessary for school success.

One important context for facilitating these important early literacy skills is that of adult-child shared storybook reading. Shared book reading between young children and adults is common in literacy-rich environments, and its contribution to reading success is well documented. In addition to building children's enjoyment of and interest in literacy, a very early outcome of shared book reading is children's acquired appreciation of how pictures and text interact to form a story (Adams, 1990). Shared book reading also helps to develop emergent literacy skills including knowledge about print concepts, letter identification, vocabulary, and storytelling ability (Bus, van IJendorn, & Pellegrini, 1995; Whitehurst & Lonigan, 1998). Of importance, SLPs can systematically utilize this context to promote children's print concept knowledge.

Shared Book Reading as an Intervention Context

Studies indicate that both the quantity and the quality of shared book reading are important to oral language and emergent literacy development (Whitehurst & Lonigan, 1998). As an interactive social activity, shared reading is most beneficial when it occurs in a safe, comfortable, relaxed, and positive context so that children can examine pictures, discuss the meaning of the book, and become familiar with the format and functions of print (Adams, 1990; Bus, 2002). Furthermore, parents and clinicians should understand that typical preschoolers do not listen passively as adults read or describe stories. Instead, children are actively involved as they point to pictures, ask questions, and label or comment on the pictures or story (Crowe, Norris, & Hoffman, 2000).

The behaviors and attitudes of both the child and the adult affect shared book reading. Specifically, children's interest in book reading is both a prerequisite to and consequence of shared reading. If children are interested in and enjoy shared book reading, adults are more likely to engage in the activity; in turn, children may become even more interested in book reading. The converse also is true: Children's lack of interest in shared book reading may lead to less shared reading by adults, which in turn leads to less interest on behalf of the children.

Although shared book reading has been shown to foster many literacy skills, the value of shared reading is controversial. Scarborough and Dobrich's (1994) finding that shared reading accounts for only 8% of the variance in children's later literacy achievement suggests that children acquire knowledge essential for literacy development in a number of contexts. Nonetheless, shared book reading is an important contributor to both language and literacy development, and it can be used instrumentally to facilitate the development of emergent literacy skill, particularly print concept knowledge (van Kleeck, 2003). For example, Neuman (1999) conducted a large study targeting economically disadvantaged children in which child care providers received training in literacy development, reading aloud to children, techniques to enhance children's responses to stories, and book maintenance. Compared with children whose providers received no such training, these children showed educationally meaningful gains in knowledge of letter names, writing, narratives, and print concepts. These gains were still evident 6 months later in kindergarten.

In an effort to integrate literacy activities into language intervention, SLPs often incorporate shared reading in their intervention protocols. To date, the primary purpose of shared reading in intervention, beyond providing children with exposure to books, has been to promote targeted oral language goals, such as vocabulary and grammatical skills. However, SLPs can systematically modify shared reading activities to address a range of literacy-related skills, which in turn may contribute to later reading achievement (Lovelace & Stewart, in press; Stahl, 2003; van Kleeck & Vander Woude, 2003). One approach that has been studied for its effectiveness is that of print referencing (e.g., Justice & Ezell, 2000, 2002; Lovelace & Stewart, in press), which involves modification in the extent to which print is a focus of adult-child shared storybook reading interactions. As discussed in the next section, SLPs can use a range of strategies to make print a more salient focus of their reading interactions with children, which result in increases in children's print concept knowledge. This can provide an important clinical strategy by which to promote children's emergent literacy skills and to reduce their risk for later reading difficulties steming from early delays in the development of print concept knowledge.

Recruiting Children's Attention to Print During Shared Book Reading

As noted, SLPs can modify the way they read books with children during clinical interventions to promote print concept knowledge while simultaneously attending to targeted oral language skills. One modification adults can make is the use of an explicit print focus to recruit children's attention to print within the storybook. This technique, called *print referencing* (Ezell & Justice, 2000), helps adults to direct children's attention explicitly to targeted print concepts during shared reading to increase the likelihood that children will attend to, and consequently learn, these concepts. The print referencing strategy is based on evidence that at-risk children often fail to acquire skills through *implicit* instructional strategies; instead, these children require *explicit* repeated, systematic, and deliberately scaffolded experiences to acquire skills and concepts (Justice, Chow, Capellini, Flanigan, & Colton, 2003; Justice & Kaderavek, 2004).

The successful use of print referencing to improve children's print concept knowledge has been demonstrated in several studies. Ezell and Justice (2000) showed that adults' use of explicit print references during shared book reading increased middle-class 4-year-old children's verbal utterances about print during reading. Results of a follow-up study indicated that when parents were taught to use nonverbal and verbal print referencing in a 4-week, home-based program, their use of explicit print-referencing behaviors increased, and their preschoolers' print concept knowledge improved more than children whose parents did not receive such instruction (Justice & Ezell, 2000). Similar findings were observed in a study of 30 children attending Head Start who were from low-income families; these children participated in 24 reading sessions with an SLP who used print referencing strategies to focus the children's attention on aspects of print. Compared with a control group of children who participated in picture-focused reading sessions, those in the print referencing group made significantly better gains on three measures of print concept knowledge: words in print; print recognition; and alphabet knowledge (Justice & Ezell, 2002).

Two studies have examined the use of print referencing for children with communication disorders. Ezell, Justice, and Parsons (2000) found that children with communication disorders made notable gains in print concept knowledge when caregivers used print referencing behaviors in a 5-week intervention featuring regular home-based storybook reading. More recently, Lovelace and Stewart (in press) studied the use of print referencing by SLPs for five children with language impairment. Important features of this study were that the clinicians used only nonevocative print referencing cues (commenting about print, tracking and pointing to print) and that print referencing was one part of a larger intervention program focused on language facilitation. All five children made gains in not only language but also print concept knowledge, indicating that print referencing can be effectively and efficiently implemented within the context of a language intervention program.

Print Referencing Procedures

Print referencing procedures are defined as adults' use of cues to recruit children's attention to print concepts embedded into book reading interactions (e.g., see Justice & Ezell, 2004). These cues direct children's attention to various forms, functions, and conventions of written language. *Cues* are behaviors that either implicitly or explicitly direct attention to a referent or concept, and print-referencing cues specifically direct children's attention to various features of print. Using these behaviors, children's attention is deliberately recruited to some aspect of written language in ways that have been found to increase print concept knowledge (Justice & Ezell, 2000). Print referencing cues can be classified according to the style of presentation: *verbal* or *nonverbal*.

Verbal cues

Verbal cues include adults' comments, questions, and requests about print. *Comments* include adults' explanations, remarks, and observations intended to recruit children's attention to print concepts. These comments do not require children to respond, and are thus considered *nonevocative*. For example, while reading aloud, the SLP may draw attention to specific print forms by commenting, "There's a letter T, just like in your name." These comments may be brief asides that inform the child on some aspect of print, although they also may sometimes incite longer discussions about print if the child chooses to take up the topic. The following excerpt demonstrates how comments can be used to heighten children's awareness of multiple book conventions while reading *If You Take a Mouse to the Movies* (Numeroff, 2000).

> *SLP*: This is the <u>front</u> of the book. The <u>title</u> of the book is *If You Take a Mouse to the Movies*.
>
> *Marty*: I like this book.
>
> *SLP*: Yes, I do too. Now let's turn the <u>page</u> and read it.

In this example, the SLP highlighted three book conventions while introducing the book: *front*, *title*, and *page*. Print-related input was provided unobtrusively and fit naturally into introductory comments about the story. To ensure that Marty attended to the salient aspects of the comments, this SLP used highlighting strategies (i.e., emphasizing the target concepts in her own speech through exaggerated stress and intonation) and pointing to the title while dramatically turning the page and commenting. The child did not "pick up" on the print-focused topic, and the SLP responded to this cue by moving on to begin reading the text.

Questions also can be used to recruit children's attention to print concepts. Use of this strategy requires children to interact with the reader and engage more openly with aspects of print. Because questioning requires the children to respond, it is considered an *evocative* strategy. For example, asking "What do you think that word is?" obligates the child to reply. Using questions to support children's learning about book and print conventions is evident in the following transcript of the interaction between an SLP and a child as they begin reading *The Napping House* (Wood, 1984).

SLP: Let's look here. The <u>author</u> is Audrey Wood. Who is the <u>author</u>?

Carlos: Audrey Wood.

SLP: Yes, Audrey Wood is the <u>author</u>. That means she wrote the book. What does <u>author</u> mean?

Carlos: She wrote the book.

SLP: Exactly. Let's read the book.

The SLP used questions to ensure that Carlos is attending to and learning the targeted print concepts. She first provided input on the concept of *author* and then asked the child to answer questions related to this concept. Unlike comments, use of questions requires that SLPs provide sufficient scaffolding for children to be successful. In this example, the SLP asked questions only after modeling the correct response because the concept of *author* was new to Carlos. The SLP will systematically reduce the scaffolding provided and ask questions without prior models and prompts only when she is confident that Carlos can answer the questions correctly.

Requests relating to print features of the text, like questions, also are considered *evocative*. They serve as turn-taking devices and require children to respond. For example, "Show me where I go next to continue reading" is a request the SLP can use to direct the child's focus on the directionality of print while fostering active engagement with the text. The following excerpt shows how requests can be used to focus on print conventions and print forms while the SLP reads *The Napping House* (Wood, 1984).

SLP: Show me where I begin reading on this page.

John: [points to the top left word on the page]

SLP: That's right. I'll begin reading right here. Let's look at this word. Point to a letter that is in your name.

John: [points to the letter O in the word]

SLP: Yes, that's the letter O and it is in your name. [The SLP reads the page aloud.] Now, show me where I will go to read next.

John: [points to the top of the next page]

SLP: Perfect. That's exactly what I will do next.

In this excerpt, the SLP uses requests to engage the child in the activity and informally assess his understanding of several print concepts. This book reading activity followed others in which the SLP used print referencing cues to focus on letters and print directionality. As with use of questions, scaffolding may be required for children to successfully engage with the print. In this example, the SLP is confident that John can correctly follow her requests without scaffolding because of his past performance, and she provides specific feedback only after he completes the task.

Nonverbal Cues

Nonverbal cues refer to instances when adults point to and track print to recruit children's attention to print concepts; these can occur in the absence of explicit verbal cues. These cues do not require children to respond and thus are considered *nonevocative*.

Pointing refers to pointing to aspects of text during shared reading. Pointing to individual words while reading aloud is an example of how this cue can be used to draw children's attention to the *concept of word* during book sharing. Pointing can be used independently or combined with other strategies. In the following excerpt, the SLP uses pointing to draw attention to words and the direction of print while reading *If You Take a Mouse to the Movies* (Numeroff, 2000).

> *SLP*: Now I will read each word on this page
>
> *Aaron*: Okay.
>
> *SLP*: [finger points to each word as she reads the page]
>
> *SLP*: I am here [points to the bottom of the page], so now I have to go here to keep reading [points to the top of the following page].

In this example, the SLP combined finger pointing with commenting to draw Aaron's attention to words. Because neither cue required a response, Aaron could focus on the task without any expectation of having to perform. The SLP continued to highlight the concept of *word* by pointing to each word while reading aloud. When she came to the bottom of the page, the SLP again combined pointing and commenting to demonstrate print directionality from one page to the next. Although pointing can be effective in helping children focus on words, Clay (1993) cautions against allowing children to use finger pointing extensively in their own reading because it may interfere with reading fluency.

Tracking print involves moving a finger beneath letters or words while reading aloud. Tracking includes such motions as moving a finger left to right below letters in a word or words in a line, making a return sweep to the next line, and then moving from the bottom of a page to the top of the next while reading. Although tracking can be used to focus on several print concepts, it is especially useful for directing children's attention to the directionality of print (Clay, 1993). In the following example, the SLP introduces the concept of directionality of print while reading *The Napping House* (Wood, 1984).

> *SLP*: Now I am going to read here and go this way [as she moves her finger in a sweeping fashion left to right, line by line].
>
> *Otis*: Okay.

> *SLP*: [draws her finger along under the text as she reads aloud]

In this instance, the SLP provided input using nonevocative strategies to introduce the concept of directionality. In a subsequent reading session, the SLP modeled the sweeping motion and then requested Otis to imitate the motion. A still later session involved tracking individual words and focusing on the first, middle, and last letters in the word.

Integrating Print Referencing Cues

By recruiting children's attention to print using print referencing strategies in the context of meaningful activities, such as shared reading, SLPs can facilitate development of critical print concepts necessary for success in reading and writing. The preceding examples show how each print referencing strategy is applied independently; however, SLPs typically address multiple print concepts using a variety of print referencing cues simultaneously. Table 10–2 demonstrates how an SLP uses a range of different print referencing cues to focus attention on several print concepts while reading the book *Wemberly Worried* (Henkes, 2000) with a child with language impairment.

Selecting Intervention Targets

Use of print referencing strategies to recruit children's attention to print concepts during shared reading can be implemented as a general facilitation strategy or as a method to address specific print concept knowledge. If the strategies are being used for facilitation, SLPs can select several concepts from Table 10-1 that are appropriate for the book being read and appear suitable for the children's developmental level. More careful assessment and monitoring will be necessary, however, if specific, individualized print concepts are targeted. Whether this approach is used as a generalized facilitation strategy or as a strategy to address specific print concepts, several print concepts can be targeted simultaneously in a single reading session (Kaderavek & Justice, 2004).

Table 10–2. Sample Book Sharing Activity Integrating Several Print Concepts and Print Referencing Behaviors

Script		Print Referencing Cues	Print Concept
SLP:	This is our new book. The title of the story is *Wemberly Worried.* [tracking print under the title while reading]	Commenting Tracking	Title Print direction
Child:	Is that mouse Wemberly?		
SLP:	Yes, that's Wemberly and this word is her name—Wemberly. [pointing to the word].	Commenting Pointing	Concept of word
Child:	W-em-ber-ly. [moving finger beneath the word]		
SLP:	Right. And do you remember what this is called? [tracking print under the title]	Questioning Tracking	Title
Child:	It's a title.		
SLP:	That's exactly right. It's the title.	Commenting	Title
SLP:	[opening book] This is the beginning of the story. I'll begin reading here [pointing to the first line of text and tracking print as it is read]	Commenting Tracking	Begin (to read) Print direction
SLP:	[SLP reads several lines and comes to a natural place to stop]. Show me where I go next to read.	Requesting	Print direction

continues

341

Table 10–2. (*continued*)

Script	Pring Referencing Cues	Print Concept
Child: [correctly points to the next line of text]		
SLP: Yes, that's where I go next. [points to place where child pointed] I will read some more.	Commenting Pointing	Print direction
SLP: [continues to read aloud and then stops] Look! There's the letter "I," just like in your name. [pointing to "I" at the beginning of a word]	Commenting Pointing	Letter (print form)
Child: Where? There it is! [pointing to the "I"] And here is a "k" just like mine. [pointing to a "k" in another word on the page]		
SLP: That's right! You are so smart. That is a "k." [pointing to the "k"]	Commenting Pointing	Letter
SLP: Tell me: Is "k" a letter or is it a word?	Questioning	Letter Word
Child: It's a letter.		
SLP: Yes, "k" is a letter.	Commenting	Letter
SLP: Let's read more! [reads aloud]		

Specific Targets

To select specific print concepts for intervention, children's skills should be carefully assessed and monitored to ensure that targeted concepts are within the children's "zone of proximal development." Skills in the zone of proximal development are those that children can perform with assistance but have not mastered to the level of independence. Skills at the lower end of the zone are those that are nearing mastery (i.e., are fairly mature), whereas skills at the upper limit are those that children can accomplish only when provided with maximum adult support (Vygotsky, 1978). When targeted skills are within children's zone of proximal development, adult scaffolding, such as modeling, demonstration, cues, explanations, and guided questions, is provided and then systematically removed as children acquire the skills.

Multiple strategies can be used to select and monitor progress on intervention targets. Observation of children engaged in literacy activities can be helpful in determining the children's knowledge of print concepts and other skills. For example, SLPs can observe how children manipulate books, notice how they track print during reading, observe whether children attempt to read words or name letters, and monitor children's questions and comments during reading. SLPs can also gain much information about children's print concept knowledge by observing their involvement in other literacy-related activities, such as writing and reading environmental print. An ongoing collection of artifacts (e.g., efforts at scribbling or writing, completed literacy-related classroom activities) also can be used to identify children's approximate skill levels and to monitor improvement over time.

SLPs also can informally assess children's print-related skills using a dynamic assessment process. They can observe children's responses to direct requests made in the context of literacy-related activities (e.g., "Write your name"; "Tell me the first letter of this word"; "Turn to the last page of the book"), identify those skills that are mastered, and experiment to determine the extent and type of support needed for the children to acquire additional print concepts.

Formal assessment instruments are available to assess children's print concept knowledge. Most of these instruments are adaptations of the Concepts about Print (CAP) assessment tool developed by Clay (2002). The CAP is used as a primary means of assessment for children in the Reading Recovery program (Clay, 1993), and it is recognized as a valid and reliable tool. However, most items on the CAP were developed for children in elementary grades who have received formal reading instruction, and its norms are relevant only for school-age children. Consequently, researchers and clinicians have found it necessary to modify the test for use with preschool children (e.g., Justice & Ezell, 2000, 2002; Lovelace & Stewart, in press). Although these modified instruments have obvious face validity (i.e., they appear to measure print concept knowledge), the reliability and validity of these instruments have not been established. In response to the need for a valid and reliable assessment instrument, Justice, Bowles, and Skibbe (2006) recently studied the validity and reliability for their instrument, the Preschool Word and Print Awareness (PWPA) tool (see Justice & Ezell, 2001), which is a modification of the CAP (Clay, 2002) that is used to assess 3- to 5-year-old children's understanding of 14 print concepts. The PWPA is individually administered during an adult-child shared book reading activity. This tool, which is reproduced in Appendix 10-A, provides a valid measure for assessing preschoolers' print concept knowledge and is sensitive to differences among children at-risk for reading problems as a result of language impairment and lower socioeconomic status (Justice et al., 2006). The PWPA and other informal and formal tools constitute important resources for clinicians who require quantitative data for selecting intervention goals and monitoring intervention effects.

Selecting Print Referencing Strategies and Contexts

Activities for recruiting children's attention to print can be carried out in many contexts using various print referencing strategies. Justice and Ezell (2004) describe the challenges and benefits of targeting print concepts in group and individual intervention settings. They suggest that all children can benefit from print referencing strategies incorporated into group shared reading activities in preschool classrooms, particularly when use of these strategies does not interrupt the flow of the shared reading activity. When identified by observation in whole-class environments and results of additional assessment, those children who lack understanding of print concepts and who are not making satisfactory progress can be enrolled in individual or small group intervention for more frequent, intense, and focused print concept instruction (Kaderavek & Justice, 2004).

Children's cultural and linguistic backgrounds, as well as their capabilities, interests and experience with books and book sharing routines, should be considered when preparing book sharing activities and selecting print referencing strategies (Kaderavek & Justice, 2002). SLPs should plan book sharing activities that are sensitive to the type of adult input and adult-child interaction most familiar to children during shared reading and to children's familiarity with books and book sharing routines. SLPs also must keep in mind that adult reading styles and child engagement exert bidirectional effects, and some types of input may actually negatively affect or reduce adult-child communication (Kaderavek & Justice, 2002; Rabidoux & MacDonald, 2000). For example, it may be more appropriate to initiate the shared book reading procedure using nonverbal print referencing strategies, such as commenting, pointing, and tracking, for children from backgrounds in which direct questioning by children is not appropriate. As another example, shared book reading that includes explicit attention to print concepts may be inappropriate for children with severe cognitive or language impairments because these children may not enjoy book reading and may respond differently to activities embedded in book reading than typical children (Crain-Thoreson and Dale, 1999). For these children, the purpose of book reading interventions may be to promote a general interest in print and books.

To encourage children's engagement, parents and clinicians can select books with children's interests in mind, let children choose books, make the book reading event brief, and reduce performance demands on the child. Some children may find shared reading enjoyable if it occurs in a special reading place or "book nook," such as an attractive reading corner with comfortable "beanbag" chairs, reading lights, and a readily available selection of children's favorite books. A special routine and time associated with book reading also can facilitate children's interest in book reading. For children who do not enjoy being read to, explicit attention to print concepts should be delayed and implemented gradually only after the children demonstrate an interest in and an ability to attend to books.

For children who lack the requisite skills to respond verbally to print cues or for whom such cues seem inappropriate, consideration should be given to the selection of evocative and nonevocative print referencing cues. Although use of evocative techniques has been found to elicit more child responses during book reading and other contexts than occurs with use of nonevocative techniques (Justice, Weber, Ezell, & Bakeman, 2002; Olsen-Fulero & Conforti, 1983; Whitehurst et al., 1994; Yoder & Davies, 1990), a study by Lovelace and Stewart (in press) demonstrated that nonevocative techniques can be effective in facilitating print concept knowledge. In their study, children with language impairment learned print concepts presented using only nonevocative cues (commenting, pointing, and tracking) during shared book reading conducted as part of language intervention. These findings are important because children with language impairment may be limited in their ability to respond orally to evocative cues during book reading interactions. For these children, use of nonevocative print referencing strategies that place fewer demands on children's expressive language facility may be as effective as evocative approaches.

Recruiting Children's Attention to Print: General Guidelines for Implementation

Achieve Balance

Strategies for recruiting children's attention to print during shared book reading should be used judiciously. The transition to implementation of print referencing activities may be gradual for some children, but even when fully implemented, the strategies should not be the primary focus of the book sharing. Instead, these activities should be embedded during story reading to complement other aspects of the story. In fact, Justice and Ezell (2004) recommend using print referencing cues a total of 3 to 5 times during storybook reading. This guideline is flexible depending on such factors as the types of print referencing strategies used, the timing of presentation of the print reference cues during the shared reading activity, the type and length of the book, and children's interests and capabilities. For example, the number of print referencing cues used can be increased if the selected cues are less intrusive (e.g., simple, nonevocative cues, such as pointing to words) or if some of the print referencing activity occurs before and after the actual book reading (e.g., showing the title of the book, identifying the author, showing the back of the book).

Some kinds of books do not lend themselves to print referencing opportunities. For example, alphabet books may be suitable for focusing attention on print forms, whereas drawing attention to print concepts while reading a poem would be disruptive to the flow of the poem. Children's behavior also may dictate the amount and type of attention given to print concepts. Because preschool children are more likely to respond to evocative than nonevocative cueing strategies (Justice et al., 2002), children who are inattentive or unengaged may benefit from evocative cues (e.g., questioning, requesting) that require them to participate more actively in the book sharing activity. Highly interactive children, on the other hand, may require relatively few print reference cues because they may comment on and ask numerous questions about book and print features spontaneously, thereby creating multiple and extended opportunities to discuss print concepts.

Involve Parents and Teachers

Book reading is a social, interactive activity that is best conducted between children and adults with whom the children have a positive attachment (Bus, 2002). By involving parents, families, and teachers, opportunities for positive and frequent shared reading events between the children and caring adults are enhanced (Justice & Pence, 2004). In their description of the embedded-explicit emergent literacy intervention approach, Justice and Kaderavek (2004) discuss the importance of SLP consultation and collaboration with parents and teachers to ensure high quality and adequate quantity of socially embedded literacy-focused experiences. By utilizing others to provide these experiences, SLPs can then focus on individualized assessment and ongoing monitoring, guide the development of intervention goals, provide expert consultation on intervention strategies, and serve as the direct provider of explicit, structured, and more intense intervention on targeted print concept–related goals.

Parent involvement can begin with an assessment of the importance placed on literacy-related activities in the home. Because home literacy environments are critical to children's attitudes and success in literacy learning, SLPs can encourage parents to create literacy-rich environments by (1) having a variety of print materials in the home; (2) reading aloud to their children often and re-reading favorite books; and (3) reading in a way that promotes children's enjoyment of books, enhances the development of language skills, and facilitates children's print concept knowledge (Ezell et al., 2000).

Although shared book reading should be encouraged, it should be noted that some adults fail to use effective book reading strategies. Fortunately, several studies (see Snow et al., 1998) have been conducted showing that adults can be taught basic strategies for enhancing storybook reading, although some adults may require extensive instruction and modeling. Parents may need instruction in how to make reading enjoyable by moving beyond reading stories verbatim and providing children with opportunities to interact and join in the reading. Such interactions may be especially important for at-risk readers because these interactions may help bridge the gap between book content and children's knowledge and interest (Bus, 2002).

Even parents who are experienced at reading aloud to their children may refer to print concepts sparingly, either verbally or nonverbally (Ezell & Justice, 2000; Phillips & McNaughton, 1990; Stahl, 2003); instead, they focus on the meaning of the story (Ezell & Justice, 2000). Several studies, however, have shown that adults can be taught to use specific print referencing strategies with relative ease. For example, Ezell and Justice (2000) found that graduate student clinicians increased their use of verbal and nonverbal print references after minimal training and that children's questions and comments about print increased when the students used these strategies. In a subsequent study, parents who were taught to use print-referencing strategies during reading and then participated in a 4-week shared reading program increased their use of print referencing cues, and their children demonstrated improvement in several areas of print and word awareness (Justice & Ezell, 2000).

Although these studies indicate that parents can learn print referencing strategies, the kinds of parental supports and scaffolding required for implementation of general and print concept-specific book reading strategies will vary according to parents' background experiences and their attitudes and skills around literacy. For some parents, home visits may be beneficial, and regular consultation and ongoing scaffolding for creating a literacy-rich environment and providing positive, beneficial book sharing experiences may be necessary (Landry & Smith, 2006; Snow et al; 1998).

Select Books With Goals in Mind

Varying the format, genre, and content of books used during book reading can help maintain children's interest and help ensure generalization of targeted print concepts. Examples of book format variations include the very small or large books, pop-up books, shape books, books with textures or buttons to push that promote direct interaction with the book, books with pages or text that vary in size, and board books. Examples of genre variations include poetry, fiction, nonfiction, predictable books, fairytales, and ABC or number books. Content can be varied to include stories about animals, people, nature, different cultures, cartoon characters, fantasy, and so forth.

It is intuitively obvious that colorful, interesting books are more likely to engage preschoolers' interest. Trade books such as *The Read-Aloud Handbook* (Trelease, 2001) provide lists of age-appropriate, high-quality books for reading aloud. The American Library Association publishes lists of award-winning books on its Web site, including winners of the prestigious Caldecott, Newbery, and Coretta Scott King awards. In selecting books for reading aloud, it should be remembered that books somewhat beyond the reading level of children may be appropriate, provided that the content is interesting and suitable, because adults will be doing the reading.

Predictable books, defined as books that contain repetitive structures that enable children to predict the next word or line or episode (Bridge, Winograd, & Haley, 1983), can be especially useful in encouraging children to attend to print concepts. Their use adds to children's enjoyment and participation by allowing children to join in the reading the familiar portions of the book, thus having the experience of being successful readers. Children often enjoy having these books read aloud repeatedly, and they can gradually turn their focus to other aspects of the book, such as print concepts, as they gain familiarity with the book content.

Big Books, or oversized books, are beneficial for reading to large groups of children (e.g., Adams, 1990; Snow et al., 1998). The novelty of Big Books appeals to young children, and the larger size allows adults to readily model and demonstrate print concepts to an entire group. Big books can be purchased in sets that also include duplicate, standard-size books so that children can mimic the adult's modeling and follow along individually while the adult reads and comments using the oversized book. A strategy for highlighting print concepts that is especially amenable to the use of Big books is "fingerpoint reading." Using this method, adults point to words in sequence while reading aloud, and children "read" the words aloud with the adults (Holdaway, 1979). This activity, which helps develop word knowledge and print directionality, can be enhanced by having children point to the words in their own books while the adult models the strategy in the accompanying big book.

The kinds of support and nature of interactions between children and adults vary naturally according to the book genre and format (Rabidoux & MacDonald, 2000; Snow et al., 1998). For example, when reading storybooks aloud, adults perceive the purpose of the reading to be entertainment and enjoyment (Teale & Sulzby, 1986), and they begin the activity with a discussion of the author, characters, and concepts, clarify vocabulary in the story, and engage children in predicting and explaining the story. However, when reading books with pictures and single words or phrases, adults are more likely to focus on print concepts, including the words and print on each page. For emphasizing print form concepts, especially concepts pertaining to letters, ABC books or books that emphasize a particular feature of the alphabet may be most appropriate (Teale & Sulzby, 1986). Similarly, print-salient books with large and distinctive print may be most suitable for emphasizing print conventions and print forms (Justice & Ezell, 2004).

Vary the Context

A comprehensive program targeting print concepts should extend beyond shared book reading to other literacy-based activities. The language experience approach (LEA) (Hall, 1987), wherein children complete an activity, dictate a story about the activity to the adult, and then join the adult in repeated oral reading of the story, provides multiple opportunities for highlighting print concepts. While writing the story, adults can talk about the parts of a story, name letters and words, and highlight letter features, such as, capital letters (Adams, 1990; Snow et al, 1998; Stewart & Page, 1992). During reading, adults can focus on directionality, pause between words, and draw attention to letters. An excellent resource for LEA activities is *Book Cooks: Literature-Based Classroom Cooking* (Bruno, 1991), which describes cooking activities associated with children's books.

Dramatic play provides rich opportunities for children to practice literacy-related activities while adults recruit children's attention to print concepts. For example, when children engage in restaurant role play, patrons "read" menus, waiters "write down" the food orders, cooks "read" the order, and waiters "write" the bill after the meal. Adults can draw attention to print concepts while enhancing children's understanding of the special uses of print and heightening their enjoyment of literacy. An excellent source of role-play activities that incorporate literacy can be found in Bunce's book (1995) on the Language-Focused Curricula.

In the natural environment, adults can recruit children's attention to print by fingerpoint reading each word on a label (e.g., Fruit Loops), pointing out distinctive letters on logos (e.g., the "tailed" *C* in Coca-Cola), or pointing to the first letter of a word on a sign (e.g., stop). Adults also can point out directionality, name letters, and discuss other print concepts as children practice writing.

Explicit instruction that focuses specifically on print concepts may be appropriate for children who do not acquire print concept knowledge through repeated exposure in more naturalistic contexts. Providing explicit instruction individually or in small groups allows SLPs to focus on print concepts more intensively within activities that may be intrusive or distracting in a large group setting. Best practice indicates that explicit instruction should be focused, intense, and brief, and that concepts targeted in direct instruction should be systematically generalized into naturalistic contexts.

Summary

This chapter presents clinicians with a description of strategies for recruiting children's attention to print using print referencing strategies during book sharing. Print referencing allows intervention to be provided in the naturalistic context of shared reading, during which adult scaffolding can be provided to meet the needs of individual children. This approach recognizes the importance of a social-interactionist approach to emergent literacy (Kaderavek & Justice, 2002). Intervention at the preschool level also recognizes that emergent literacy skills are critical to later academic success, and represents a means for SLPs to include attention to emergent literacy development within the context of language intervention. Of importance, instruction in print concepts should be conducted in tandem with other skills known to be important to emergent literacy development, including development of oral language, comprehension and production of narratives, enjoyment of and appreciation for the uses of print, recognition of environmental print and beginning word reading, emergent writing, and phonological awareness. By using the strategies discussed in this chapter as part of a comprehensive language and literacy program, SLPs can help improve children's learning outcomes, thus contributing to children's overall school success and quality of life.

References

Adams, M. J. (1990). *Beginning to read: Thinking and learning about print*. Cambridge, MA: MIT Press.

American Speech-Language-Hearing Association. (2001). *Roles and responsibilities of speech-language pathologists with respect to reading and writing in children and adolescents (guidelines)*. Rockville, MD: Author.

Bridge, C., Winograd, P., & Haley, D. (1983). Using predictable materials vs. preprimers to teach beginning sight words. *The Reading Teacher, 38*, 884–891.

Bruno, J. (1991). *Book cooks: Literature-based classroom cooking*. Cypress, CA: Creative Teaching Press.

Bunce, B. (1995). *Building a language-focused curriculum for the preschool classroom. Vol. II: A planning guide*. Baltimore: Paul H. Brookes.

Bus, A. G. (2002). Joint caregiver-child storybook reading: A route to literacy development. In S. B. Neuman, & D. K. Dickinson (Eds.), *Handbook of early literacy research* (pp. 179–191). New York: Guilford Press.

Bus, A., Van IJendorn, M., & Pellegrini, A. (1995). Joint book reading makes for success in learning to read: A meta-analysis on intergenerational transmission of literacy. *Review of Educational Research, 65*, 1–21.

Catts, H. W., & Kamhi, A. G. (Eds.). (1999). *Language and reading disabilities*. Boston: Allyn & Bacon.

Chaney, C. (1998). Preschool language and metalinguistic skills are links to reading success. *Applied Psycholinguistics, 19*, 433–446.

Clay, M. M. (1993). *Reading recovery: A guidebook for teachers in training*. Portsmouth, NH: Heinemann Education.

Clay, M. M. (2002). *An observation survey of early literacy achievement* (2nd ed.). Portsmouth, NH: Heinemann Education.

Crain-Thoreson, C., & Dale, P. S. (1999). Enhancing linguistic performance: Parents and teachers as book reading partners for children with language delays. *Topics in Early Childhood Special Education, 19*(1), 28–40.

Crowe, L. K., Norris, J. A., & Hoffman, P. R. (2000). Facilitating storybook interactions between mothers and their preschoolers with language impairment. *Communication Disorders Quarterly, 21*, 131–146.

Dickinson, D. K., & Neuman, S. B. (2006). *Handbook of early literacy research* (Vol. 2). New York: Guilford Press.

Ezell, H. K., & Justice, L. M. (2000). Increasing the print focus of shared reading through observational learning. *American Journal of Speech-Language Pathology, 9*, 36–47.

Ezell, H. K., Justice, L. M., & Parsons, D. (2000). Enhancing the emergent literacy skills of preschoolers with communication disorders: A pilot investigation. *Child Language Teaching and Therapy, 16*(2), 121–140.

Gillam, R. B., & Johnston, J. R. (1985). Development of print awareness in language-disordered preschoolers. *Journal of Speech and Hearing Research, 28*, 521–526.

Hall, N. (1987). *The emergence of literacy*. Portsmouth, NH: Heinemann.

Henkes, K. (2000). *Wemberly worried*. New York: Greenwillow Books.

Holdaway, D. (1979). *The foundations of literacy*. Sydney, Australia: Ashton Scholastic.

Justice, L. M., Bowles, R, & Skibbe, L. (2006). Measuring preschool attainment of print concepts: A study of typical and at-risk 3- to 5-year-old children. *Language, Speech, and Hearing Services in Schools, 37*, 1–12.

Justice, L. M., Chow, S. M., Capellini, C., Flanigan, K., & Colton, S. (2003). Emergent literacy intervention for vulnerable preschoolers: Relative effects of two approaches. *American Journal of Speech-Language Pathology, 12*, 1–14.

Justice, L. M, & Ezell, H. K. (2000). Enhancing children's print and word awareness through home-based parent intervention. *American Journal of Speech-Language Pathology, 9*, 257–269.

Justice, L. M., & Ezell, H. K. (2001). Written language awareness in preschool children from low-income household: A descriptive analysis. *Communication Disorders Quarterly, 22*, 123–134.

Justice, L. M., & Ezell, H. K. (2002). Use of storybook reading to increase print awareness in at-risk children. *American Journal of Speech-Language Pathology, 11*, 17–29.

Justice, L. M., & Ezell, H. K. (2004). Print referencing:An emergent literacy enhancement strategy and its clinical applications. *Language, Speech, and Hearing Services in Schools, 35*, 185–193.

Justice, L. M., & Kaderavek, J. N. (2004). Embedded-explicit emergent literacy intervention I: Background and description of approach. *Language, Speech, and Hearing in Schools, 35*, 201–211.

Justice, L. M., & Pence, K. L. (2004). Addressing the language and literacy needs of vulnerable children: Innovative strategies in the context of evidence-based practice. *Communication Disorders Quarterly, 25*, 173–178.

Justice, L. M., Weber, S. E., Ezell, H. K., & Bakeman, R. (2002). A sequential analysis of children's responsiveness to parental print references during shared book-reading interactions. *Language, Speech, and Hearing Services in Schools, 11*, 30–40.

Kaderavek, J. N., & Justice, L. M. (2002). Shared storybook reading as an intervention context: Practices and potential pitfalls. *American Journal of Speech-Language Pathology, 11*, 395–406.

Kaderavek, J. N., & Justice, L. M. (2004). Embedded-explicit emergent literacy intervention II: Goal selection and implementation in the early childhood classroom. *Language, Speech, and Hearing Services in Schools, 35*, 212–228.

Landry, S. H., & Smith, K. E. (2006). The influence of parenting on emerging literacy skills. In D. K. Dickinson, & S. B. Neuman (Eds.), *Handbook of early literacy research* (Vol. 2, pp. 135–148). New York: Guilford Press.

Lomax, R. G., & McGee, L. M. (1987). Young children's concepts about print and reading: Toward a model of word reading acquisition. *Reading Research Quarterly, 22*, 237–256.

Lovelace, S., & Stewart, S. R. (in press). Increasing print awareness in preschoolers with language impairment using non-evocative print referencing. *Language, Speech, and Hearing Services in Schools*.

Marvin, C., & Mirenda, P. (1993). Home literacy experiences of preschoolers enrolled in Head Start and special education programs. *Journal of Early Intervention, 17*, 351–367.

Marvin, C., & Wright, D. (1997). Literacy socialization in the homes of preschool children. *Language, Speech, and Hearing Services in Schools, 28*, 154–163.

Neuman, S. B. (1999). Books make a difference: A study of access to literacy. *Reading Research Quarterly, 34*(3), 286–311.

Neuman, S. B., & Dickinson, D. K. (Eds.). (2002). *Handbook of early literacy research*. New York: Guilford Press.

Numeroff, L. (2000). *If you take a mouse to the movies*. New York: Harper Collins.

Olsen-Fulero, L., & Conforti, J. (1983). Child responsiveness to mother questions of varying type and presentation. *Journal of Child Language, 10,* 495–520.

Phillips, G., & McNaughton, S. (1990). The practice of storybook reading to preschool children in mainstream New Zealand families. *Reading Research Quarterly, 25,* 196–212.

Rabidoux, P. C., & MacDonald, J. D. (2000). An interactive taxonomy of mothers and children during storybook interactions. *American Journal of Speech-Language Pathology, 9,* 331–344.

Scarborough, H. S. (1998). Early identification of children at risk for reading disabilities: Phonological awareness and some other promising predictors. In B. K. Shapiro, P. J. Accardo, & A. J. Capute (Eds.), *Specific reading disability: A view of the spectrum* (pp. 75–119). Timonium, MD: York Press.

Scarborough, H .S. (2002). Connecting early language and literacy to later reading (dis)abilities: Evidence, theory, and practice. In S. B. Neuman, & D. K. Dickinson (Eds.), *Handbook of early literacy research* (pp. 97–110). New York: Guilford Press.

Scarborough, H. S., & Dobrich, W. (1994). On the efficacy of reading to preschoolers. *Developmental Review, 14*(3), 245–302.

Schuele, C., & van Kleeck, A. (1987). Precursors to literacy: Normal development. *Topics in Language Disorders, 7*(2), 13–31.

Snow, C. E., Burns, M. S., & Griffin, P. (Eds.). (1998). *Preventing reading difficulties in young children*. Washington, DC: National Academy Press.

Stahl, S. A. (2003). What do we expect storybook reading to do? How storybook reading impacts word recognition. In A. van Kleeck, S. A. Stahl, & E. B. Bauer (Eds.), *On reading books to children* (pp. 363–383). Mahwah, NJ: Lawrence Erlbaum Associates.

Stanovich, K. E. (1988). *Children's reading and the development of phonological awareness*. Detroit: Wayne State University Press.

Stewart, S. R., & Page, J. L. (1992, November). *Using language experience to improve oral and written language*. Short course presented at the annual convention of the American Speech-Language-Hearing Association, San Antonio, TX.

Storch, S. A., & Whitehurst, G. J. (2002). Oral language and code-related precursors to reading: Evidence from a longitudinal structural model. *Developmental Psychology, 38,* 934–947.

Teale, W., & Sulzby, E. (1986). *Emergent literacy: Writing and reading*. Norwood, NJ: Ablex.

Trelease, J. (2001). *The read-aloud handbook* (5th ed.). New York: Penguin Books.

van Kleeck, A. (2003). Research on book sharing: Another critical look. In A. van Kleeck, S. A. Stahl, & E. B. Bauer (Eds.), *On reading books to children* (pp. 271–320). Mahwah, NJ: Lawrence Erlbaum Associates.

van Kleeck, A, & Vander Woude, J. (2003). Book sharing with preschoolers with language delays. In A. van Kleeck, S. A. Stahl, & E. B. Bauer (Eds.), *On reading books to children* (pp. 58–92). Mahwah, NJ: Lawrence Erlbaum Associates.

Vygotsky, L. (1978). *Mind in society*. Cambridge, MA: Harvard University Press.

Whitehurst, G. J., Epstein, J. N., Angell, A. L., Payne, A. C., Drone, D. A., & Fischel, J. E. (1994). Outcomes of an emergent literacy intervention in Head Start. *Journal of Educational Psychology, 86*(4), 542–555.

Whitehurst, G. J., & Lonigan, C. J. (1998). Child development and emergent literacy. *Child Development, 69*, 848–872.

Wood, A. (1984). *The napping house*. San Diego, CA: Harcourt.

Yoder, P. J., & Davies, B. (1990). Do parental questions and topic continuations elicit replies from developmentally delayed children? A sequential analysis. *Journal of Speech and Hearing Research, 33*, 563–573.

APPENDIX 10–A

Preschool Word and Print Awareness (PWPA) Assessment Tool

PRESCHOOL WORD AND PRINT AWARENESS—*Print Concepts*
L. M. Justice & H. K. Ezell (2001)

DIRECTIONS: Present the following tasks in the order depicted below. Use the book *Nine Ducks Nine* (Hayes, 1990). Read the text presented on the page and then administer the task. Each item may be repeated one time. Do not prompt, reinforce, or provide feedback to the child in any way. Score 0 for items to which the child does not respond or provides an answer that does not meet scoring criteria.

SAY: *We're going to read this book together, and I need you to help me read.*

Score/Item	Page: *Examiner Script*	Scoring Criteria
_____ 1. Front of book	**Before administering task:** Give book to child with spine facing child. **Cover: *Show me the front of the book.***	1 pt: turns book to front or points to front
_____ 2. Title of book	**Cover: *Show me the name of the book.***	1 pt: points to one or more words in title
_____ 3. Role of title	**Cover: *What do you think it says?***	1 pt: says 1 or more words in title or relevant title
_____ 4. Print vs. pictures	**Pages 1–2: *Where do I begin to read?*** **After administering task:** Put finger on first word in top line and say: ***I begin to read here***	2 pts: points to first word, top line 1 pt: points to any part of narrative text
_____ 5. Directionality	**Pages 1–2: *Then which way do I read?***	2 pts: sweeps left to right 1 pt: sweeps top to bottom

continues

APPENDIX 10–A. *continued*

Score/Item	Page: *Examiner Script*	Scoring Criteria
____ 6. Contextualized print	**Pages 3–4:** *Show me where one of the ducks is talking.*	1 pt: points to print in pictures
____ 7. Directionality (left/right)	**Pages 5–6:** *Do I read this page (point to left page) or this page (point to right page) first?*	1 pt: points to left page
____ 8. Directionality (top/bottom)	**Pages 7–8:** *There's four lines on this page (point to each). Which one do I read first?* **After administering task:** Put finger on first line and say: *I read this one first.*	1 pt: points to top line
____ 9. Directionality (top/bottom)	**Pages 7–8:** *Which one do I read last?*	1 pt: points to bottom line
____10. Print function	**Pages 9–10:** *Point to the words spoken by the ducks in the water, and say:* **Why are there all these words in the water?**	1 pt: tells that words are what ducks say or similar (e.g., "because they are talking")
____11a. Letter concept	**Pages 11–12:** *Show me just one letter on this page.*	1 pt: points to one letter
____11b. First letter	**Pages 11–12:** *Show me the first letter on this page.*	1 pt: points to first letter
____11d. Capital letter	**Pages 11–12:** *Now show me a capital letter.*	1 pt: points to capital letter
____12. Print function	**Pages 23–24:** *And the fox says "stupid ducks." Where does it say that?*	2 pts: points to fox's words 1 pt: points to other print on page

OBSERVATIONS	SCORING INSTRUCTIONS

___ Difficulty attending

___ Asked for repetition

___ Timid or reticent

___ Difficult to understand

Other:

Total Raw Score: _____

Add the numbers to the left of each item in the Item column.

Print-Concept Knowledge Estimate: _____

Use the scale provided below to convert total raw scores to PCK Estimates

Raw Score	PCK Estimate	Raw Score	PCK Estimate	Raw Score	PCK Estimate
0	46	6	97	12	118
1	63	7	100	13	123
2	74	8	104	14	128
3	82	9	107	15	134
4	88	10	111	16	145
5	92	11	115	17	161

From Justice, L. M., & Ezell, H. K. (2001). Word and print awareness in 4-year-old children. *Child Language Teaching and Therapy, 17*, 207–226. Reprinted with permission of Arnold Publishers.

Chapter Eleven

Integrating Beginning Word Study into Clinical Interventions

Latisha L. Hayes

Overview

The accumulated empirical evidence indicates that reading disabilities, over and above difficulties caused by inadequate reading experience and instruction, are caused by linguistic deficiencies in the area of phonological awareness—namely, phonological coding (for reviews, see Adams, 1990; Chall, 1996; Stanovich, 2000; Vellutino et al., 1996). Phonological coding is the ability to code abstract representations of the sounds in spoken and written words into the form of phonemes (i.e., the individual components of the speech stream). An impressive line of research has proven the strong relationship between language deficits and reading problems (Bishop & Adams, 1990; Catts, 1993; Lewis & Freebairn, 1992; Magnusson & Naucler, 1993). In fact, Catts and colleagues (Catts, Fey, Tomblin, & Zhang, 2002) found that children with language impairment in kindergarten were at a high risk for diagnosed reading disabilities in second and fourth grades, with about 50% of kindergartners exhibiting significantly poor reading skills. This rate of prevalence is consistent with that reported in previous studies (Aram, Ekelman, & Nation, 1984; Catts, 1993; Menyuk, Chesnick, Liebergott, Korngold, D'Agostino, & Belanger, 1991). The Catts et al.

(2002) study also corroborated earlier assertions by Bishop and Adams (1990) that children with language impairment in earlier grades who had experienced language improvement were less likely to have reading problems in later grades than those with persistent language impairments.

Mounting evidence over the past two decades indicates that deficits in phonological coding can be eliminated in younger children through appropriate instruction (Ball & Blachman, 1988; Bradley & Bryant, 1983; Bus & van IJzendoorn, 1999; Byrne & Fielding-Barnsley, 1995; Vellutino et al., 1996). Many of these studies have shown such instruction to have sustained positive effects over time. For children with language impairment specifically, there is a burgeoning line of research investigating speech-language therapy that incorporates systematic attention to improving phonological awareness. For example, Gillon (2000) found that an intervention emphasizing phoneme awareness and letter-sound knowledge for children with spoken language impairment improved not only speech production but also literacy-related performance. Such evidence provides an important inroad into ensuring that children with language impairment receive systematic attention to those literacy skills that will reduce their risks for reading difficulties. This chapter provides an introduction to methods and foci used in beginning reading instruction, including description of an approach to instruction termed *word study*. Word study is a method of instruction used in many beginning reading programs that systematically improves children's orthographic, phonological, and alphabetic skills. Of importance, word study as a method can readily be incorporated into clinical interventions for children with language impairment to promote their skills in these areas as a supplement to the traditional domains of speech and language addressed by speech-language pathologists (SLPs). In fact, this practice is recommended by the American Speech-Language-Hearing Association (2002).

Beginning Reading: Targets of Instruction

Many policy documents (e.g., National Reading Panel, 2000) emphasize the importance of providing children with "balanced" reading programs. In this context, "balanced" refers to the need to address both the code- and meaning-related aspects of reading development. Although beginning reading instruction necessarily includes a systematic focus on building children's reading comprehension skills, it also must provide children with the skills for a natural, comfortable transition from learning to read to reading to learn. In other words, they must be able to read words automatically and fluently so that they can focus their cognitive resources on comprehension.

The focus of this section is on the importance of ensuring that children who are learning to read receive instruction that effectively ensures their progress toward reading automatically and fluently—by emphasizing mastery of the alphabetic code.

Numerous correlational studies have found a strong relationship between early decoding ability and phonological awareness, and that poor phonological awareness often is what keeps children from becoming effective decoders (for review, see National Reading Panel, 2000). Of importance, evidence from over the past two decades also indicates that phonological awareness deficits in younger children can be eliminated through appropriate instruction (Ball & Blachman, 1988; Bradley & Bryant, 1983; Bus & van Ijzendoorn, 1999; Byrne & Fielding-Barnsley, 1995; Vellutino et al., 1996). Many of these studies have shown sustained positive effects over time using longitudinal research designs. All of these studies have included explicit instruction in phonological awareness or systematic phonics, or a combination of the two. It is thus logical to conclude that phonological awareness, alphabet knowledge, and explicit instruction in the consistent relationship between letters and sounds (i.e., phonics) are critical elements of beginning reading instruction, which is exactly the conclusion drawn by the National Reading Panel (2000) in its synthesis of effective beginning reading instruction.

A discussion of phonics (decoding) cannot exist without its sidekick, spelling (encoding). Whereas phonics instruction focuses on helping children to decode written language, spelling instruction focuses on helping children to encode written language; of importance, the two are highly inter-related during beginning reading development, and Ehri (2000) tagged phonics and spelling as "two sides of the same coin." Ehri's (2000) review of correlational studies in which students of various ages (first grade through college) were asked to read and spell words found that correlations between reading and spelling ranged from .68 to .86, suggesting that both skills draw on similar processes. In other studies, spelling measures have accounted for as much as 40% to 60% of the variance in oral reading performance (Zutell, 1992; Zutell & Rasinski, 1989). In a 2-year study that followed students from first through third grade, Ellis and Cataldo (1992) reported spelling to be the most consistent predictor of reading achievement. Not surprisingly, intervention studies exploring the value of spelling instruction have repeatedly found that spelling instruction improves not only spelling but also performance in oral reading, reading comprehension, and other reading-related measures (Berninger et al., 1998; Goulandris, 1992; Graham, Harris, & Chorzempa, 2002; McCandliss, Beck, Sandak, & Perfetti, 2003). These findings suggest that effective, balanced reading instruction should include a focus not only on decoding but also on encoding.

Phonics and spelling instruction, not unlike instruction in other academic areas, should be developmental in nature, especially for children at risk for reading difficulties. Thus, instruction responds to children's developmental levels and specific needs at a given time. This often is called "differentiated instruction," meaning that instruction is differentiated to respond to children's developmental status in reading. Juel and Minden-Cupp (2000) found that differentiated phonics instruction was especially beneficial for primary-age students with the lowest levels of literacy skill, and Foorman and Torgesen (2001) reported that differentiated instruction comprises one of the critical instructional elements in promoting literacy success for at-risk children.

In providing differentiated instruction in beginning reading, it is essential that professionals identify the child's developmental level so that instruction can be tailored to the child's needs. One approach to doing so is considering children's spelling development to identify "instructional levels." Analysis of students' spellings uses qualitative analysis of the error types contained in spelling, which can provide important insights into children's knowledge of orthography, phonology, and phonics (Morris, Blanton, Blanton, Nowacek, & Perney, 1995; Morris, Blanton, Blanton, & Perney, 1995; Morris, Nelson, & Perney, 1986). Even within a specific grade, children can vary tremendously in their spelling development (see Hayes, 2004), as shown by Schlagal (1982), who found a spread of at least three grade levels in spelling achievement in virtually every class in grades 1 through 6.

Developmental Reading and Spelling Stages: The Pivotal Factors of Word Study Instruction

"To teach well is to know what and whom you teach."—*Author unknown*

Word study instruction is a systematic approach used in beginning reading programs to promote children's decoding and encoding abilities—reading and spelling. For children who are having difficulty developing a firm base of orthographic, phonological, and phonics knowledge, such as children with a history of language difficulties, word study can be readily integrated into speech-language intervention to provide an added boost to reading instruction received in the classroom.

The general principle of word study, as suggested by its name, is to improve children's orthographic, phonological, and phonics knowledge through their own systematic study and analysis of features of words, particularly the patterns of print and sound within words. For instance, word study can be used to help a child learn to attend to the initial sounds in words. A common word study technique is *sorting*, in which children sort words on the basis of a specific orthographic or phonological feature. As a technique, sorting requires children to carefully analyze features of words. For the child who is learning to attend to the initial sounds in words, an effective sorting activity is for the child to sort pictures of items according to whether they start with an /s/ sound or an /m/ sound.

Successful implementation of the word study approach requires professionals to become experts in developmental spelling theory. Knowledge of the developmental sequence of spelling acquisition helps guide professionals in their instructional decision-making, particularly identifying the level at which to provide instruction so that it matches a child's developmental needs. Vygotsky theorized that educators must not only determine the developmental level (i.e., instructional level) of their students but also ascertain instructional goals that are appropriately challenging for their students (Dahl, Scharer, Lawson, & Grogan, 2001; Hedegaard, 1990). Snow, Burns, and Griffin (1998), in fact, argued that effective literacy teaching techniques include "adjusting the mode (grouping) and explicitness of instruction to meet the needs of individual students" (p. 196).

Learning to read is a process that spans many years of a child's academic life, and children go through distinct stages in the process of learning to read. The *emergent stage* is the first stage. Children in this stage are learning about the sound structure of the English language and developing a concept of the printed word and other aspects of print such as directionality. They also are learning about the nuances of the alphabet, including letter-sound correspondences. As children acquire a concept of the printed word and a working knowledge of the alphabetic code, children move into a stage called *beginning reading*; here, they solidify their knowledge of the sound structure of language and begin to collect a store of words they know by sight. Once children have a sizable number of words known by sight and are reading fluently with attention to the meaning of the text, they are in the *intermediate (proficient) stage* of reading.

This chapter focuses on emergent and beginning readers, who typically are preschool and primary grade children. The challenges for emergent and beginning readers differ from those for proficient readers. Proficient readers are working to make sense of the texts they are reading, whereas emergent readers are just striving to grasp the concept that spoken language corresponds to print and can be broken into phonemes that correspond to letters. Beginning readers, having established the connection between spoken language and print, are working to apply their developing letter-sound knowledge to recognize words. In this stage of development, readers tackle words by viewing the individual letters of words as "phonemic maps" that provide pronunciations of each corresponding letter (Ehri, 1997). Phonics and spelling instruction help children make the necessary connections between letters and sounds so that they can commit words to memory; consequently reading gradually becomes more automatic. Phonics instruction allows children to practice blending sounds into words as they read (decoding), whereas spelling instruction allows children to practice segmenting the sounds in words as they write (encoding).

Researchers have consistently demonstrated a developmental progression of spelling skills, which also appears to relate highly to children's developmental progression of decoding skills (Bear & Barone, 1989; Ganske, 1999; Invernizzi, 1992; Viise, 1994). The word study approach to phonics and spelling instruction is a systematic approach based on a scope and sequence of phonetic and spelling features that parallel students' growing knowledge of English orthography. The word study approach to phonics instruction differs from traditional, systematic basal programs in that the content of word study is determined by predictable developmental differences based on developmental spelling theory and research (Bear, Invernizzi, Templeton, & Johnston, 2004; Chall, 1996; Dahl et al., 2001; Henderson, 1990). Within the word study approach, students are assessed to determine their instructional level (i.e., where they fit in the developmental sequence of orthographic development), and instruction is designed to mirror where children are along that developmental sequence.

There are five conceptual stages of orthographic knowledge (i.e., spelling development) that emerge in a developmental sequence (see Henderson, 1990). As children move through these stages, they learn about letter-sound relationships, spelling patterns, and morphemes, such as prefixes, suffixes, Greek roots, and Latin stems (Bear et al., 2004). This same developmental progression has been found in students with learning disabilities (Worthy & Invernizzi, 1989) and in students identified as dyslexic (Sawyer, Wade, & Kim, 1999). The five stages are *preliterate, letter name, within word pattern, syllables and affixes,* and *derivational relations.* The first two stages, which reflect spelling achievements in the emergent and beginning reading stages of development, are discussed here; readers desiring information on the latter stages may wish to consult *Words Their Way* by Bear et al. (2004) for a comprehensive discussion.

Preliterate spellers are in the emergent literacy stage of development, and they are not yet reading. Their spelling attempts do not represent any letter-sound correspondences. For example, a preliterate speller may spell the word *elephant* with scribbles or even a random string of letters or symbols. Beginning readers are in the letter name spelling stage, which follows the preliterate phase. The *letter name speller* relies on the names of letters to spell words. For example, when spelling the word *jet*, the letter name speller may write *gat*. The sound of the *j* in *jet* sounds like the name of the letter *g*; the short *e* sound is close to the name of the letter *a*; and the sound of *t* leads the letter name speller to the letter name *t*. These children typically progress along a continuum by which they master the following features in their spellings: initial, single letter sounds (e.g., apple, balloon, comb); short-vowel families (e.g., cat, cap, can); initial consonant blends and digraphs (e.g., frog, ship); final consonant blends and digraphs (e.g., dish, belt); and short medial vowels including consonant blends and digraphs (e.g., mash, sled). Preconsonantal nasals, a particularly difficult ending blend (e.g., jump, sing), round out this stage. See Figure 11–1 for a more detailed explanation of this progression.

Establishing Word Study Instructional Levels

The system of word study instruction revolves around the instructional levels or stages and the specific orthographic features negotiated by student within those levels or stages. Identifying a child"s instructional stage is the first step to providing effective word study instruction that is differentiated to a child's developmental stage. For instance, a first-grade student may be a letter name speller whose instruction is focused on the short-vowel families, whereas another student may be learning how to represent final blends in short-vowel words. These students are very different in terms of their orthographic development and require differentiated instruction that meets their needs. Qualitative spelling inventories such as the Developmental Spelling Analysis (Ganske, 2000) and the Primary Spelling Inventory (Bear et al., 2004) are important tools for identifying where a child is in terms of the general stage of spelling development (e.g., letter name speller) and where the child is within that stage (e.g., learning to represent short-vowel families). The aforementioned assessments are appropriate for children who have some knowledge of sound-letter correspondence and are within the letter name spelling stage (or beyond). For children without solidified letter-sound knowledge, some tools that examine the emerging orthographic skills of emergent spellers are available (e.g., the Phonological Awareness Literacy Screening: Kindergarten; Invernizzi et al., 2003). Regardless of the specific tool used, developmental spelling inventories focus not simply on calculating the number of words spelled correctly but rather on conducting a careful feature analysis to study children's orthographic, phonological, and phonics knowledge as displayed by their spelling.

Feature analysis is a critical tool for determining the instructional levels of students, so as to place students within the developmental continuum and then to provide word study instruction that

Preliterate Spellers

Letter Names	A B C D E F G H I J K L M N O P Q R S T U V W X Y Z
Initial Sounds	s m a t f r i d o l g h u c b n k v e w j p y z

Letter Name Spellers

Features	Feature Examples	Sort Examples
II. Word Families		
Short a	-at -an -ad -ap -ag	-at vs. -an; -at vs. -an vs. -ap; -ap vs. -ag
Short i	-it -in -ip -ig	-it vs. -in; -it vs. -in vs. -ig; -ig vs. -ig
Short o	-og -ox -op -ot	-og vs. -op; -og vs. -op vs. -ot; -op vs. -ot vs. -ox
Short u	-un -ug -um -ut -ud	-un vs. -ug; -un vs. -ut vs. -ud
Short e	-ed -et -en	-ed vs. -et; -ed vs. -et vs. -en
Review all families	Mixed short a, i, o, u, e families	-ap vs. -ip vs. -op; -ack vs. -ick vs. -ock; -et vs. -ut vs. -it

continues

Figure 11–1. Progression of features for emergent and beginning readers. Please note that this chart was made and modified by many persons affiliated with the McGuffey Reading Center at the University of Virginia in Charlottesville, Virginia. *continues*

Letter Name Spellers

Features	Feature Examples	Sort Examples
III. Digraphs	sh ch th	s vs. h vs. sh; c vs. h vs. ch; sh vs. ch vs. th
IV. Blends		
L blends	sl fl bl cl pl gl	s vs. l vs. sl; b vs. l vs. bl; sl vs. bl vs. fl; fl vs. cl vs. pl
S blends	sm sp st sn sc sw sk	s vs. m vs sm; s vs. t vs. st; sm vs. st vs. sw
R blends	fr gr br tr dr cr pr	g vs. r vs. gr; t vs. r vs. tr; gr vs. tr vs. br; dr vs. cr vs. pr
Affricates	dr tr	dr vs. j; tr vs. ch; dr vs. j; tr vs. ch
V. Final Blends and Digraphs	-ch -th -sh -st -ft -sk	-ch vs. -th vs. -sh -t vs. -st vs. -ft; -st vs. -ft vs. -sk
VI. Medial Short Vowels	a, i, o, u, e	short a vs. short o words short o vs. short u words short e vs. short i words short a vs. short e words Review medial short vowels
VII. Preconsonantal Nasals	-mp -nd -nk -ng	-m vs. -p vs. mp; -n vs. -d vs. -nd; -mp vs. -nd vs. -ng

Figure 11–1. *continued*

370

will move them along that continuum. Consider the spelling sample for Penny presented in Figure 11–2. Penny is a kindergarten child whose spelling performance clearly shows her to be a preliterate speller and an emergent reader. She displays no letter-sound connections in her writing and, instead, uses mock-linear scribbles to represent the target words. The SLP who has collected this sample recognizes that Penny has very limited phonological awareness and alphabet knowledge and does not have a concept of word in print (i.e., the understanding that words are basic units of printed language that correspond with spoken units of meaning). For Penny, word study instruction needs to emphasize developing phonological awareness (e.g., rhyme and syllable awareness), with specific attention to attending to single consonants in words by sorting words on the basis of specific sounds contained in the words. For instance, Penny can sort cards with pictures using the initial sounds /t/ and /n/.

David, on the other hand, is a letter name speller and a beginning reader (see Figure 11–3). His spelling sample epitomizes the

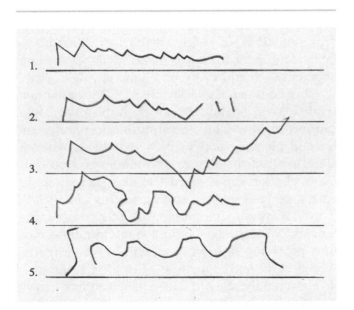

Figure 11–2. Penny's spelling sample: jam, rob, fun, sip, let.

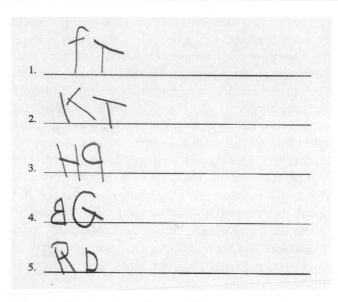

Figure 11–3. David's spelling sample: fit, cat, hop, bug, red.

early letter name speller in that he is making very linear, sound-by-sound representations of single-syllable, short-vowel words. As should be evident, the early letter name speller is not consistently able to segment each and every phoneme in single-syllable words and is therefore considered to rely only partially on phonemic cues. For example, David spelled *fit* as *ft*. Appropriate word study instruction for David will include attention to phoneme-level segmentation and blending activities so that he can develop skills in attending to all of the sounds and letters in words, as well as comparisons of short-vowel word families, such as -at versus -an versus -ag. Figure 11–4 shows a sorting activity in which David will analyze words sharing a short vowel but that come from different "word families." Word families offer a stable pronunciation for the vowel, thus providing support for David as he moves to include medial vowels in his representations of single-syllable words. Once David has mastered these word families, he can move to analysis of other short-vowel patterns through a systematic sequence of instruction, as shown in Figure 11–5.

_at cat	_an can	_ag tag
_at	_an	_ag
pat	man	bag
sat	fan	rag
bat	van	nag
fat	ran	wag

Figure 11–4. Sorting activity for David: -at versus -an versus -ag words.

Week	Sort Sample
1	-at vs. -an vs. -ag
2	-ag vs. -ap
3	-an vs. -at vs. -ap
4	-in vs. -it
5	-in vs. -it vs. -ip
6	-ip vs. -in vs. -ig
7	-op vs. -ot
8	-op vs. -ot vs. -og

Figure 11–5. Sample 8-week progression for analysis of short vowel patterns for David.

An additional example is that of Lydia, who is a second grader and a solid letter name speller, as shown in Figure 11–6. Consider Lydia's spelling of "bet," which she spelled *bat*, probably because the place of articulation for the short vowel *a* is close by that for the short vowel *e*. She also spelled "drip" *jrip* (with a reversed p),

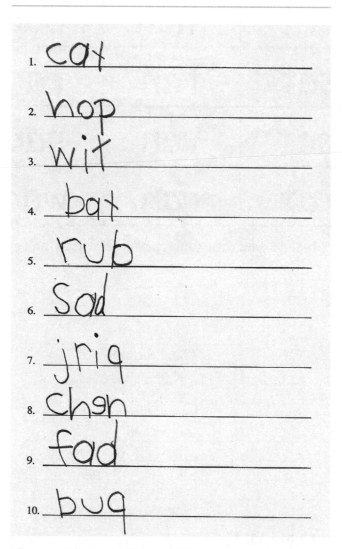

1. cat
2. hop
3. wit
4. bat
5. rub
6. sad
7. jriq
8. chgn
9. fad
10. buq

Figure 11–6. Lydia's spelling sample: cat, hop, went, bet, rub, sad, drip, chin, fed, bump.

in which she shows difficulty with representing the initial affricate in this word. Affricates often confuse letter name spellers. Lydia's spelling of "bump," with the exclusion of the m (also with a reversed p), indicates difficulty representing the preconsonantal nasal. These types of errors are instrumental for designing word study goals and activities for Lydia, which will include promoting her representation of affricate sounds, specifically her confusions with dr- blends. Figure 11–7 illustrates a sorting activity to help Lydia to differentiate dr- blends from words beginning with similar-sounding phonemes, and Figure 11–8 provides a sample sequence of orthographic and phonological comparisons to take Lydia through the letter name stage.

dr_ 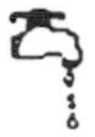 drip	d_ 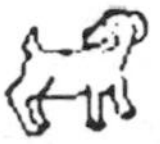 dog	j_ 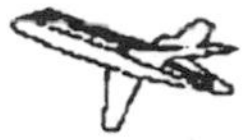 jet
dr_	d_	j_
drop	dug	jug
drag	dig	jab
drug	did	jog
drum	dock	job
drat	deck	jack

Figure 11–7. Sorting activity for Lydia: dr- versus d- versus j-words.

Week	Sort Sample
1	dr- vs. d- vs. j-
2	tr- vs. t- vs. ch-
3	short i vs. short e
4	short a vs. short e
5	short a vs. short e vs. short i
6	-m vs. -p vs. -mp
7	-n vs. -g vs. -ng
8	-sh vs. -st vs. -nt vs. -nd

Figure 11–8. Sample 8-week progression of orthographic and phonological comparisons to take Lydia through the letter name stage.

Word Study Instruction

Word study instruction is not an "off-the-shelf" program featuring a series of scripted routines; rather, it involves sophisticated decision making by the professional to identify children's instructional spelling levels and to provide word study opportunities that are suited to the children's developmental needs at a specific point in time. In this way, word study instruction is similar to other clinical activities familiar to the SLP, such as designing effective interventions for addressing disorders of expressive phonology, in which careful phonological analysis is followed by systematic instruction that is tailored to a child's phonological development and current patterns of errors. This section maps out the explicit instructional routines that are used in word study instruction, to include a detailed day-by-day description of a week of instruction.

Word Sorting as an Instructional Fulcrum

Word study is viewed as a conceptual process that requires children to recognize and analyze the similarities and differences among words (Zutell, 1992). This idea is not unlike the "associative nets" proposed by Kintsch, whereby a concept's complete meaning is acquired by exploring its relations to other components (i.e., nodes) of the associative net (Kintsch, 1974, 1994). Word study draws heavily on sorting, or categorizing, words on the basis of similarities and differences. Categorization is a fundamental cognitive activity that leads to forming the concepts that make up our knowledge base (Gillet & Kita, 1980). Categorization allows us to create order in the stimuli that we receive by considering new stimuli in relation to things that are already familiar and making generalizations about the characteristics of all members of a certain category (Bruner, Goodnow, & Austin, 1966). Anglin (1977) purports that categorization is a "ubiquitous cognitive act" that is involved in almost all linguistic acts.

Word study also seeks to "mimic basic cognitive learning processes" by guiding students to compare and contrast features of words through the instructional activity of sorting (Bear et al., 2004, p. 2). In sorting, children must examine words to learn the regularities of written and spoken English and make categorical judgments about words, such as that the *-at* phonogram is a shared feature of such words as *pat*, *mat*, and *chat*.

Explicit sorting requires students to explore the relationships (i.e., similarities and differences) among words, and professionals must guide them in that process. Specifically, word sorting requires the professional to determine categories of investigation (e.g., the ending phonograms *-at* and *-an*) and key words to exemplify these categories (e.g., c<u>at</u>; s<u>at</u>; b<u>at</u>; c<u>an</u>; t<u>an</u>; f<u>an</u>). Chall and Popp (1996) contend that a "problem-solving atmosphere" during phonics instruction is more effective and more motivating for students. Word sorting creates this type of atmosphere by providing hands-on opportunities for students to make cognitive connections about the similarities and differences among the targeted features. Bear et al. (2004) noted the applicability of the ancient proverb "I hear and I forget, I see and I remember, I do and I understand" (p. 62). In part, these problem-solving opportunities provided by active sorting contribute to the positive effects of word sorting compared with more traditional methods of spelling instruction (Hall, Cunningham, & Cunningham, 1995; Joseph, 2000).

Sorting is thus the central element of a typical weekly routine for the study of targeted orthographic or phonics features using preselected words that exemplify them. When students are engaged in these sorting activities, the professional provides explicit directions and guidance to focus students' attention on the targeted features. For example, when sorting words with initial digraphs (e.g., s̲h̲ip, c̲h̲op, t̲h̲at), the professional discusses the sounds of each digraph, as well as their corresponding letter patterns (e.g., "The /sh/ in ship is spelled with the letters s-h") and their positions in the words (e.g., "The /sh/ in ship is at the beginning of the word").

In organizing a week of word study instruction, the typical starting point is a teacher-led introduction of the orthographic features to be studied that week. This introduction may be an analogy-based activity comparing the two phonograms *-at* and *-an* in which children categorize sets of words written on individual cards that exemplify the targeted phonograms. During this time, instruction includes explicit teaching about the sounds and patterns of the targeted features, as well as the features' positions in the words. For student reference, the teacher can use a word card displaying the feature, a key word emphasizing the feature, and a picture clue. For example, when introducing a word card for the phonogram *-at* showing *cat* as the key word, the teacher can provide the following explanation:

> "When you see the letters a-t, you know that these two letters together say /æt/ as in *cat*. So, when you see the word *cat*, you can take what you know—*c* and *at*—and put them together to make *cat*. You can hear the /æt/ at the end of the word *cat*. You can see a-t at the end of the word *cat*, too."

The teacher then models sorting a few words while thinking aloud. The remaining words can be sorted as a group while the teacher provides any necessary support.

Children then sort their own words with guidance by the teacher. For instance, they may sort *mat, sat, rat, bat, man, pan, fan*, and *van* under the two phonograms -at and -an, thereby providing hands-on practice with reading, sorting, and analyzing their own sets of words. Along with sorting the word cards, children can record their word sorts on paper to practice writing these words, as well as to provide additional practice reading them as they check their work for accuracy.

Phoneme Segmenting and Blending: The Perfect Complement to Sorting

Phoneme segmenting and blending activities are an important part of word study routines. As children investigate the similarities and differences among words at the orthographic level, they also examine and manipulate these words at the level of the phoneme. Explicit instruction involving segmentation and blending of phonemes is widely accepted as effective in early reading development (Adams, 1990; Chall, 1996; Ehri & Nunes, 2002; Juel & Minden-Cupp, 2000). In the word study approach, letter tiles often are used for these segmenting and blending activities so that the children are continually reviewing letters and their corresponding sounds. Segmenting and blending activities also can include explicit talk about each sound, and any individual letters or letter patterns can be highlighted to emphasize larger spelling units. For example, while segmenting and blending the word *ship*, the professional may talk about each sound in the word—/sh/, /ɪ/, /p/—and the larger spelling units within the word—*sh* and *ip*. These tiles can be individually placed in boxes (i.e., Elkonin boxes) to further emphasize the phonemes, and multiple tiles can be placed within one box to emphasize the larger spelling units. Placing *sh*, *i*, *p* in separate boxes will emphasizes the phonemes, while placing *sh* in one box and *ip* in another box will emphasize the phonogram or the -ip spelling unit.

Analogous Connections Among Words: An Activity for the Long Haul

Word study also can help children learn to make analogies between words on the basis of orthographic and phonological features—for instance, that two words are analogous in their rime unit (shack, back). Instruction using analogies requires professionals to emphasize larger spelling units that children can draw on in making analogies among words (e.g., c-at; sh-ack; h-and). Intervention studies have reinforced the assertion that beginning readers can use analogies when systematically helped to do so (Bruck & Treiman, 1992; Greaney, Tunmer, & Chapman, 1997; Santa & Hoien, 1999). In analogy-based instruction, children are taught key words, or clue words, for targeted phonics features. These words can be used as exemplars (key words) during sorting instruction. Students use the key words to decode and spell by comparing unknown words and the known key words, and the professional can provide an explicit explanation of the process by verbalizing, "If I know *can*, then I know *fan*, *man*, and *pan*." This practice obviously involves using explicit talk about how words are alike, how they are different, and how children can use what they know about one word to help them read and spell other words.

Analogy-based instruction, such as that just described, is adapted from the Benchmark Word Identification Program developed by Gaskins and her colleagues (Gaskins, Ehri, Cress, O'Hara, & Donnelly, 1997; Gaskins, Gaskins, & Gaskins, 1991). This approach involves teaching key words to emphasize common phonograms (e.g., h-im) through explicit instruction that follows a teacher modeling and guided practice format. Lovett and her colleagues' (1994) intervention studies have demonstrated substantial gains for students using an adaptation of the Benchmark program.

Application to Reading and Writing: Ensuring That Instruction "Sticks"

A consistent weekly routine with daily planned activities must include opportunities for application of word study to reading and writing tasks (National Reading Panel, 2000; Pressley, 2002; Snow, Burns, & Griffin, 1998). Bear et al. (2004) operationalize this requirement through activities such as word hunts, dictated sentences, and word study games in which the skill's application is made explicit. In a word hunt, students search through previously read texts for words that contain the same spelling features they have just sorted and written. Word hunts help children make connections between spelling words and reading words. Students hunt in familiar texts to collect exemplars of the week's features, recording found words in their notebooks. Children hunt in "easy" books they have already read in order to eliminate the competing needs for decoding and reading to glean meaning.

Children also are encouraged to apply learned orthographic features in their writing. To initiate students' application of certain features, teachers can dictate sentences that include preselected words representing current and past features of study. This practice does not, of course, take the place of writing instruction. It is instead a quick check of application to a contextual writing task, and a way to encourage students in making such an application. For example, David's study of short *a* families can be complemented with the dictated sentence "I <u>had</u> a <u>tag</u> in my <u>hat</u>."

A Sample Word Study Routine: A Bird's Eye View of a 5-Day Plan

A sample weekly word study instructional routine for beginning readers involves these key components: sorting words, manipulating words, and connecting words to authentic reading and writing. This weekly routine takes approximately 30 minutes to complete each day. These routines are guided by a specific sequence of explicit instruction to ensure carefully planned, systematic lessons; specifically, each lesson should involve the following sequence (Duffy, 2003; Winograd & Hare, 1988):

1. Review previously learned features
2. Explicitly present new content using declarative, procedural, and conditional knowledge through explanation and modeling
3. Support student practice
4. Provide feedback on performance
5. Provide student independent practice

Day One

The first day of the week begins with an introduction of the features to be studied using a set of key words. If the targeted features are -it and -in, for instance, the key words may be *sit* for -it and *pin* for -in. The children first categorize pictures of words containing -it and -in patterns; then they categorize the written words using a set of cards developed for this purpose, such as *fit, hit, pit, kit, bin, tin, fin, win*. These words are studied by the children each day during the entire week. After children have sorted their cards into two categories (-it words, -in words), they must review and justify each decision. Last, a brief writing activity using children's individual notebooks is completed to focus children on analogies among words. Specifically, children are asked to complete this phrase: "If I know _____ [key word from the day], then I know _____." This activity is included to further emphasize the similarities among words, scaffolding the children in their discovery that by manipulating the onset and holding the ending rime constant, they can produce new words. "If I know . . . " is revisited later in the week and is described in more detail in the Day Four section.

Day Two

The students begin the day sorting again those words from the previous day. A manipulation activity follows. Students are given individual sets of letter tiles (e.g., tiles on cardstock or magnetic tiles) that they manipulate with guidance from the teacher. The manipulation task involves changing letters and sounds in words (e.g., *sit* to *fit*, *fit* to *bit*, *bit* to *bin*) using the tiles. These activities always include explicit talk by the teacher about the part of the words to be changed and what parts should be kept constant. After manipulating words, the students record in their notebooks the words they have manipulated. As a final activity, the teacher dictates a sentence to the children to write in their notebooks that includes words that follow the current features, as well as features of past study.

Day Three

The students begin the day reviewing the individual word sorts from day one, followed by a manipulation activity similar to the letter tile manipulation activity described in Day Two's routine. After manipulating words, the students (with teacher direction or support) hunt in familiar texts to collect exemplars of the week's features, furthering the conceptual connection to *real* reading tasks. For instance, students may look through books to find words containing the rime units -it and -in, which they record in their notebooks. The lesson ends with a teacher-dictated sentence as described in Day Two's routine.

Day Four

The students begin the day by reviewing their individual word sorts. This is followed by an analogy-based activity that focuses children's attention on "chunks" that are similar among words—namely, rime units. The key words for the week are used as a guide (e.g., sit for -it and pin for -in). The children have individual booklets with a standard introduction on each page: "If I know _____ [in this case *sit*], then I know _____." A list of words that can be read and spelled on the basis of their knowledge of the word *sit* is generated. This practice involves explicit talk by the teacher about how the words are alike, how they are different, and how the children can use what they know about one word to help them read and spell other words. The lesson is concluded with a writing sort, during which children are dictated a list of words and must write them under one of two headings (e.g., -it words, -in words). The students must write the words in their appropriate categories and attempt to spell the words correctly. After the children have written their words, they can look back through their notebooks at previous lists of these words to check their own work.

Day Five

The students begin the day with their individual word sorts. A "spell check" activity follows, during which children are asked to write a series of words studied during the week as well as words that haven't been studied but follow the same featured patterns. The spell check activity ends with a dictated sentence to check the transfer of knowledge in the context of a sentence. Previously studied features are included in the dictated sentence for reinforcement. On Fridays after the spell check activity, students can play games to review both previously and currently studied features.

Summary

As the sequence of instruction discussed in the previous section shows, word study involves engaging children in a series of systematic activities in which they are guided to carefully study words for specific orthographic, phonological, and phonics features. The specific features of words studied are carefully determined through analysis of where a child is on the developmental continuum of spelling and decoding abilities, which are highly interrelated.

Of importance, the principles and approaches of word study instruction can be readily integrated into speech-language interventions, provided that the professional develops a strong understanding of how to conduct developmental spelling analysis to design instructional activities that are responsive to children's needs. SLPs can, for instance, utilize the sequence of activities described in the five-day weekly plan in the previous section, embedding these into their clinical sessions with children. Alternatively, SLPs also can serve as important collaborators in the general education environment by working with small groups of pupils in differentiated instruction that involves word study.

Regardless of the method of service delivery, word study instruction offers an effective approach to ensuring that children with language impairment have systematic opportunities to develop and refine their orthographic, phonological, and phonics abilities. Word study instruction can have an important place within a more comprehensive, well-balanced literacy "diet" that also includes attention to writing, reading comprehension, vocabulary, and reading fluency (Pressley, 2002). Ensuring the quality of this literacy diet for children with language impairment specifically and all children generally is essential to reducing the prevalence of reading difficulties among schoolchildren.

References

Adams, M. J. (1990). *Beginning to read: Thinking and learning about print*. Cambridge, MA: MIT Press.

American Speech-Language-Hearing Association. (2002). Knowledge and skills needed by speech-language pathologists with respect to reading and writing in children and adolescents. *ASHA 2002 Desk Reference, 3*.

Anglin, J. M. (1977). *Word, object, and conceptual development*. New York: W. W. Norton.

Aram, D. M., Ekelman, B. L., & Nation, J. E. (1984). Preschoolers with language disorders: 10 years later. *Journal of Speech and Hearing Research, 27*, 232–244.

Ball, E. W., & Blachman, B. A. (1988). Phoneme segmentation training: Effect on reading readiness. *Annals of Dyslexia, 38*, 208–224.

Bear, D., & Barone, D. (1989). Using children's spellings to group for word study and directed reading in the primary classroom. *Reading Psychology, 10*, 275–292.

Bear, D. R., Invernizzi, M., Templeton, S., & Johnston, F. (2004). *Words their way: Word study for phonics, vocabulary, and spelling instruction* (3rd ed.). Upper Saddle River, NJ: Prentice-Hall.

Berninger, V. W., Vaughan, K., Abbott, R. D., Brooks, A., Abbott, S. P., Rogan, L., et al. (1998). Early intervention for spelling problems: Teaching functional spelling units of varying size with a multiple-connections framework. *Journal of Educational Psychology, 90,* 587–605.

Bishop, D. V. M., & Adams, C. (1990). A prospective study of the relationship between specific language impairment, phonological disorders and reading retardation. *Journal of Child Psychology and Psychiatry, 31,* 1027–1050.

Bradley, L., & Bryant, P. E. (1983). Categorizing sounds and learning to read: A causal connection. *Nature, 301,* 419–421.

Bruck, M., & Treiman, R. (1992). Learning to pronounce words: The limitations of analogies. *Reading Research Quarterly, 27,* 374–387.

Bruner, J. S., Goodnow, J. J., & Austin, G. A. (1966). *A study of thinking.* New York: John Wiley.

Bus, A. G., & van IJzendoorn, M. H. (1999). Phonological awareness and early reading: A metaanalysis of experimental training studies. *Journal of Educational Psychology, 91,* 403–414.

Byrne, B., & Fielding-Barnsley, R. (1995). Evaluation of a program to teach phonemic awareness to young children: A 2- and 3-year follow-up and a new preschool trial. *Journal of Educational Psychology, 87,* 488–503.

Catts, H. W. (1993). The relationship between speech-language impairments and reading disabilities. *Journal of Speech and Hearing Research, 36,* 948–958.

Catts, H. W., Fey, M. E., Tomblin, J. B, & Zhang, X. (2002). A longitudinal investigation of reading outcomes in children with language impairments. *Journal of Speech, Language, and Hearing Research, 45,* 1142–1157.

Chall, J. S. (1996). *Learning to read: The great debate* (3rd ed.). New York: McGraw-Hill.

Chall, J. S., & Popp, H. M. (1996). *Teaching and assessing phonics: A guide for teachers.* Cambridge, MA: Educators Publishing Service.

Dahl, K. L., Scharer, P. L., Lawson, L. L., & Grogan, P. R. (2001). *Rethinking phonics: Making the best teaching decisions.* Portsmouth, NH: Heinemann.

Duffy, G. G. (2003). *Explaining reading: A resource for teaching concepts, skills, and strategies.* New York: Guilford Press.

Ehri, L. C. (1997). Sight word learning in normal readers and dyslexics. In B. Blachman (Ed.), *Foundations of reading acquisition and dyslexia: Implications for early intervention* (pp. 163–187). Mahwah, NJ: Lawrence Erlbaum Associates.

Ehri, L. C. (2000). Learning to read and learning to spell: Two sides of a coin. *Topics in Language Disorders, 20,* 19–36.

Ehri, L. C., & Nunes, S. R. (2002). The role of phonemic awareness in learning to read. In A. E. Farstrup & S. J. Samuels (Eds.), *What research has to say about reading instruction* (3rd ed., pp. 110–139). Newark, DE: International Reading Association.

Ellis, N., & Cataldo, S. (1992). Spelling is integral to learning to read. In C. M. Sterling & C. Robson (Eds.), *Psychology, spelling, and education* (pp. 122–142). Clevedon, UK: Multilingual Matters Ltd.

Foorman, B. R., & Torgesen, J. (2001). Critical elements of classroom and small-group instruction promote reading success in all children. *Learning Disabilities Research & Practice, 16,* 203–212.

Ganske, K. (1999). The developmental spelling analysis: A measure of orthographic knowledge. *Educational Assessment, 6,* 41–70.

Ganske, K. (2000). *Word journeys: Assessment-guided phonics, spelling, and vocabulary instruction.* New York: Guilford Press.

Gaskins, I. W., Ehri, L. C., Cress, C., O'Hara, C., & Donnelly, K. (1997). Procedures for word learning: Making discoveries about words. *The Reading Teacher, 50,* 312–327.

Gaskins, R. W., Gaskins, J. C., & Gaskins, I. W. (1991). A decoding program for poor readers: And the rest of the class, too! *Language Arts, 68,* 213–225.

Gillet, J. W., & Kita, M. J. (1980). Words, kids, and categories. In E. H. Henderson & J. W. Beers (Eds.), *Development and cognitive aspects of learning to read: A reflection of word knowledge* (pp. 120–126). Newark, DE: International Reading Association.

Gillon, G. T. (2000). The efficacy of phonological awareness intervention for children with spoken language impairment. *Language, Speech, and Hearing Services in Schools, 31,* 126–141.

Goulandris, N. K. (1992). Alphabetic spelling: Predicting eventual literacy attainment. In C. M. Sterling & C. Robson (Eds.), *Psychology, spelling, and education* (pp. 143–158). Clevedon, UK: Multilingual Matters Ltd.

Graham, S., Harris, K. R., & Chorzempa, B. F. (2002). Contribution of spelling instruction to the spelling, writing, and reading of poor spellers. *Journal of Educational Psychology, 94,* 669–686.

Greaney, K., Tunmer, W., & Chapman, J. (1997). Effects of rime-based orthographic analogy training on the word recognition skills of children with reading disability. *Journal of Educational Psychology, 89,* 645–651.

Hall, D. P., Cunningham, P. M., & Cunningham, J. W. (1995). Multilevel spelling instruction in third grade classrooms. In K. A. Hinchman, D. L. Leu, & C. Kinzer (Eds.), *Perspectives on literacy research and practice* (pp. 384–389). Chicago: National Reading Conference.

Hayes, L. (2004). *A comparison of two systematic approaches to phonics and spelling instruction in beginning reading: A basal phonics program and word study.* Unpublished doctoral dissertation, University of Virginia, Charlottesville, VA.

Hedegaard, M. (1990). The zone of proximal development as basis for instruction. In L. C. Moll (Ed.), *Vygotsky and education: Instructional implications and applications of sociohistorical psychology* (pp. 349–371). Cambridge, UK: Cambridge University Press.

Henderson, E. H. (1990). *Teaching spelling* (2nd ed.). Boston: Houghton Mifflin.

Invernizzi, M. (1992). The vowel and what follows: A phonological frame of orthographic analysis. In S. Templeton & D. Beers (Eds.), *Development of orthographic knowledge and the foundations of literacy: A memorial Festschrift for Edmund H. Henderson* (pp. 106–136). Hillsdale, NJ: Lawrence Erlbaum Associates.

Invernizzi, M., Swank, L., Juel, C., & Meier, J. (2003). *Phonological awareness literacy screening (PALS-K)*. Charlottesville, VA: University of Virginia Press.

Joseph, L. M. (2000). Developing first graders' phonemic awareness, word identification and spelling: A comparison of two contemporary phonic instructional approaches. *Reading Research and Instruction, 39*, 160–169.

Juel, C., & Minden-Cupp, C. (2000). Learning to read words: Linguistic units and instructional strategies. *Reading Research Quarterly, 35*, 458–492.

Kintsch, W. (1974). *The representation of meaning in memory*. Hillsdale, NJ: Lawrence Erlbaum Associates.

Kintsch, W. (1994). The role of knowledge in discourse comprehension: A construction integration model. In R. B. Ruddell, M. R. Ruddell, & H. Singer (Eds.), *Theoretical models and processes in reading* (4th ed., pp. 951–995). Newark, DE: International Reading Association.

Lewis, B.A., & Freebairn, L. (1992). Residual effects of preschool phonology disorders in grade school, adolescence, and adulthood. *Journal of Speech and Hearing Research, 35*, 819–831.

Lovett, M. W., Borden, S. L., DeLuca, T., Lacerenza, L., Benson, N. J., & Brackston, D. (1994). Treating the core deficits of developmental dyslexia: Evidence of transfer of learning after phonologically- and strategy-based reading training programs. *Developmental Psychology, 30*, 805–822.

McCandliss, B., Beck, I., Sandak, R., & Perfetti, C. (2003). Focusing attention on decoding for children with poor reading skills: Design and preliminary tests of the word building intervention. *Scientific Studies of Reading, 7*, 75–103.

Magnusson, E., & Naucler, K. (1993). The development of linguistic awareness in language-disordered children. *First Language, 13*, 93–111.

Menyuk, P., Chesnick, M., Liebergott, J. W., Korngold, B., D'Agostino, R., & Belanger, A. (1991). Predicting reading problems in at-risk children. *Journal of Speech and Hearing Research, 34*, 893–903.

Morris, D., Nelson, L., & Perney, J. (1986). Exploring the concept of "spelling instruction level" through the analysis of error-types. *Elementary School Journal, 87,* 181–2000.

Morris, D., Blanton, L., Blanton, W. E., Nowacek, J., & Perney, J. (1995). Teaching low achieving spellers at their "instructional level." *Elementary School Journal, 96,* 163–177.

Morris, D., Blanton, L., Blanton, W. E., & Perney, J. (1995). Spelling instruction and achievement in six classrooms. *Elementary School Journal, 92,* 145–162.

National Reading Panel. (2000). *Teaching children to read: An evidence-based assessment of scientific research literature on reading and its implications for reading instruction.* Rockville, MD: National Institute of Child Health and Human Development.

Pressley, M. (2002). *Reading instruction that works: The case for balanced teaching* (2nd ed.). New York: Guilford Press.

Santa, C., & Hoien, T. (1999). An assessment of Early Steps: A program for early intervention of reading problems. *Reading Research Quarterly, 27,* 54–79.

Sawyer, D. J., Wade, S., & Kim, J. K. (1999). Spelling errors as a window on variations in phonological deficits among students with dyslexia. *Annals of Dyslexia, 49,* 137–159.

Schlagal, R. (1982). A qualitative inventory of word knowledge: A developmental study of spelling grades one through six (Doctoral dissertation, University of Virginia, 1982). *Dissertation Abstracts International, 47*(03), 915.

Snow, C. E., Burns, M. S., & Griffin, P. (1998). *Preventing reading difficulties in young children.* Washington, DC: National Academy Press.

Stanovich, K. E. (2000). *Progress in understanding reading.* New York: Guilford Press.

Vellutino, F. R., Scanlon, D. M., Sipay, E., Small, S., Pratt, A., Chen, R., & Denckla, M. (1996). Cognitive profiles of difficult-to-remediate and readily remediated poor readers: Early intervention as a vehicle for distinguishing between cognitive and experiential deficits as basic causes of specific reading disability. *Journal of Educational Psychology, 88,* 601–638.

Viise, N. (1994). *Feature word spelling list: A diagnosis of progressing word knowledge through an assessment of spelling errors.* Unpublished doctoral dissertation, University of Virginia, Charlottesville, VA.

Winograd, P. N., & Hare, V. C. (1988). Direct instruction of reading comprehension strategies: The nature of teacher explanation. In C. E. Weinstein, E. T. Goetz, & P. A. Alexander (Eds.), *Learning and study strategies: Assessment, instruction, and evaluation* (pp. 121–139). New York: Academic Press.

Worthy, M. J., & Invernizzi, M. (1989). Spelling errors of normal and disabled students on achievement levels one through four: Instructional implications. *Bulletin of the Orton Society, 40,* 138-149.

Zutell, J. (1992). An integrated view of word knowledge: Correlational studies of the relationships among spelling, reading, and conceptual development. In S. Templeton & D. Bear (Eds.), *Development of orthographic knowledge and the foundations of literacy: A memorial festschrift for Edmund H. Henderson* (pp. 213-230). Newark, DE: International Reading Association.

Zutell, J., & Rasinski, T. (1989). Reading and spelling connections in third and fifth grade students. *Reading Psychology, 10,* 137-155.

Chapter Twelve

Literacy Intervention in a Culturally and Linguistically Diverse World: The Linking Language and Literacy Project

Peggy Rosin

> It is clear from the research on emergent literacy that important experiences related to reading begin very early in life. Primary prevention steps designed to reduce the number of children with inadequate literacy-related knowledge (e.g., concepts of print, phonemic awareness, receptive vocabulary) at the onset of formal schooling would considerably reduce the number of children with reading difficulties and, thereby, the magnitude of the problem currently facing schools. (Snow, Burns, & Griffin, 1998, p. 317)

Several groups of children are likely to begin school inadequately prepared to learn to read and therefore may be less likely to be-come successful readers (Snow et al., 1998). One such group consists of children from culturally and linguistically diverse back-grounds (Culatta, Aslett, Fife, & Setzer, 2004; Justice, Chow, Capellini, Flanigan, & Colton, 2003; Snow et al., 1998; Thomas-Tate, Washington, & Edwards, 2004). In 2005, the National Assessment for Educational Progress reported that by fourth grade, 59% of African American children and 56% of Latino/Hispanic children read below basic levels, compared with 25% of majority-culture children. This national study also found that 54% of children living in poverty demonstrated reading proficiency below basic reading levels. Dual-language learners also perform significantly poorer than their

English-speaking counterparts on measures of reading (Lutkus, Rampey, & Donahue, 2005). For those preschool children who are known to be at risk for language and literacy problems, it is prudent to provide appropriate interventions so that they may enter kindergarten on par with other children.

In today's diverse society, children should be provided with emergent literacy opportunities that respect and build on their home culture while simultaneously preparing them to succeed in the majority culture. (The importance of this approach is discussed in Chapter 2.) However, making evidence-based decisions about how best to promote the language and literacy skills of preschoolers from culturally and linguistically diverse backgrounds is challenging. This chapter provides specific guidance regarding clinical approaches to be used to promote emergent literacy development in preschool children who are English language learners, who live in poverty, and whose cultural backgrounds differ from the majority culture. For this purpose, the *Linking Language and Literacy Project* is introduced as a model program that combines current evidence and recommended practice to promote the emergent literacy skills of children from diverse backgrounds.

Challenges to Providing Evidence-Based Practice

It is crucial to acknowledge the challenges encountered in developing an evidence-based program for at-risk preschoolers from diverse backgrounds. Johnston and Wong (2002) warn practitioners that "it will be difficult, if not impossible, for professionals to fully understand the practice implications inherent in the culture of client families" (p. 923). Indeed, several major challenges to providing evidence-based language and emergent literacy programs for culturally and linguistically diverse preschool children are recognized. For both the researcher and the practitioner, a foremost challenge is defining what is meant by children who are "culturally and linguistically diverse." Additional challenges include finding a sufficient research base characterizing literacy development and effective interventions for these children, synthesizing research across studies, and applying existing research to practice. Specifics of these challenges are described next.

Challenge 1: Defining the Population of Children

The term *culturally and linguistically diverse* generally is applied to persons who are not from the majority culture. Children who are *linguistically* diverse are defined as those whose first language is either a language other than English or a language other than "middle-class" mainstream English (Perez, 1998), which represent the majority culture in the United States. Children who are *culturally* diverse are distinguished by ethnicity and socioeconomic status differences from those of the majority culture. Describing or comparing children who are culturally and linguistically diverse is no simple matter. Numerous influences shape children's culture, including individual characteristics of the child (gender, communication skill, socioemotional status, motor skills, and so on) and his or her family (values and beliefs, structure and organization, socioeconomic status, educational status, language, race, and ethnicity). Culture is the consequence of the beliefs, values, and attitudes that underlie the behaviors of those groups of which the children are a part. Culture is not a fixed phenomenon; rather, it is learned and evolves in accordance with the child's collective life experiences.

Challenge 2: Lack of a Research Base and Difficulty Synthesizing Research across Studies

Demographic trends indicate that a growing number of preschool children in the United States are learning English as a second language. Monolingualism, an exception in most countries, is becoming less common in the United States. The latest U.S. census (U.S. Census Bureau, 2000) reported 322 languages spoken across the country, with more than 100 languages spoken in greater than half of the states. Language and literacy issues related to research, assessment, and intervention with children who are linguistically diverse are complex. Even with a surge in research related to bilingualism and English language learning, Goldstein and Kohnert (2005) see workers in this field as "just beginning to know what we do not know" (p. 267).

There is a paucity of literature documenting the typical language and literacy skills of linguistically diverse preschoolers and even less research about English language learning in preschoolers with communication disorders (Kohnert, Yim, Nett, Fong Kan, & Duran, 2005). Without clear developmental expectations for typically developing, non–English-speaking children, it is difficult to distinguish language impairment from differences due to English language learning. Associated challenges in the assessment and intervention process are (1) defining a child's level of proficiency in a language other than English; (2) establishing whether there is a language delay or disorder versus a language difference due to English language learning; (3) determining whether English or the first language is the dominant language to be used for intervention; and (4) facilitating English language learning while maintaining the home language.

Children who are bilingual may be equally proficient in both languages, or they may know one language better than the other. Usually, proficiency in the dominant language depends on the context and the opportunities the child has to use the language. Bilingualism and second language learning are affected by numerous factors in the child's life, including whether both languages are learned together from infancy (i.e., simultaneous bilingualism) or learned after the first language is established (i.e., second language learning); and whether or not the language is widely used, valued, and associated with economic power in the community (Genesee, Paradis, & Crago, 2004). The consequence for researchers (and those who seek research to guide their practice) is that it is difficult to control for and compare degrees of bilingualism in children. Some authors argue that bilingualism, in and of itself, is not a liability for children's developing language and literacy skills and may even offer advantages in aspects of learning (Goldstein & Kohnert, 2005; Genesee et al., 2004; McLaughlin, 1995; Oller & Pearson, 2002). It also is not clear what effect, if any, bilingualism has on emergent literacy. With preschool dual-language learners, a major emergent literacy concern is that children develop a strong language base on which to map code-related skills. Additionally, children also require intentional and supportive interactions with the code-related aspects of emergent literacy to ensure that these skills are developed in a timely manner.

Complicating any assessment of the effects of bilingualism on language and literacy development are the effects of poverty. Many bilingual or dual-language learners in the United States live in low-income families, a circumstance that places children at risk for language and learning problems (Oller & Pearson, 2002). It can be very difficult to disentangle the effects of poverty and ethnicity in studying dual-language acquisition. A major group of children at risk for language and literacy problems, whether they are second language learners or not, comprises those living in low-income families. Unfortunately, the incidence of poverty is on the rise in the United States. The National Center for Children in Poverty (2004) reported that between 2000 and 2004, the number of children younger than 6 years of age who were poor increased by 14%. Approximately 43% of the 24 million children in the United States under age 6 live in low-income families, and 21% of these live in poor families. A disproportionate number of people of color live in poverty, in comparison with families who are white, and rates are significantly greater for African American and Latino families (Rosin, 1996). According to the National Center for Children in Poverty, the percentages of preschoolers under age 6 living in low-income families based on race/ethnicity are as follows:

66% of Latino children—3.4 million

64% of black children—2.2 million

25% of Asian children—0.2 million

30% of white children—4.0 million

Justice and colleagues (2003) summarized the potentially detrimental effects of poverty on the development of emergent literacy skills, reporting that children living in poverty tend to have limited exposure to language and literacy experiences and do less well on measures of print production, book reading concepts, environmental print decoding, alphabetic knowledge, and phonological awareness. However, an unexpected finding from an investigation by Craig, Connor, and Washington (2003) was that, among the African American preschoolers they studied, those from from low-socioeconomic-status backgrounds outperformed African American children from middle-income families by third grade. These investigators hypothesized that perhaps the educational opportunities available for preschool children from low-income families mediated the potential negative effects of poverty on their literacy learning. Because poverty was not seen as a sufficient explanation for lower literacy performance in African American children, Craig, Thompson, Washington, and Potter (2004) examined other possible contributing factors to account for this finding, including dialect density, differences in shared cultural knowledge leading to biased assessment, and a mismatch between home and school language. There are no clear answers about how this combination of factors or others may contribute to the "cycle of illiteracy" (Snow et al., 1998; Washington, 2006) for African American or other children living in poverty. Nonetheless, ample evidence suggests that early proactive interventions that focus intensively on promoting emergent literacy and language skills can positively affect the developmental trajectories of children who live in poverty.

Challenge 3: Relevance of Existing Research

Research findings should be the foundation for choices and approaches in provision of language and literacy intervention. This consideration is particularly timely in view of the current emphasis on evidence-based practice. The past decade has witnessed a surge in professionals' access to empirical research describing emergent literacy development and intervention strategies for prekindergarten children. However, the complex, multifaceted, and evolving nature of culture makes conducting and applying research with preschoolers from culturally and linguistically diverse backgrounds rather complicated. Also, interpreting and applying findings of research may be difficult with children who have multiple risk factors associated with language and literacy problems, who infrequently are studied in larger-scale intervention research. To further complicate matters, research about one cultural group cannot be generalized to other groups; in addition, intracultural variation and individual differences make application of research findings difficult even within cultural groups.

Implications for Practice

Of necessity, the design and implementation of programs aimed at developing and supporting emergent literacy for culturally and linguistically diverse children will require translation of research to practice. Because of current limitations in available research, however, such programs must be flexible and adaptable to reflect emerging research findings. Future empirical evidence and personal experience must continue to shape recommended practice.

It is crucial that researchers and practioners continue to build an evidence base to provide the best possible services based on the best available evidence. Because there is a lack of scientific evidence about emergent literacy intervention with culturally and linguistically diverse learners, it is recommended that practitioners integrate existing evidence with theoretical, practical, and personal knowledge (Dollaghan, 2004; Justice & Pence, 2004). This recommendation was a central tenet in the design and implementation of the Linking Language and Literacy Project (Rosin, Schraeder, & DeFelice, 2005), a program that was developed at the University of Wisconsin–Madison to integrate developmentally appropriate and culturally competent practice with available empirical information to promote language and literacy skills in at-risk preschool children.

The Linking Language and Literacy Project

Risk is not destiny. (Shore, 1997, p. 61)

Through the Linking Language and Literacy Project, University of Wisconsin–Madison undergraduate students worked directly with at-risk pupils in Head Start programs to promote their early achievements in literacy and language. The Linking Language and Literacy Project built on an existing undergraduate service-learning course during which, each semester, the students performed volunteer service under the supervision of a clinical professor in the University's Department of Communicative Disorders. Student clinicians were assigned to Head Start programs to implement an evidence-based 12-week emergent literacy intervention, with their typical assignment comprising 2-hour sessions twice per week, for a total service-learning commitment of about 48 hours. Funds for language and literacy kits were provided through a Kemper K. Knapp 2004–2005 award (Rosin, Schraeder, & Miller, 2004). This program was designed to incorporate the accumulated research literature on providing effective emergent literacy interventions to at-risk preschoolers; thus, the student volunteers gained valuable exposure to this literature in tandem with translating research into effective practices through service learning. The remainder of this chapter provides details concerning this evidence-based program, including its design principles and sample activities, all of which can be readily applied to other programs serving similar populations of children.

Project Participants

The 37 preschoolers involved in this project during its first year of implementation attended Head Start programs in Madison, Wisconsin. The children qualified for the Head Start program on the basis of family income, and most children lived in households below the poverty threshold. The 3- to 5-year-olds were primarily African American children who spoke African American English or children who were Latino and Spanish-English bilinguals, although several children spoke the Asian language Hmong in addition to English. The children were selected for participation in the project on the basis of their at-risk status for later literacy problems due to early deficits in language performance in one or more domains. Identification of participants for the program was made through a collaborative decision by the Head Start's speech-language pathologist, program site directors, and classroom teachers in consulta-tion and with permission from the children's parents. Table 12–1 summarizes the demographic characteristics of the program participants.

Project Principles

The Linking Language and Literacy Project was founded on five key principles.

Principle 1: Language and Literacy Skills Should Be Promoted Together

Considerable evidence shows that there is a strong and reciprocal link between language and emergent literacy development in preschool children (American Speech-Language-Hearing Association [ASHA], 2001 Justice, Invernizzi, and Meier, 2002; Montgomery,

Table 12–1. Demographics for Participants in the Linking Language and Literacy Project

Characteristic	Number/Value
Number of children	37
Age	
Range	3 years 3 months to 5 years 1 month
Mean	51 months
Gender	
Boys	24
Girls	13
Primary language	
African American English	23
Standard American English*	7
Spanish	6
Asian (Hmong)	1

*Does not imply racial/ethnic background.

2005; Whitehurst & Lonigan, 2001); nonetheless, the precise nature of this relationship is not well defined (Nathan, Stackhouse, Goulandris, & Snowling, 2004). One well-documented expression of this link is the frequent co-occurrence of language and literacy problems. Several longitudinal and numerous other studies show that young children with speech and language difficulties are at risk for later literacy problems (Aram & Hall, 1989; Boudreau & Hedberg, 1999; Catts, Fey, Tomblin, & Zhang, 2002; Snowling, Bishop, & Stothard, 2000; Stothard, Snowling, Bishop, Chipcase, & Kaplan, 1998). According to Catts (1997), many cases of "reading disability" are actually language-based disorders. In a review by Flax, Realpe-Bonilla, Hirsch, Brzustowicz, Bartlett, and Tallal (2003) of studies on the co-occurrence of language and reading impairments in children, as many as half of the children had both impairments. Many experts suggest that early interventions for children with language difficulties, rather than focusing exclusively on language acquisition for children, should include a reciprocal and similarly intensive focus on emergent literacy development (e.g., Justice et al., 2002).

Principle 2: Children Should Participate Actively in Their Learning

The National Association for the Education of Young Children (NAEYC) (1998) established the concept of *developmentally appropriate practice* for promoting young children's language and literacy development based on theories and research about how children learn. Children are seen as "active constructors of meaning," with adults playing a critical role in children's literacy development by engaging their interest, creating challenging but achievable goals and expectations, and supporting their learning. Being responsive to children's individual differences, such as temperament and learning style, also is needed to engage children in language and literacy learning.

Principle 3: Language and Literacy Activities Should Be Meaningful

Neuman and Roskos (2005) emphasize that children should be engaged in meaningful experiences that respect their home language, and that these experiences act as a base on which to build and extend children's language and literacy. Research has documented that cultures vary in the frequency, uses, and types of literacy events, as well as the interactional styles used during literacy activities (Hammer, Miccio, & Wagstaff, 2003; Johnston & Wong, 2002; Tabors & Snow, 2001; Vernon-Feagans, Scheffner Hammer, Miccio, & Manlove, 2001). A premise of the Linking Language and Literacy Project was that co-constructing meaningful experiences, while being alert to the effects on the child of adult interaction style and facilitation techniques, materials, and activities used, can mitigate any cultural differences between the student clinicians and the children.

Principle 4: Direct Instruction Should Co-occur With Embedded Opportunities for Learning

In addition to increasing more naturalistic exposure to language and literacy for at-risk children, Justice and colleagues (Justice & Kaderavek, 2004; Justice & Lankford, 2002; Justice & Pullen, 2003; Justice et al., 2003) argue that explicit or direct instruction also should be used for promoting emergent literacy skills in at-risk preschoolers. Two rationales for incorporating explicit instruction into a language and literacy program are offered by Justice and colleagues (2003): (1) explicit instruction may be the most efficient route to skill learning, and (2) because at-risk children often are not learning at the same rate or in the same manner as for their typically developing peers, they need a more direct and systematic approach to skill learning. Thus, an embedded-explicit model of emergent literacy intervention (Justice & Kaderavek, 2004; Kaderavek & Justice, 2004), consistent with "balanced instruction" recommended by the National Institute of Child Health and Human Development (NICHD) (2000), was implemented both in classroom-based activities and in individual sessions of the Linking Language and Literacy Project.

Principle 5: Prevention of Language and Literacy Problems is the Goal

Consistent with the premise that "early prevention may be the best weapon we have to combat reading failure" (Craig et al., 2003, p. 31), research has shown that the prevention of reading problems is more effective than attempting to remediate a reading disability after it is manifested (Juel, 1988). Those children who experience difficulties in learning to read are unlikely to catch up with their peers (NICIID, 2000; Watson, Layton, Pierce, & Abraham, 1994; Whitehurst & Lonigan, 2001), and the most effective way to prevent reading difficulties is to accurately identify children who are at risk and to intervene *before* failure. Implementing prevention programs in preschool may decrease the need for remedial services in later school years (Justice et al., 2004; Snow et al., 1998). Nonetheless, it is not feasible to provide intervention to every child who lives in poverty or has limited English proficiency. Justice and colleagues (2002) elaborate on the risk factors described by Snow and coauthors (1998) and offer a means to refine the "risk factors" associated with later reading difficultie, to identify those children most in need of additional literacy supports. They suggest analyzing the nature and history of any existing language problem the child may exhibit while also attending to other associated child and family risk factors. These risk factors were considered as part of the selection criteria for enrollment in the Linking Language and Literacy Project. The rationale for including these preschoolers in the project was to mitigate potential future reading problems.

The Project's Components

The Linking Language and Literacy Project consisted of three integrated program components: (1) assessment of communication and literacy abilities; (2) selection of language and/or literacy goals for intervention, and (3) promotion and monitoring of skills within the classroom, during individual sessions, and through home-based opportunities. The remainder of this chapter describes the Linking Language and Literacy Project and offers the evidence base used for decisions about literacy goals targeted for these preschool children and the methods and activities used to enhance their language and literacy skills.

Component 1: Assessing Children's Language and Literacy Abilities

To set specific goals for individual children in speech and language development, each child's communication skills were evaluated in English to develop a communication profile for speech (comprehensibility, speech sound development, fluency, prosody, voice) and language (production, comprehension, social skills). Evaluation procedures included collecting information from teachers and caregivers, conducting authentic assessment (e.g., Stockman, 1996) within the classroom, and collecting and analyzing a 15-minute speech and language sample. Additional assessment using criterion-referenced measures, informal elicitation tasks, dynamic assessment, and standardized measures was performed as needed to develop the communication profile for each child. Analysis and interpretation of the evaluation data took into account features of African American or Spanish-influenced English (Long, 2005) so that these features could be differentiated from those requiring intervention. If the child was found to exhibit specific speech or language impairments, goals were developed to address these areas. In children who were found to exhibit typical speech and language skills, additional assessment was completed to measure preacademic and emergent literacy skills to set goals for facilitation.

Complementing the communication assessment was assessment focused on characterizing children's preacademic and emergent literacy skills. Few standardized or criterion-referenced tools are available that offer information about literacy expectations for preschoolers, especially children from culturally and linguistically diverse backgrounds. To identify preschool children who may benefit from emergent literacy intervention, it is essential to understand what literacy skills typical children demonstrate. In the Linking Language and Literacy Project, several informal criterion-referenced tools were selected to measure emergent literacy skills, to include examining for a range of early reading behaviors (see Table 12-2) and indicators of phonological awareness (see Table 12-3), which were used as frameworks for setting expectations and selecting criteria for emergent literacy goals. Also utilized were two informal published tools, the Early Reading Checklist (Crowe & Reichmuth, 2001) and the Ladders to Literacy checklist (Notari-Syverson, O'Connor, & Vadasy, 1998); for some children, the Phonological Awareness Literacy Screening—PreK (Invernizzi, Sullivan, & Meier, 2001) also was administered to gain more specific information on various aspects of phonological awareness.

Thus, each child was given a range of assessments to identify areas of identified weakness (i.e., clinically significant problems or areas of relative weakness within the assessment profile), with a profile for each child developed to represent abilities in language comprehension, language expression, pragmatics, speech/phonology, literacy and preacademic skills, hearing, and social/behavioral competence. Table 12-4 identifies the areas of significant weakness in specific domains of language and literacy among children who participated in the program. As these data show, the participants were a heterogeneous group, although all of them had identified weaknesses that constituted risk factors for later literacy difficulties.

Component 2: Selecting Language and Emergent Literacy Goals

Emergent literacy depends on the development of two broad classes of skills identified for later reading success (as discussed in Chapter 1): code-related skills and oral language (meaning-related) skills. *Code-related skills* include phonological awareness, print awareness, letter naming, and emergent writing. *Oral language skills* include receptive and expressive vocabulary, syntactic and

Table 12–2. Examples of Early Reading Behaviors

Book Awareness	Concepts of Print	Story Sense	Rereading Familiar Books	Phonemic Awareness	Sound Symbol and Word Identification
Front/back	Read environmental print	Beginning, middle, and end sequences	Use own oral language to comment or label objects while referring to pictures	Rhyme awareness (onset and rime)	Letter names
Left/right	Understand that print carries a message	Main ideas/concepts	Use own oral language to tell story while referring to pictures	Initial consonant awareness (soap, sick, sad, man)	Letter sounds
Top/bottom	Match print to speech	Make inferences or conclusions	Use mixture of own language and print to tell story while referring to pictures	Blending and segmenting syllables and words	Sound-letter association
Title/author	Identify letter, word, sentence	Characters	Refer to print, may refuse to read if cannot identify words	Blending and segmenting phonemes	Sight words
Where to begin reading		Problem, events, and resolution			

Source: From Valencia, S. W. (1977). *Authentic assessment of early reading: Alternatives to standardized tests.* Reprinted with permission of the Helen Dwight Reid Educational Foundation. Published by Heldref Publications, 1319 Eighteenth St., NW, Washington, DC 20036-1802. Copyright © 1997.

Table 12–3. Phonological Awareness Development

Age (years)	Behavior
By age 3, children typically can	• Recite familiar rhymes (e.g., "Pat-a-cake") • Recognize alliteration
By age 4, children typically can	• Spontaneously use rhyming word combinations • Produce multisyllabic words while separating the syllables
By age 5, children typically can	• Count the number of syllables in a word
By age 6, children typically can	• Tell a word that rhymes with a given word • Blend 2 or 3 sounds to form a word • Count the number of sounds in a word • Segment the initial sound from words to match with other words • Segment the initial sound from words to create a new word
By age 7, children typically can	• Blend more than 3 sounds to form a word • Segment 3 or 4 sounds in words • Spell simple words phonetically • Remove phonemes from words to make new words (e.g., "date" without /t/ is "day")

Source: Reprinted with permission from Peura-Jones, R., & DeBoer, C. (2000). *More story making: Using predictable literature to develop communication.* Eau Claire, WI: Thinking Publications.

Table 12–4. Frequency of Weakness in Specific Domains of Language and Literacy Among Participating Children

Assessment Domain	Number of Children with Identified Weakness
Language comprehension	5
Language expression	16
Pragmatic skills	2
Speech/phonology	10
Early literacy/preacademic skills	8
Hearing	11*
Social/behavioral	9†

*These children failed hearing screening because of middle ear problems (none had confirmed hearing loss).
†Based on teacher report.

semantic knowledge, and narrative discourse processes (NICHD Early Child Care Research Network, 2005). All of these skills needed to be addressed within effective emergent literacy interventions, because all conribute to later reading success (Justice et al., 2002; Roth & Baden, 2001; Scarborough, 2001; Whitehurst and Lonigan, 2001).

Scarborough (2001) proposed several components for an emergent literacy intervention program. Phonological awareness training was recommended because these skills have been demonstrated to play a pivotal role in learning to read and also because they target achievements directly linked to achievement of the alphabetic principle of letter recognition and sound-letter correspondence. Other suggested components for an intervention program come from correlational research and include increasing oral language abilities and enhancing early decoding and print awareness skills. Craig and colleagues (2003) also suggest targeting complex syntax skills and abstract pattern matching as part of emergent literacy intervention. These skills areas were the focus for goal development in the Linking Language and Literacy Project, which targeted both code-related and language-related skills, including the following:

- Written language awareness (print, awareness book conventions)
- Phonological awareness (rhyming, alliteration, blending, segmentation)
- Alphabetic principle (letter name knowledge, grapheme-phoneme awareness)
- Early writing experiences (scribbling, drawing, production of letter-like forms, use of invented spelling, production of conventional forms)
- Development of oral language (vocabulary, syntax, morphology, narration)
- Literacy motivation (interest in and ability to focus on books and other print material)

In the Linking Language and Literacy Project, student clinicians carefully considered each child's communication profile to select goals from among these six to address those areas of significant need. Generally, two goals were selected per child (e.g., oral language and phonological awareness), with a range of one to four goals. The specific goals established for individual children were addressed in large-group classroom-based instruction, in individual sessions, and in the development of language and literacy kits for each child in the program. Although not every child had specific literacy goals established, it is important to note that all communication goals were addressed within the context of literacy activities, to provide a general enhancement of all children's literacy abilities even when specific weaknesses were not identified.

For instance, goals for one child participant, Ronald, focused specifically on speech intelligibility and vocabulary, with limitations in both areas making his communication in the classroom extremely compromised. Intervention to promote intelligiblity and vocabulary was conducted within the context of a range of literacy-focused activities that also emphasized development of print awareness, alphabet knowledge, and phonological awareness, as summarized in Table 12–5. Thus, although two specific goals were identified for Ronald to pursue in the program, attention to literacy development was an additional feature of all intervention activities.

Table 12–5. Clinical Example: Activities to Increase Speech and Language Goals While Simultaneously Promoting Literacy Skills

---

Case Report: Ronald

Identified Speech/Language Areas of Weakness

Ronald was 3 years 7 months old at the time of participation. Both Ronald's classroom teacher and his mother were concerned about his speech intelligibility and wondered whether some of his behavioral problems in the classroom were related to his difficulty making himself understood. Ronald's communication profile showed significant weaknesses in his length of utterance and vocabulary diversity, as well as his speech intelligibility in connected speech.

Interventions: Speech/Language Areas

To increase Ronald's intelligibility and vocabulary, weekly themes were selected including color, vehicles, animals, and body parts. Books and extension activities were selected that incorporated the targeted vocabulary. Scripts were developed for games and activities and books with repeated phrases were selected that were modeled and used for "choral reading" or simultaneous production. These scripts were practiced until Ronald produced the scripts and phrases using an appropriate rate to increase comprehensibility.

Interventions: Literacy-Based Activities

Simultaneously, literacy goals were promoted during all intervention sessions by using evidence-based techniques designed to facilitate print awareness, alphabet knowledge, phonological awareness, and motivation toward literacy. These literacy activities included (1) print referencing as a means to demonstrate parts of the books read, such as front, cover, back, title, and pages; (2) using books with rhyme, nursery rhymes, songs, and finger plays that used cloze techniques and encouraged choral productions; (3) encouraging and modeling writing and drawing in extension activities; and (4) offering choices of books with high interest and appeal.

Outcome

In ten sessions, Ronald's intelligibility increased from 78% to above 90% when transcribed by an unfamiliar listener. In addition, Ronald increased his identification of the targeted vocabulary by correctly identifying new vocabulary words in three out of four trials.

Component 3: Promoting Language and Emergent Literacy Skills

The embedded-explicit model of emergent literacy intervention (Justice & Kaderavek, 2004; Justice et al., 2003) underlying the Linking Language and Literacy Project emphasized that children's learning opportunities combine *skill-based instruction* within a *meaningful* context. This model also can be considered meaning-based instruction (Culatta et al., 2004) in that it incorporates "systematic, repeated experience with literacy targets in literature or social contexts so that children acquire needed skills and simultaneously construct an understanding of the purpose and function of print" (p. 80). In their work with Spanish-speaking children, Culatta and colleagues stressed several important considerations for working with culturally and linguistically diverse learners: (1) integrate meaning and skill-based instruction; (2) provide engaging, interactive instruction, (3) have varied and increased exposure to literacy practice; (4) use relevant texts and materials; and (5) develop integrated theme-based units. These considerations also were included as core operating principles of the Linking Language and Literacy Project. All of the activities, materials, and procedures that were employed were relevant and sensitive to children's previous cultural and linguistic experiences and were drawn from current evidence-based practice on emergent literacy. A sampling of and rationale for activities and procedures used in the project follow.

Promoting Language and Literacy: Evidence-Based Contexts and Strategies

At the time the Linking Language and Literacy Project was conducted, the Head Start programs used the High/Scope curriculum in their classrooms (Hohmann & Weikart, 2002). The project's student volunteers were provided with didactic information about the central principles of the curriculum as part of a 3-week (6-hour) workshop on campus. A key point emphasized in the workshop was that children were to be active learners while adults manipulated the environment to incorporate 58 key learning experiences identified by High/Scope to facilitate learning. Specific focus via discussion and videotape viewing was on the six language and literacy key High/Scope experiences: (1) talking with children about personally meaningful experiences; (2) describing objects, events, and relations; (3) having fun with language: listening to and making up stories and rhymes; (4) writing in various ways: drawing, scribbling, production of letter-like forms, use of invented spelling, production of conventional forms; (5) reading in various ways: storybooks, signs, symbols, the child's own writing, and constructed books; and (6) dictating stories. Specific techniques to enhance language (e.g., follow the child's attentional lead, comment on ongoing action, echo and echo-expand, recast) were discussed, demonstrated, and practiced by the student clinicians.

The project's student volunteers also were provided with more specific training on how to incorporate attention to language and literacy within individual sessions with the children and across a range of large-group activities, including shared storybook reading, language experience sessions, and extension activities. After assessment and goal setting for each of the 37 children who participated in the Linking Language and Literacy Project, an individualized program was developed and implemented for each child. On average, children had approximately 13 20- to 30-minute, individual sessions over the 12 weeks of the program. However, there were frequent absences for some children, with the total number of sessions per child ranging from 2 to 22.

Individual Intervention Sessions

Individual sessions for the children were designed and delivered by the student clinicians through a careful preplanning activity that involved selecting specific themes, activities, procedures, and materials to promote language and literacy goals (see Table 12–6). Preplanning involved the following:

- Choosing a theme based on the child's strengths, interests, language and literacy goals, and the theme's associated vocabulary and cultural appropriateness
- Employing shared book reading, language experience, and/or extension activities (e.g., toys, props, puppets, crafts, games, constructing books, writing in journals)

Table 12–6. Preplanning for Individual Intervention Sessions in the Linking Language and Literacy Project

Choose:	*Consider:*
Theme	• Language and literacy goal • Child's strengths and interests • Associated vocabulary • Culturally appropriate • Relevance to classroom activities • Prior knowledge and experience
Activity type	• Shared book reading • Language experience • Extension • Combination of activities
Procedures/strategies	• Focusing • Elicitation • Scaffolding • Feedback
Materials	• Language and literacy goal • Relevance to theme • Link to activity • Targeted vocabulary • Developmentally appropriate • Culturally appropriate

■ Choosing appropriate facilitation strategies or techniques to focus, elicit, scaffold, and reinforce targeted goal behaviors, as illustrated in Table 12–7
■ Selecting appropriate materials and books related to the theme that reflected the child's experiences and world knowledge and were at an appropriate developmental level (e.g., pictures, amount of text on the page, length of book) and were appropriate to the goal (e.g., if the goal was to increase participation, flap book with repetition of words or phrases or books that encouraged gesture or pantomine were appropriate choices).

Table 12–7. Strategies for High-Quality Shared Storybook Reading

Type of Strategy	Examples of Strategies
Before Reading	
Focusing	Physical proximity
	▪ Have child sit next to you or on your lap
	▪ Sit so book is easy to view
	▪ Use a "big" book
	Preparatory set
	▪ Introduce author
	▪ Read title
	▪ Show cover and discuss illustrations
	▪ Introduce setting, characters, when it takes place
	▪ Ask child to listen for word or action
	▪ Introduce vocabulary
	Paraphrase
During Reading	
Focusing	▪ Vary voice to fit characters (register, pitch, loudness)
	▪ Move your finger under the words as you read
	▪ Point out pictures
Scaffolding	▪ Add information to clarify content
	▪ Rephrase confusing content
	▪ Explain new vocabulary
	▪ Encourage child to elaborate on ideas and communicate them to others
	▪ Ask child to predict action
	▪ Relate story to child's experience
	▪ Discuss pictures
	▪ Share your own reactions
	▪ Use props

Table 12-7. *continued*

Type of Strategy	Examples of Strategies
	▪ Provide feedback – Acknowledge or confirm child's comment – Expand or reword what child says – Extend or link ideas – Request clarification – Recast and clarify incorrect responses ▪ Use open-ended questions (e.g., "I wonder if . . . ?" "How do you think . . . ?" "What happened when . . . ?") ▪ Regulate the task for success ▪ Point out or ask about consequences, associations, similarities, and differences ▪ Use cloze procedure
Elicitation	▪ Gesture or pantomime ▪ Phonemic cue ▪ Binary choice question ▪ Constituent question ▪ Relational tie ▪ Semantic cue ▪ Comprehension or summarization question ▪ Provide feedback (as above)

After Reading

Elicitation	▪ Ask child to recall story events, characters, and so on ▪ Relate the story to the child's experiences ▪ Review the new vocabulary ▪ Elicit the child's reaction ▪ Extension activities (e.g., language experience activity, craft, props, or construction/creation of a book, journal, song, skit)

Source: Adapted with permission from Crowe, L., & Reichmuth, S. (2001). *The source for early literacy development* (pp. 42–46). East Moline, IL: LinguiSystems.

To introduce each session, a schedule of possible events to be covered in the session, called the "Daily Activity List," was developed. The child's name was displayed prominently at the top of a list of numbered activities, each depicted with a word and graphic symbol. This list was used to assist children in recognizing, spelling, and writing the letters in their name; to preview and establish the session's agenda with the child; to encourage choice making by selecting from the menu of activities; to mark transitions between activities; and to achieve closure by reviewing the session after completion of the selected activities. The Daily Activity List also served as a way to communicate the day's events with family members.

Shared Book Reading Activities

Shared book reading frequently was used within individual sessions to facilitate children's language and literacy goals in the Linking Language and Literacy Project. Shared book reading is a collaborative context in which to increase language and emergent literacy skills with preschoolers (Cutspec, 2004; Justice & Pullen, 2003; Kirchner, 1991; Lonigan & Whitehurst, 1998; van Kleeck, Vander Woude, & Hammett, 2006). Whitehurst and Lonigan (1998) demonstrated that a program of shared book reading called *dialogic reading* can produce substantial changes in preschool children's language skills (Chapter 8 provides more extensive details concerning this approach). In dialogic reading, the adult assumes the role of an active listener and partner in the activity, by asking questions, adding information, and prompting the child to increase the sophistication of descriptions of the material in the picture book. A child's responses to the book are encouraged through praise and repetition, and more sophisticated responses are encouraged by expansions of the child's utterances and by more challenging questions from the adult reading partner. Engaging children in favorite and familiar books makes the predictable, repetitive nature of shared book reading an ideal context for learning language and literacy skills.

Four research principles extracted from the extant literature on shared reading by Coyne, Simmons, & Kame'enui (2004) were applied in engaging children in joint book reading during the program: (1) using interesting and engaging storybooks; (2) engaging in rich dialogic discussion; (3) encouraging multiple readings of storybooks; and (4) reading with small groups of children (primarily dyadic reading interactions were used in the individual sessions). A fifth principle recommended by Coyne and associates—use of a performance-oriented adult book reading style—was adopted for some but not all children. Rather, a reading style that was most responsive to each child's abilities and interactive style and appropriate for the goals of the activities was selected, drawing from the three adult styles of book reading described by Reese and Cox (1999). These book reading styles are differentiated by the level of demand from the child, the type of adult input, and the timing of the adult comments or questions during reading:

- *Describer style*—lower demand, with the adult requesting the child to describe and label pictures throughout the book reading
- *Comprehender style*—higher demand, with the adult requesting the child to give reason-based answers and to make inferences related to the story throughout the book reading
- *Performance-oriented style*—higher demand, with adult reading the story without interruption and direction of adult comments and questions to children before or after book reading

Book types were matched to children's level of ability and the goals of the activity. Several resources for selecting books for inclusion in the program were used, including Web sites available for this purpose (such as http://www.earlyliterature.ecsd.net). Several books were made available during each session to encourage children to choose which book to read. Multiple readings of the same book were also used to help children learn vocabulary and to promote comprehension of the narrative. Pattern books or predictable books, which include patterned text, repetitive words and phrases, and predictable plots also were used liberally to increase children's active participation in the reading session; children often exhibited heightened interest when they were able to remember the story and enjoyed saying the repetitive words and phrases because this allowed them to participate in the telling of the story. Patterns were used to promote choral "reading" that emphasized vocabulary, grammatical structures, rate control, and speech sound development. Patterns included the following:

- Repetition of phrase or sentence (e.g., "Brown Bear, Brown Bear, What do you see?" [Martin, 1970])
- Addition of a repetitious phrase or sentence (e.g., "I know an old lady who swallowed a fly" [Wescott, 1980])
- Rhyming pattern with frequent repetition (e.g., *Green Eggs & Ham* [Dr. Seuss, 1960])
- Occurrence of events in a manner to foster prediction (e.g., *Good Night Gorilla* [Rathmann, 1994]).

Language Experience Activities

Language experience activities employ the child's own experiences to improve oral language and emergent literacy skills. Generally, language experience activities involve engaging children in an authentic learning activity (e.g., taking a walk, going on a nature hunt), followed by a mediated writing experience that details aspects of the experience. Gonzalez and Stewart (1999) described this highly flexible approach in a four-step process (see Table 12–8) that was adapted in the Linking Language and Literacy Project. In this program, the language experience activities were centered on a theme to help build vocabulary. While engaged in the language experience approach with the children, the student clinicians applied the same strategies used during shared book reading, including focusing, scaffolding, and eliciting. Focused stimulation, a frequently used procedure within the classroom and individual sessions, is thought to be applicable to culturally and linguistically diverse children (Ellis-Weismer & Robertson, 2006); therefore, this strategy also was utilized. Student clinicians preselected linguistic targets and manipulated the context and their input to the child to increase the saliency of the target during language experience activities.

Extension Activities

Theme-based extension activities usually were paired with the shared book reading to extend concepts learned within the reading context. These activities took many forms, depending on the child's strengths,

Table 12–8. Development of Language Experience Activities for Improving Language and Literacy

Step	Activities
Planning	▪ Choose theme-based activity, associated script, and materials. ▪ Link to language and literacy goals.
Implementing	▪ Guide the activity to focus on established goals. ▪ Structure multiple opportunities for practice. ▪ Highlight targets verbally (state target specifically; to emphasize placement of target in sentence, use inflection, emphatic stress). ▪ Use visual aids (photos, picture from a book, template, drawings, sequence cards).
Generating the story	▪ Select and organize content (use the selected photos, pictures, or objects, or use graphic organizers, outline, recipe, or shopping list). ▪ Write the story. ▪ Scaffold the writing by offering support as needed (e.g., fill in the blank using a pattern). ▪ Stories comprise 3 to 5 sentences including an opening and a closing sentence. For example, after the children make "silly soup" (different objects are placed into a pot and stirred), the sentence starters might be: We made silly soup. We put in _____. Then we put in _____. It tasted _____. ▪ Write the first draft and create a final draft for next session. ▪ Alternatively, set up clear steps to the activity's sequence, with a page per step; illustrate each page with a picture; and ask the child to dictate the story.
Providing practice	▪ Review story and practice "reading" the story together; then the child reads it independently. ▪ Use multiple occasions to review and read the story. ▪ Vary the audience (peers, puppets, teachers, parents).

Source: Adapted with permission from Gonzalez, L., & Stewart, S. (1999). *Literacy-based strategies for improving speech and language skills in young children.* Psi Iota Sorority Interactive Television Series on Individuals with Communication Disabilities. Lexington, KY: University of Kentucky.

interests, learning style, and needs, and often used procedures similar to those for the language experience activities described previously. For instance, after a book was read, the student clinicians completed a meaningful activity with the children that was related to the book's topic or vocabulary. Owocki (2001) suggested the use of a variety of extension activities including visual retellings (painting, drawing, craft); story webs to discuss characters, setting, problem, and resolution; flow maps or templates used to represent a story with a sequence; and prop retellings using toys, puppets, flannelboard pieces, or materials developed by the student clinicians. For example, a reading of the *The Very Hungry Caterpillar* (Carle, 1969) may be extended by making or coloring a caterpillar, introducing food-related vocabulary and discussing the child's favorite foods, or using a flannelboard with a caterpillar and recalling the sequence of the story.

Explicit Intervention Approaches Across Contexts and Activities

Regardless of the instructional activities or context utilized (e.g., shared storybook reading, language experience activities), an important principle for effective intervention is the use of explicit teaching (Justice et al., 2003). Justice and colleagues (2003) suggested that an explicit approach may be the most efficient route to skill development, particularly for children who have not learned sufficiently from more informal, naturalistic literacy-based interactions. Accordingly, the Linking Language and Literacy Project combined meaningful activities with direct and explicit instruction via shared book reading, language experience, and extension activities. Explicit and direct instruction was provided to pupils participating in the project for the six goals: written language awareness, phonological awareness, alphabetic principle, early writing, oral language, and literacy motivation.

Goal 1: Increasing Written Language Awareness

A principal strategy used to increase written language awareness was that of print referencing. *Print referencing* is defined as the nonverbal (pointing and tracking print) and verbal (comments, questions, requests about print) cues used by an adult to direct a child's attention to the forms, features, and functions of written language (Justice & Ezell, 2004). Print referencing during shared book reading is a promising intervention for promoting written language awareness (Justice & Pullen, 2003). Encouraging children to be interested in print is an early metalinguistic milestone; according to Whitehurst and Lonigan (2001), such interest serves as a cornerstone for all subsequent literacy achievements. Justice and Lankford (2002) found that children infrequently attend to print in storybooks, but that use of storybooks with larger print size, salient print features, and less text was helpful for drawing children's attention to print. Justice and Ezell (2004) documented that explicitly drawing children's attention to print (e.g., prompting) by talking and questioning about print enhanced children's development of print awareness.

Targeted skills: The following specific skills within written language awareness were targeted for all children:

- Alphabet knowledge: the ability to discriminate letters on the basis of distinctive features and to recognize or label letters of the alphabet
- Print conventions: the understanding of how books are to be held and how a book is organized
- Print concepts: recognition of words as distinct from other print categories

Sample activities: A Daily Activity List was used in each individual session to build a routine and to increase written language awareness. During shared book reading, the student clinicians pointed to and commented on the text using such prompts as:

Alphabet knowledge

"I spy with my little eye a . . . "

"I see the P that's in my name. Where is the M like in your name?"

Print conventions

"Look what's on the cover/front of the book."

"This is the name of the book. It's the title. The title says . . . "

"Let's find a word on this page."

Print concepts

"How many words are in the name of this book? Let's count."

"Where's Spot? This word says the dog's name. Let's find the word Spot."

Goal 2: Increasing Phonological Awareness

Extensive research suggests that phonological awareness is related to later reading and spelling success in mainstream children and that phonological awareness skills can be systematically taught and learned (National Reading Panel, 2000; Snow et al., 1998). It is not clear how dialect and bilingualism affect phonological awareness (Vernon-Feagans et al., 2001), and it is important to consider how the child's first language and dialect may influence English language learning, especially as it relates to phonological awareness. Standard American English was modeled during project activities, and children's use of African American English or Spanish-influenced English was not targeted or pointed out in conversational contexts or activities unless related specifically to the goal (e.g., "'Hat' has three sounds, listen, h-a-t, hat"). Characteristics of effective intervention for phonological awareness are summarized by Sterling-Orth (2004) as being explicit, systematic, supportive, and intensive. She stressed that phonological awareness training is most effective when age-appropriate "meta" strategies (e.g., explanations of tasks and strategies, use of mediated learning) are used with children.

Targeted skills: Targets were based on a developmental continuum involving primitive awareness of speech sounds and rhymes to rhyme awareness and sound similarities and, at the highest level, awareness of syllables or phonemes. In the Linking Language and Literacy Project, phonological awareness tasks related to rhyme, alliteration, and word awareness with a more limited focus on blending, and segmentation were emphasized; the selection process drew from several commercially available curricula, such as Ladders to Literacy (Notari-Syverson et al., 1998) and Sound Foundations (Byrne & Fielding-Barnsley, 1991). Project activities were individualized for each child.

Sample activities:

Rhyme awareness: Short familiar poems, fingerplays, songs or nursery rhymes were used and often paired with clapping or movement and corresponding exaggeration of the rhyming words.

Rhyme match: A variety of games were devised, such as concentration involving matching words on the basis of rhymes.

Alliteration: Children made up sentences that involved organizing words sharing beginning sounds (e.g., for mouse, monkey, and mitten: "Monkey's mittens are missing" or "Mouse makes the monkey mittens").

Word awareness: Words were pointed out individually in reading books using print-referencing strategies (e.g., "Let's count the number of words in the title of the book").

Blending: Children moved picture cards corresponding to each syllable in multisyllable words (e.g., blending "cow" and "boy" for "cowboy").

Segmenting: Children engaged in "say it silly" games in which they had to break words into their onset and rime (c-at) or phonemes (c-a-t).

Goal 3: Increasing Knowledge of the Alphabetic Principle

Whitehurst and Lonigan (2001) have suggested that emergent knowledge of the alphabet principle, including the individual letters of the alphabet as well as some sound-to-letter pairings, is one of the best predictors of children's later achievements in decoding. However, they caution against conducting alphabetic instruction (particularly that featuring rote repetition and drill) in the absence of meaningful activities and instruction in other emergent literacy skills, especially phonological awareness.

Targeted skills: A range of skills were addressed within this domain of learning: knowledge of the alphabet string (through song); matching, recognizing, and labeling some letters, especially the letters in the child's first name; and learning some letter-sound correspondences. Generally, the first letter of the child's first name was introduced in uppercase, followed by teaching the remaining letters of the name in lowercase.

Sample activities: The Daily Activity List that introduced each session featured the child's name. Name booklets were made with a letter per page. These booklets generally included space for the child to write, trace, or dot-to-dot the targeted letters. All crafts, worksheets, or "make-n-takes" were labeled with the child's name, and the student clinicians supported each child to write and spell his or her name. Direct practice games included bingo, memory, mazes, "Go Fish," scavenger hunts, and writing letters in mixed media such as shaving cream, sand, play dough, or fingerpaint. Writing on "wipe boards" with markers often was particularly motivating. Language experience activities included making a grocery list, shopping list, menu, and job lists; for each type, the student clinician included explicit discussion of the letters and their sounds.

Goal 4: Increasing Early Writing Experiences

Writing experiences constitute an additional route to helping children understand and practice the code-related skills of emergent literacy, and children's writing development is intrinsically linked to other areas of emergent literacy and oral language achievement. Writing experiences allow children an opportunity to express written language versus simply experiencing written language as occurs when children listen to storybooks.

Targeted skills: An emphasis was placed on improving children's written expression along a continuum represented by the following modes of expression: scribbles, draws, writes letter-like forms, begins invented spelling, and produces conventional forms.

Sample activities: The shared book reading and language experience extension activities provided a rich context for encouraging meaningful writing attempts. For example, children were asked to fill in parts of a journal concerning themselves:

My name is _____.

I am _____ years old.

I live with _____.

I like to _____.

The children also were encouraged to regularly sign their names on the works they produced (books, crafts, worksheets).

Goal 5: Increasing Oral Language

Two aspects of oral language were explicitly targeted within the program: vocabulary and narrative.

Vocabulary. Children living in poverty may not have had the same amount or quality of input from adults related to vocabulary and vocabulary elaboration in comparison with children in middle-income households (Hart & Risley, 1995). Coyne and associates (2004) express the need for research-based, intensive vocabulary interventions for young children at risk for later reading difficulties; they advocate the use of explicit instruction in building vocabulary skills during shared book reading. Nonetheless, shared book reading alone may not have a large measurable impact on building the vocabulary of preschoolers with low vocabulary skills. Justice, Meier, and Walpole (2005) found that at-risk kindergarten children's use of target vocabulary did not increase as a result of repeated practice with these words during shared book reading sessions, and increased only modestly through the use of elaboration (e.g., providing definitional information or synonyms). These investigators therefore suggest a "mixed-method" approach to teaching vocabulary, with repeated practice of target vocabulary during shared reading that features (1) increasing the number of occurrences of the word in the text; (2) making the child an active partner through dialogic reading; (3) providing the meaning of novel words in salient, contextualized activities; and (4) encouraging exposure to words outside of book reading. In their review of the literature on ways to increase vocabulary through shared-book reading, Gormley and Ruhl (2005) also suggest use of seven strategies (including some of the aforementioned strategies) to achieve "optimal success": (1) questioning and prompting; (2) modeling; (3) praising and encouraging; (4) defining; (5) labeling; (6) using follow-up activities; and (7) summarizing.

Targeted skills: Vocabulary targets were selected on the basis of the results of the child's individualized assessments. Selection factors for vocabulary included the targeted language and literacy goal, the child's strengths and interests; cultural appropriateness;

relevance to classroom and functional activities; and the child's prior knowledge and experience. Most often, dynamic assessment (i.e., test-teach-retest) established the child's receptive and expressive vocabulary for a specific themed unit. Between 5 and 10 words were preselected that were associated with the theme, baseline abilities were established, intervention focused on words that the child did not know, progress was monitored, and a new vocabulary or theme was introduced when the child demonstrated competence.

Sample activities: With the vocabulary selected, children were explicitly told their "special words" of the day. These words were presented in a variety of shared reading, language experience, and extension activities using the principles as described, with a particular focus on the storybook reading context as a means to provide exposure to new words. Student clinicians presented vocabulary *before* the activity, *during* the activity by defining or elaborating on the word at the point in the story where it is needed, and *after* the story to review the words. Multiple opportunities to see (e.g., pictures with printed word, objects), hear (e.g., definitions, elaborated explanations, associations and synonyms, focused stimulation, auditory bombardment), and say the word (e.g., model-mand, contingent questions, scripts) were provided throughout individual sessions.

Narrative. Narrative development influences children's language, literacy, and social development and may even affect academic success at a more basic level: Some scholars propose that narratives "form the foundation of human thinking" (Gillam, McFadden, & van Kleeck, 1995). That children from different cultural and linguistic backgrounds vary from mainstream children in their production of narratives is not surprising, but research has not clearly identified the specific factors resulting in these differences (e.g., bilingualism, home experiences with storytelling). Several differences in narrative production for children from non–majority-culture backgrounds are cited by Fiestas and Peña (2004): story length, level of description, content, sequence and structure of the story, and predominant verb forms used (e.g., past tense versus present progressive).

Vernon-Feagans and colleagues (2001) hypothesize that "cultural clashes" between home and school practices have negative effects on poor children, who may fall farther behind in language and literacy development after beginning school. In their discussion of the narrative skills of African American children from low-income families, these authors implicate a potential mismatch between school and home in strategies (e.g., fewer question-asking routines in the home), story grammars, and experiences and associated vocabulary compared with other children. Even children with excellent language skills, when narratives were collected in naturalistic settings, were not demonstrating these skills at school. Paradoxically, some of the children's positive abilities (e.g., joint storytelling) were negatively related to literacy and school ratings by teachers. Children in poverty did worse in paraphrasing a story that they previously demonstrated they understood and were less able to answer abstract questions (e.g., why, how). More "out of category" responses by the children found teachers unsure how to respond and therefore less likely to give corrective feedback for incorrect responses.

Targeted skills: For the preschoolers in the Linking Language and Literacy Project, narrative skills to be targeted were determined by assessing their productive language abilities. Supports were then provided for children's movement along a continuum of narrative development from labeling pictures with a single word to telling and retelling stories based on shared book reading, language experience activities, or personal accounts about family or other salient events (e.g., field trip to the zoo). Specific skills promoted included attending to and labeling pictures in books; making comments and asking questions about an individual picture in a book; telling a story and linking events based on pictures using conversational language; providing explanations and making predictions about a story; sequencing story pictures into beginning, middle, and end events; relating and organizing elements of a story structure in a coherent sequence (setting, theme, episodes, resolution); and making interpretations and judgments about the story.

Sample activities: Story narratives were promoted by reading and re-reading books together; retelling a story with puppets, a flannelboard, or toys as props; making "books" as part of a language experience activity; and using templates or other graphics to sequence story action.

Goal 6: Increasing Literacy Motivation

The Linking Language and Literacy Project repeatedly stressed that reading is fun! Research has associated several instructional features with increasing literacy motivation for elementary school children such as access to books, opportunities for choice, provision of books with interesting content, and building on the familiar (Gambrell, 1996; Guthrie & Humenick, 2003; Turner, 1995).

Targeted skills: Not all children required systematic attention to improve motivation, but for those who did require this focus, the goal was to increase their attention, engagement, and persistence toward shared book reading and related activities. This was measured by time on task, interaction with the book, and engagement with the student clinician in dialogic book reading.

Sample activities: Successfully motivating children who initially rejected books depended on careful prior planning by selecting highly interesting, developmentally appropriate activities, materials, and procedures that invited verbal and nonverbal interaction and matched the child's learning style. The student clinicians took care to be responsive to child cues and to scaffold the activity to ensure child success. Liberally encouraging active participation, ensuring close proximity during reading (usually laps), and ensuring a positive adult affect and comments about reading were key features of the activities.

Language and Literacy Kits

An important feature of the Linking Language and Literacy Project was to provide each child with a literacy kit at the end of the program to ensure generalization of strategies used and goals addressed to the children's home environment. The intent was to offer children and caregivers access to materials linked to the six emergent literacy goals emphasized throughout the program. Each kit provided materials and suggestions for having conversations while focusing on books, making crafts, practicing writing, and playing with toys. This home-based component was added to the program because Hammer and coauthors (2003) report that bilingual preschoolers benefit from increased exposure to literacy materials and literacy events during the preschool years. Also, Roberts, Jurgens, and Burchinal (2005) have indicated that the overall responsiveness and support of the home environment constituted strong and consistent predictors of later language and literacy outcomes among at-risk preschoolers. The goal in providing the literacy kits was to increase the opportunity for children to be exposed to language and literacy activities in the home.

Thus, at the end of the project, student clinicians developed and presented to each child a language and literacy kit (sample kits are shown in Appendix 12–A). A theme of high interest to the child was paired with the child's goals, and books and materials were selected. Each kit included introductory information; two or three books on a theme of interest to the child that were culturally sensitive and provided exposure to a variety of book types (e.g., predictable, flaps, alphabet/counting, narrative, classic); suggestions about promoting language and literacy specific to the theme; a list of "Top Ten Ways for Helping Your Child to Read" (see Appendix 12–B); toys consistent with the bag's theme that encouraged parent-child play; writing materials (e.g., markers, crayons, scissors, paper, sticky notes); and a simple craft activity, based on the theme, that the caregiver and the child could perform together.

Outcomes of an Evidence-Based Emergent Literacy Program

For the 37 children who participated in the Linking Language and Literacy Project, a total of 69 language and literacy goals were set, averaging approximately two per child. Baseline information was collected during the language and literacy assessment, and a criterion for documenting whether an individual goal was met was set. Twenty children met all of their goals, whereas nine children met one or two goals, and eight children met none of their goals. Although some goals were not met and some children met none of their established goals, this does not indicate that progress was not made toward these goals. In most cases, although the *criterion* for achieving a specific goal was not met, progress was evident toward the goal. Additionally, in terms of the service-learning experience for the student clinicians, the successful design and implementation of an evidence-based intervention, and the overall progress observed among the children served, the outcomes of the Project were unequivocally positive.

Continued refinements of the focus and effectiveness of this program will draw from lessons learned during this initial period of implementation. The following key precepts based on these lessons are offered for all professionals with an interest in developing and implementing programs similar to the Linking Language and Literacy Project:

- The evidence base is sparse—draw on what is known about children's language and literacy development and the evidence that is available.
- Focus on skills predictive of better communicators and readers, until research and practice provide alternatives.
- There may be several paths to literacy—not all children may follow the same route.
- Work to be culturally competent—it is a lifelong process of learning about self and others.
- Follow developmentally appropriate practice—look to how children generally learn.
- Individualize—use the child's abilities, strengths, interests, and learning style as a guide.
- Use a responsive teaching style—reflect on the child's successes and difficulties with activities and procedures.
- Embed meaningful, socially relevant activities into teaching.
- Use explicit or direct instruction within these activities— make obvious the skill to be learned.
- Set high expectations but support children's success—no one likes to fail.
- Increase the exposure to language and literacy experiences —opportunities for learning abound if the professional remains aware of the language and literacy skill areas.
- Build shared cultural knowledge through joint experiences—these are the basis for conversations.
- Few resources exist to guide decision making in planning and implementing intervention—there is a strong impetus for developing resources.
- Use books, materials, and activities that are culturally relevant and depict and broaden children's experiences.
- Support the home language of English language learners— provide book options in the child's home language, or use bilingual or wordless books to promote conversational interaction between the child and family members.

- With some English language learners, focus on input, not output—some children may be in a silent period as they are learning the new language.
- Expect children to code switch—encourage communication in any language.
- Offer multiple modalities for language and literacy learning—pair action, visual, and written support with verbal input.
- For professionals who don't already speak the child's home language, learn words and phrases in that language—children often respond more readily and enthusiastically to an interventionist who uses their language.
- Build a child's first language first, especially for children with language and learning problems—the services of a bilingual teacher, bilingual speech-language pathologist, or interpreter may be required for assistance in this area.
- Assess children's abilities in their home language if there are concerns about communication—rule out language impairment versus language learning.
- *Have fun* with these children—they are preschoolers, and play is their business!

References

American Speech-Language-Hearing Association. (2001). Roles and responsibilities of speech-language pathologists with respect to reading and writing in children and adolescents (position statement, executive summary of guidelines, technical report). *ASHA Supplement, 21,* 17–27.

Aram, D., & Hall, N. (1989). Longitudinal follow-up of children with preschool communication disorders: Treatment implications. *School Psychology Review, 18*(4), 487–501.

Boudreau, D., & Hedberg, N. (1999). A comparison of early literacy skills in children with specific language impairment and their typically developing peers. *American Journal of Speech-Language Pathology, 8*(3), 249–260.

Byrne, B., & Fielding-Barnsley, R. (1991). *Sound foundations.* Sydney, New South Wales, Australia: Peter Leyden Educational.

Carle, E. (1969). *The hungry caterpillar*. New York: Philomel Books, A division of Young Readers Group.

Catts, H. (1997). The early identification of language-based reading difficulties. *Language, Speech, and Hearing Services in Schools, 28*, 86–89.

Catts, H. Fey, M., Tomblin, B. & Zhang, X. (2002). A longitudinal investigation of reading outcomes in children with language impairments. *Journal of Speech, Language, and Hearing Research, 45*, 1142–1157.

Coyne, M., Simmons, D., & Kame'enui, E. (2004). Vocabulary instruction for young children at risk of experiencing reading difficulties. In J. Baumann & E. Kame'enui (Eds.), *Vocabulary instruction: Research to practice* (pp. 41–58). New York: Guilford Press.

Craig, H. K., Connor, C., & Washington, J. (2003). Early positive predictors of later reading comprehension for African American students: A preliminary investigation. *Language, Speech, and Hearing Services in Schools, 34*, 31–43.

Craig, H., Thompson, C., Washington, J., & Potter, S. (2004). Performance of elementary-grade African American students on the Gray oral reading tests. *Language, Speech, and Hearing Services in Schools, 35*, 41–154.

Crowe, L., & Reichmuth, S. (2001). *The source for early literacy development*. East Moline, IL: LinguiSystems.

Culatta, B., Aslett, R., Fife, M., & Setzer, L. A. (2004). Project SEEL: Part I. Systematic and engaging early literacy instruction. *Communication Disorders Quarterly, 25*, 79–88.

Cutspec, P. (2004). Influences of dialogic reading on the language development of toddlers. *Bridges, 2*, 1–12.

Dollaghan, C. (2004, April 13). Evidence-based practice: Myths and realities. *The ASHA Leader*, 4–5, 12.

Dr. Seuss. (1960). *Green eggs and ham*. New York: Random House Beginner's Books.

Ellis-Weismer, S., & Robertson, S. (2006). Focused stimulation approach to language intervention. In R. McCauley & M. Fey (Eds.), *Treatment of language disorders in children* (pp. 75–202). Baltimore: Paul H. Brookes.

Fiestas, C., & Pena, E. (2004). Narrative discourse in bilingual children: Language and task effects. *Language, Speech, and Hearing Services in Schools, 35*, 155–168

Flax, J., Realpe-Bonilla, T., Hirsch, L., Brzustowicz, L., Bartlett, C., & Tallal, P. (2003). Specific language impairment in families: Evidence for co-occurrence with reading impairments. *Journal of Speech, Language, and Hearing Research, 46*, 530–543.

Gambrell, L. B. (1996). Creating classroom cultures that foster reading motivation. *The Reading Teacher, 50*(1), 14–25.

Genesee, F., Paradis, J., & Crago, M. (2004). *Dual language development and disorders: A handbook on bilingualism and second language learning.* Baltimore: Paul H. Brookes.

Gillam, R. B., Mc Fadden, T., & van Kleeck, A. (1995). Improving the narrative abilities of children with language disorders: Whole language and language skills approaches. In M. Fey, J. Windsor, & J. Reichle (Eds.), *Communication intervention for school-aged children* (pp. 145-182). Baltimore: Paul H. Brookes.

Goldstein, B., & Kohnert, K. (2005). Speech, language, and hearing in developing bilingual children: Current findings and future directions. *Language, Speech, and Hearing Services in Schools, 36*(3), 264-267.

Gonzalez, L., & Stewart, S. (1999). *Literacy-based strategies for improving speech and language skills in young children.* Psi Iota Sorority Interactive Television Series on Individuals with Communication Disabilities. Lexington, KY: University of Kentucky.

Gormley, S., & Ruhl, K. (2005). Shared storybook reading: Increasing vocabulary skills in an inclusive classroom setting. *Perspectives on School-based Issues.* American Speech-Language-Hearing Association Division 16, 6(1), 11-14.

Guthrie, J. T., & Humenick, N. M. (2003). Motivating students to read. In P. McCardle & V. Chhabra (Eds.), *The voice of evidence in reading research.* Baltimore: Paul H. Brookes.

Hammer, C., Miccio, A., & Wagstaff, D. (2003). Home literacy experiences and their relationship to bilingual preschoolers' developing English literacy abilities: An initial investigation. *Language, Speech, and Hearing Services in Schools, 34,* 20-30.

Hart, B., & Risley, T. (1995). *Meaningful differences in the everyday experience of young American children.* Baltimore: Paul H. Brookes.

Hohmann, M., & Weikart, D. (2002). *Educating young children* (2nd ed.). Ypsilanti, MI: High/Scope Press.

Invernizzi, M., Sullivan, A., & Meier, J. (2001). *Phonological awareness literacy screening for preschool (PALS)—PreK.* Charlottesville, VA: The Virginia State Department of Education, University of Virginia Curry School of Education.

Juel, C. (1988). Learning to read and write: A longitudinal study of 54 children from first through fourth grades. *Journal of Educational Psychology, 80,* 437-447.

Johnston, J., & Wong, M.-Y. A. (2002). Cultural differences in beliefs and practices concerning talk to children. *Journal of Speech, Language, and Hearing Research, 45,* 916-926.

Justice, L., Chow, S., Capellini, C., Flanigan, K., & Colton, S. (2003). Emergent literacy intervention for vulnerable preschoolers: Relative effects of two approaches. *American Journal of Speech-Language Pathology, 12*, 320–332.

Justice, L., & Ezell, H. (2004). Print referencing: An emergent literacy enhancement and its clinical applications. *Language, Speech, and Hearing in Schools, 35*, 185–193.

Justice, L., Invernizzi, M., & Meier, J. (2002) Designing and implementing an early literacy screening protocol: Suggestions for the speech-language pathologist. *Language, Speech, and Hearing Services in Schools, 33*(2), 84–101.

Justice, L., & Kaderavek, J. (2004). Embedded-explicit emergent literacy intervention I: Background and description of approach. *Language, Speech, and Hearing in Schools, 35*, 201–211.

Justice, L., & Lankford, C. (2002). Preschool children's visual attention to print during storybook reading: Pilot findings. *Communication Disorders Quarterly, 24*, 1, 11–21.

Justice, L., Meier, J., & Walpole, S. (2005). Learning new words from storybooks: An efficacy study with at-risk kindergartners. *Language, Speech, and Hearing Services in Schools, 36*, 17–32.

Justice, L., & Pence, K. (2004). Addressing the language and literacy needs of vulnerable children: Innovative strategies in the context of evidence-based practice. *Communication Disorders Quarterly, 25*, 173–178.

Justice, L., & Pullen, P. (2003). Promising interventions for promoting emergent literacy skills: Three evidence-based approaches. *Topics in Early Childhood Special Education, 23*(3), 99–113.

Kaderavek, J., & Justice, L. (2004). Embedded-explicit emergent literacy intervention II: Goal selection and implementation in the early childhood classroom. *Language, Speech, and Hearing Services in Schools, 35*, 212–228.

Kirchner, D. (1991). Reciprocal book reading: A discourse-based intervention strategy for the child with atypical language development. In T. Gallagher (Ed.), *Pragmatics of language: Clinical practice issues* (pp. 307–332). San Diego, CA: Singular Publishing Group.

Kohnert, K., Yim, D., Nett, K., Fong Kan, P., & Duran, L. (2005). Intervention with linguistically diverse preschool children: A focus on developing home language(s). *Language, Speech, and Hearing Services in Schools, 36*, 251–263.

Long, S. (2005). Language and linguistically-culturally diverse children. In Vicki A. Reed (Ed.), *An Introduction to Children with Language Disorders* (3rd ed., pp. 301–334). Boston: Pearson Allyn and Bacon.

Lonigan C. J., & Whitehurst G. J. (1998). Relative efficacy of parent and teacher involvement in a shared-reading intervention for preschool children from low-income backgrounds. *Early Childhood Research Quarterly, 13*(2), 263–290.

Lutkus, A. D., Rampey, B. D., & Donahue, P. (2005). *The nation's report card: Trial urban district assessment reading 2005* (NCES 2006-455). U.S. Department of Education, National Center for Education Statistics. Washington, DC: U.S. Government Printing Office.

Martin, B. (1970). *Brown bear, brown bear*. New York: Henry Holt.

McCabe, A., & Bliss, L. (2003). *Patterns of narrative discourse: A multicultural life span approach*. Boston: Allyn & Bacon, Pearson Education.

McLaughlin, B. (1995). *Fostering second language development in young children: Principles and practice*. Santa Cruz, CA: National Center for Research on Cultural Diversity and Second Language Learning, University of California.

Montgomery, J. (2005). What SLPs might learn about EBP from reading research. *ASHA Magazine, 13*.

Nathan, L., Stackhouse, J., Goulandris, N., & Snowling, M. (2004). The development of early literacy skills among children with speech difficulties: A test of the "critical age hypothesis." *Journal of Speech, Language, and Hearing Research, 47*, 377–391.

National Assessment of Educational Progress (NAEP). The Nation's Report Card. (2005). Available at: http://nces.ed.gov/nationsreportcard/reading/

National Association for the Education of Young Children. (1998). *Learning to read and write: developmentally appropriate practices for young children. A joint position statement adopted by the International Reading Association and NAEYC*. Washington, D.C.

The National Center for Children in Poverty. (2006). Basic Facts about low-income children: Birth to age 6, Columbia University Mailman School of Public Health. Web site: http://www.nccp.org

National Institute of Child Health and Human Development (NICHD) Early Child Care Research Network. (2005). Pathways to reading: The role of oral language in the transition to reading. *Developmental Psychology, 41*, 428–442.

National Reading Panel: Teaching Children to Read. (2000). National Institute of Child Health and Human Development (NICHD). NIH Publication No, 00-4754; Washington, D.C.

Neuman, S. B., & Roskos, K. (2005). Whatever happened to developmentally appropriate practice in early literacy? *Beyond the Journal: Young Children on the Web*. Available at: http://www.journal.naeyc.org

Notari-Syverson, A., O'Connor, R., & Vadasy, P. (1998). *Ladders to literacy*. Baltimore: Paul H. Brookes.

Oller, D. K., & Pearson, B. (2002). Assessing the effects of bilingualism: A background. In D. K. Oller & R. Eilers (Eds.), *Language and literacy in bilingual children*. Clevedon, England: Multilingual Matters.

Owocki, G. (2001). *Make way for literacy.* Washington, DC: National Association for the Education of Young Children.

Pérez, B. (1998). Literacy, diversity and programmatic response. In B. Pérez, T. McCarty, L. Watahomigie, M. Torres-Guzmán, J. M. Chang, H. Smith, & A. Dávila de Silva (Eds.), *Sociocultural contexts of language and literacy.* Mahwah, NJ: Lawrence Erlbaum Associates.

Puera-Jones, R., & DeBoer, C. (2000). *More story making: Using predictable literature to develop communication.* Eau Claire, WI: Thinking Publications.

Rathmann, P. (2005). *Good night gorilla.* J.P. Putnam & Sons Juvenile.

Reese, E., & Cox, A. (1999). Quality of book reading affects children's emergent literacy. *Developmental Psychology, 35,* 20–28.

Roberts, J., Jurgens, J., & Burchinal, M. (2005). The role of home literacy practices in preschool children's language and literacy skills. *Journal of Speech, Language, and Hearing Research, 48,* 345–359.

Rosin, P. (1996). The diverse American family. In P. Rosin, A. Whitehead, L. Tuchman, G. Jesien, A. Begun, & L. Irwin (Eds.), *Partnerships in early intervention.* Baltimore: Paul H. Brookes.

Rosin, P., Schraeder, T., & Miller, J. F. (2004). *Linking language and literacy project.* Madison, WI: University of Wisconsin–Madison, Kemper Knapp Bequest.

Rosin, P., Schraeder, T., & DeFelice, H. (2005, November). *Linking language and literacy: A project for culturally-linguistically diverse preschoolers.* Presentation at the American Speech-Language Association Convention, San Diego, CA.

Roth, F., & Baden, B. (2001). Investing in emergent literacy intervention: A key role for speech-language pathologists. *Seminars in Speech and Language, 22,* 163–173.

Scarborough, H. S. (2001). Connecting early language and literacy to later reading (dis)abilities: Evidence, theory, and practice. In S. B. Neuman & D. K. Dickinson (Eds.), *Handbook of early literacy research* (pp. 97–110). New York: Guilford Press.

Shore, R. (1997). *Rethinking the brain: New insights into early development.* New York: Families and Work Institute.

Snow, C., Burns, M. S., & Griffin, P. (1998). *Preventing reading difficulties in young children.* Washington, DC: National Academy Press.

Snowling, M., Bishop, D. V. M., & Stothard, S. E. (2000). Is preschool language impairment a risk factor for dyslexia in adolescence? *Journal of Child Psychology and Psychiatry and Allied Disciplines, 41,* 587–600.

Sterling-Orth, A. (2004). *Go-to guide for phonological awareness.* Eau Claire, WI: Thinking Publications.

Stockman, I. (1996). The promises and pitfalls of language sample analysis as an assessment tool for linguistic minority children. *Language, Speech, and Hearing Services in Schools, 27,* 355–366.

Stothard, S. E., Snowling, M., Bishop, D. V. M., Chipchase, B. B., & Kaplan, C. A. (1998). Language-impaired preschoolers: A follow-up into adolescence. *Journal of Speech, Language, and Hearing Research, 41,* 407–418.

Tabors, P., & Snow, C. (2001). Young bilingual children and early literacy development. In S. B. Neuman & D. K. Dickinson (Eds.), *Handbook of early literacy research* (pp. 159–178). New York: Guilford Press.

Thomas-Tate, S., Washington, J. & Edwards, J. (2004). Standardized assessment of phonological awareness skills in low-income African American first graders. *American Journal of Speech-Language Pathology, 13,* 182–190.

Turner, J. (1995). The influence of classroom contexts on young children's motivation for literacy. *Reading Research Quarterly, 30,* 410–441.

U.S. Census Bureau. (2000). *Your gateway to Census 2000.* Washington, DC: Author. Available at: http://www.census.gov/

van Kleeck, A., Vander Woude, J., & Hammett, L. (2006). Fostering literal and inferential language skills in Head Start preschoolers with language impairment using scripted book-sharing discussions. *American Journal of Speech-Language Pathology, 15,* 85–95.

Vernon-Feagans, L., Scheffner Hammer, C., Miccio, A., & Manlove, E. (2001). Early language and literacy skills in low-income African American and Hispanic children. In S. B. Neuman & D. K. Dickinson (Eds.), *Handbook of early literacy research* (pp. 192–210). New York: Guilford Press.

Washington, J. (2006). *Emergent Literacy in High-Risk Communities: Research Considerations.* Presentation at the Department of Communicative Disorders, University of Wisconsin-Madison; Madison, WI.

Watson, L., Layton, T., Pierce, P., & Abraham, L. (1994). Enhancing emerging literacy in a language preschool. *Language, Speech, and Hearing Services in Schools, 25,* 136–145.

Wescott, N. B. (1980). *I know an old lady who swallowed a fly.* Boston: Little, Brown.

Whitehurst, G., & Lonigan, C. (1998). Child development and emergent literacy. *Child Development, 69,* 848–872.

Whitehurst, G., & Lonigan, C. (2001). Emergent literacy: Development from preschoolers to readers. In S. B. Neuman & D. K. Dickinson (Eds.), *Handbook of early literacy research.* New York: Guilford Press.

APPENDIX 12–A

Literacy Kits

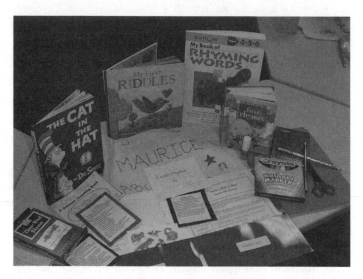

A focus on rhyme

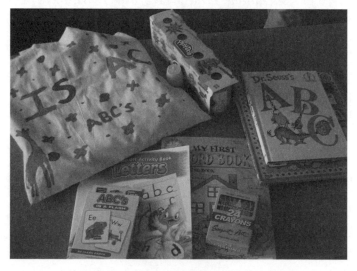

A focus on the alphabetic principle

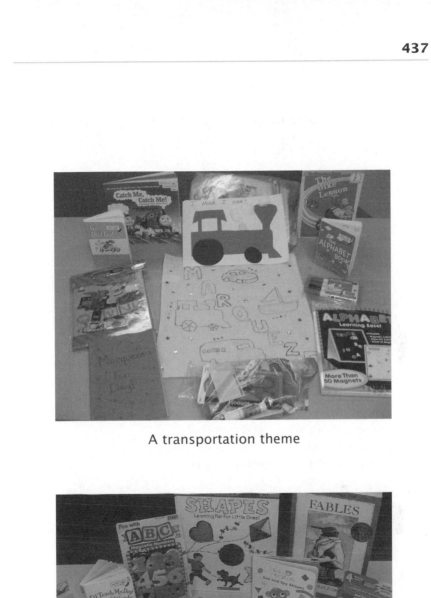

A transportation theme

An animal theme

APPENDIX 12–B

Top Ten Ways of Helping Your Child to Read

1. Talk, sing, and play with your child.
   - Say the names of the things your child sees.
   - Listen to your child.
   - Sing, chant, and use rhyme.

2. Read aloud to your child each day.
   - Set up a reading routine.

3. Surround your child with reading materials.

4. Read different types of books.
   - Check out the library for books and materials.

5. Read at a leisurely pace.
   - Sit close to your child.
   - Touch the words and point to pictures.
   - Pause and let your child talk.
   - Ask questions about the pictures on the page.
   - Ask your child to retell the story.

6. Read it again . . . and again.
   - Encourage reading together.
   - Leave pauses for your child to fill in the word.

7. Look for reading and writing opportunities everywhere.
   - Point out signs with letters that appear in your child's name.
   - Provide readily available materials for play with print and letters (for example, magnetic letters on the refrigerator, old mail, TV schedules).

8. Help your child learn about letters.
   - Sing the alphabet song, read alphabet books, play with alphabet puzzles.
   - Encourage your child to write.
   - Show your child how to "write" his/her name. (Don't expect the child to be able to actually do it.) You can use dot-to-dot for copying the letters, or ask the child to trace the letters.

9. Limit and monitor TV.
   ■ Watch with your child and talk about favorite programs.

10. Talk with your child's teacher.
    ■ Ask the teacher what's best for your child to help with reading and writing.

Of course, have fun and enjoy whatever activities you share with your child!

Index